Take the next step

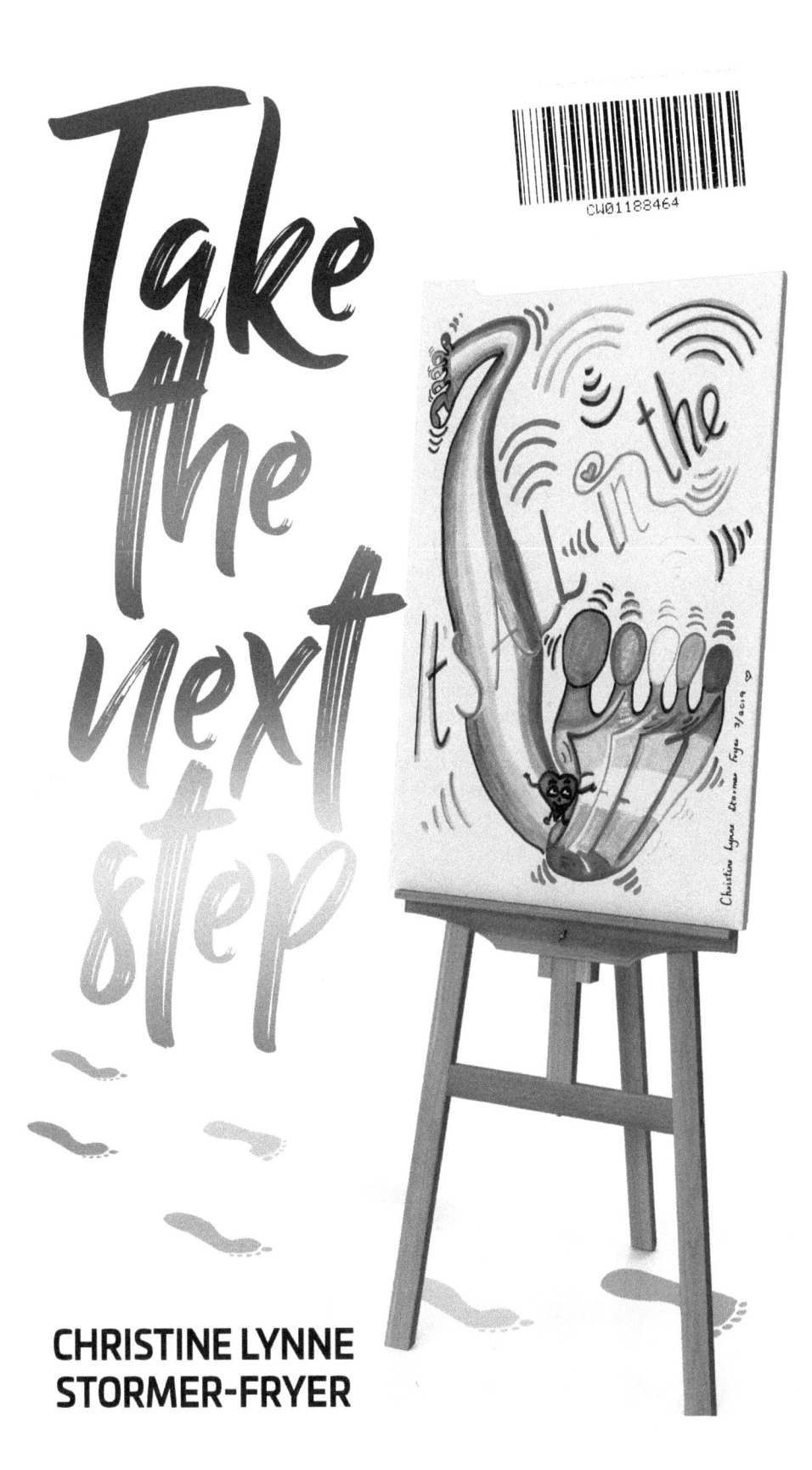

CHRISTINE LYNNE STORMER-FRYER

First published by Christine Lynne Stormer-Fryer, 2020
www.alwaysb.com

978-0-620-89695-5 (Print)
978-0-620-89696-2 (e-book)

Editor: Phillipa Mitchell
(www.phillipamitchell.com)

Proofreader: Linda Kaye
(www.writerslittlehelper.com)

Photographer & Image Editor: Naomi Anne Estment
(www.naomiestment.com)

Cover Design by Gregg Davies
(www.greggdavies.com)

All rights reserved
The moral right of the author has been asserted

Additional copies of this book can be purchased
from all leading book retailers worldwide

For all my organisers and delegates worldwide who have been such a vital and enriching part of my Soul and Sole's journey – thank you!

CONTENTS

INTRODUCTION 1

UNDER-STAND-ING THE CHARTS 3

    THIS IS IT – YOUR LIFE! PATHETIC OR OUTSTANDING? 7

    BE-ING HU-MAN 9

    INCLINATION – THE APPROACH TO LIFE 11

    ENERGETIC CONNECTIONS 13

    FEARFUL 15

    BRINGS OUT THE WORST – SO UPSETTING 17

    SYMPTOMS OF DISTRESS 19

    VICTIM OR VICTOR – IT'S A CHOICE 21

    DIS-EASE IS A FRI-END – TREAT IT BETTER 23

    HEALTH PRACTITIONER 25

THINK ON YOUR FEET – STAND UP FOR YOURSELF 27

    ONE AND ONLY – WHAT'S THE SENSE 29

    JOURNEY OF SELF-DISCOVERY 31

    COMPUTING NOTIONS 33

    WHAT DO YOU BELIEVE? GOOD FOR YOU OR NOT? 35

    BRAIN WAVE - ATTRACTORS 37

    BRAINS BEHIND IT 39

    A PAIN IN THE BRAIN 41

    WHAT'S YOUR PROBLEM? 43

    WHAT'S SO BAD? 45

    LABELLED FOR LIFE 47

    IN-JURY - JUDGE 49

    NERVOUS RESPONSES 51

    WEATHER CONDITIONS 53

COMING FROM THE PAST	55
EVOKING MEMORIES – SUCH NON-SENSE	57
ARCH-ENE-MY OR ALLY – BACK TO THE FUTURE	59
METAMORPHIC TECHNIQUE	61
DIGITAL DE-LIGHTS	63
LET'S FACE IT	65
FACING THE FACTS	67
STRIKE ACCORD – ORCHESTRATE MOVES	69

A FOOT AT THE NECK 71

CROSSING THE BRIDGE – EXPRESSWAYS – STIFLING EXPRESSION	73
GETTING IN THE WAY – MIND OUT	75
GOING WITH THE FLOW – EMPHATIC LYMPHATIC	77

GRASS GROWING UNDER FEET – FEELINGS GET IN THE WAY! 79

'E-MOTIONAL' JOURNEY - WILLINGNESS TO FEEL	81
ENERGY-IN-MOTION	83
COLOURFUL EMOTIONS – JOG MEMORIES	85
EYES – OPINIONS AND INSIGHTS – MAKING A SCENE!	87
LOOK AT THE SIGNS – WATCH OUT!	89
ON THE BALL	91
ENTERTAIN – CONTAIN	93
BLAME – SO DISEMPOWERING	95
COMPLAIN – COME PAIN	97
WHAT A PAIN – FEEL SOUL ISSUES	99
EMOTIONAL DISTRESS – HARD TO BREATHE	101
UP IN SMOKE – SELF ABUSE	103
AUTOIMMUNE DIS-EASE – LOOK FOR BEAUTY WITHIN	105
AIDS – EXTREME VULNERABILITY	107
ADDRESS ISSUE – FEEL LIKE WEARING?	109
AT ARM'S LENGTH	111
OUT ON A LIMB – EMBRACE / EMBARK	113

GIFT OF LOVE 115

FROM THE HEART	117
HEART OF THE MATTER	119
TRANSPORT – CONVEYANCE	121
BLOWING HOT AND COLD	123
KID YOU KNOT	125

GETTING OFF ON THE WRONG FOOT – INFLUENCES THE NEXT STEP....127

INCIDENTS AND ADVENTURE	129
PASSION – DESTRUCT – CONSTRUCT	131
WHAT HAPPENS OR HAPPENED - CONSIDER THE BULK OF EACH PRODUCTION	133
S-NOT AND TRA-U-MA NON-SENSE	135
BUY INTO	137
WORKING IT OUT – GENERATION TO GENERATION	139
DISHING UP – TO ONESELF AND OTHERS	141
EVEN MORE DISHING UP	143
DIGESTIVE UPSETS	145
TOO TOLERANT – NO TOLERANCE	147
SUPPRESSED URGES	149
FUEL ALL URGES	151
ANIMATED FEARS, INTOLERANCES AND ALLERGIES	153
ADDICTIONS – DESPERATE FOR MORE	155
INTERNALISE REACTIONS	157
THE SHOW MUST GO ON	159
VITAMINS - ENERGY	161
BLOSSOM AND BLOOM	163

KNOW THE LENGTH OF THE FEET - MEASURE UP TO EXPECTATIONS............165

CONVERSATIONS EN ROUTE	167
CHEMICAL MAKE-UP	169
OUT OF THE MOUTH	171
TELLING YOUR-SELF AND OTHERS – IT SHOWS	173
AFTER WHAT WAS SAID – IN-TEST-IN-ES	175

PROVERBIAL TWISTS	177
SMALL INTESTINAL YARNS	179
COLONIC CHRONICLES – ENOUGH TO GO AROUND THE BEND	181
COME ON - BE A SPORT	183
THAT'S THE SPIRIT – DROWN SORROWS OR CELEBRATE	185
FOLLOWING IN ANOTHER'S FOOTSTEPS	**187**
FAMILY WAY – KEEP IMPROVING	189
ROOT CAUSE OF DISTRESS AND DIS-EASE	191
HINGES ON THE CHIN	193
URINE – YOUR INNER EXPRESSIONS	195
WHAT'S THE DIFFERENCE? MAN-I-FEST/WOMB-MAN	197
REPRODUCE NEW CONCEPTS	199
GETS UNDER THE SKIN	201
BANKING ON CREDIT	203
INNER RESOURCES	205
WILLING TO TRANSFORM	207
BOOTS MADE FOR WALKING	209
LIVING IN THE PRESENT	211
ABOUT THE AUTHOR	**212**

IT'S ALL IN THE FEET - THE NEXT STEP IN REFLEXOLOGY

INTRODUCTION

Never in my wildest dreams did I ever imagine that one day my handmade flip charts would be published. Wow!

Initially, the charts were extremely basic – a few poignant words within outlined feet, acting as cues for me and visuals for others during my presentations worldwide. As time went on, I felt that a bit more energy and excitement were needed to help get the message across in a more lively fashion, so I challenged myself to be a tad more adventurous and produce at least thirty new charts a year. In time, the charts started evolving to contain more colour and humour.

For over thirty years, my much loved 'cue cards' have been my loyal travelling and presentation companions. Of the now 1,000+ handmade flip charts, up to eighty travel with me as I move rapidly from one presentation venue to the next. With the charts tightly rolled together in a camp chair bag and slung over my shoulder, I was rarely stopped at customs. I did, however, get a few 'odd glances' from fellow passengers that seemed to say, "Isn't she too old to be camping?" or "She doesn't look like the yoga type to me!"

The original charts stayed at home, lovingly stored in well-marked tubes. Never copyrighted, they have been shared far and wide with delegates, with the sole request to honour the many hours dedicated to creating them. Those wishing to use this method as a 'teaching tool' were encouraged to do so on the under-standing that they used their own experiences and insights instead of mine.

Choosing the best charts for this publication – and even redoing some of them – made me realise just how incredible they are in sharing life-changing Universal insights. I have been urged to publish them for decades, but my biggest concern was the huge expense of printing in colour – not just for me but for my readers as well. It was my wonderful colleague Michelle Sachs who wisely suggested using black and white images and putting the coloured ones onto a CD or something similar.

The decision to finally publish happened around the same time as the decision to sell our home in Johannesburg. The estate agent advised locking all valuables away from prying eyes. My charts, being super valuable to me, were given VIP treatment. I lovingly rolled them up in groups and stowed them safely away in a large plastic bag in a secure storeroom outside the house. I never zipped the bag up, thinking there was no need to. Who knew that a massive African storm would come along and destroy the roof of the storeroom and that the heavens would end up pouring water directly into the bag?

We had to act fast. Each of the 1,000+ charts was tenderly unrolled and placed on any flat surface available throughout our home and studio, be it a floor, a table, a bed, or a desk. Some charts were affected more than others, giving them a funkier look. Some have been kept that way, while others have received some tweaking.

It took an entire day of ironing to straighten out the crumpled charts. I was about to launch into touching up the most affected ones when, as fate would have it, I broke my right arm. I became more ambidextrous as time went on, but not enough to reinstate the charts. In March of 2020, my fabulous photographer, Naomi Estment, had a brilliant idea to shoot the chosen few and touch them up on her computer. This plan was completely derailed when South Africa was suddenly put under "lockdown" after COVID-19 hit our shores. After packing up our Johannesburg home, we moved to our beautiful farm in the Waterberg. The charts, of course, had priority.

Fortunately, in the process, I discovered that most of the charts had been scanned and saved onto discs and memory sticks by my printers when initially copied. Hallelujah, I thought, I can download them onto my laptop during lockdown. Wrong! In the rush of loading our two cars with goodies and supplies – and our beloved doggie – the bag containing storage devices was left behind, only to be retrieved four weeks later.

Out at the farm, I found myself thrust into the world of computer technology, doing 'Zoom' presentations to the Reflexology Book Club on Facebook and acquainting myself with WeTransfer so that I could send Naomi the few charts I had previously downloaded for her to start weaving her magic to digitise the images. Everything was working like clockwork while there was a respectable network signal, but then it decided to disappear for a whole five weeks.

During this time, I had to postpone two fabulous overseas tours, as well as planned trips to Portugal and Hawaii that were to be my seventieth birthday gift to myself. It was quite a task to postpone twenty-six flights and several hotel bookings – thank goodness for WhatsApp, my son David in London, my travel agent in Johannesburg, and my fabulous British, Irish, American and Canadian organisers who were left with the task of sorting out venues and contacting all the delegates.

Waking up between 1 am and 4 am every morning proved to be the best time to compose the explanations accompanying the charts. I religiously saved the files every few minutes, making copies of everything in other directories on my computer, but, without the internet, all the hours of editing just disappeared. To further compound an already desperate situation, my printer, which had been repaired shortly before lockdown, decided to 'lock down' too! It's no wonder that it took me a while to remember that I had the memory sticks – only to realise that I'd left them behind in Johannesburg.

My faith was waning fast. I even contemplated aborting the whole project. Pulling myself towards myself, I told myself that yes, there had been many challenges en route, but I had come too far and invested far too much love and energy to give up now. Besides, with the charts offering so many valuable insights, it was up to me to honour my Soul commitment of serving the planet.

I was egged on by the fact that, despite being booked for a year, my awesome editor Phillipa Mitchell was going to 'squeeze' my publication in for mid-July. Furthermore, I was greatly encouraged to know that my talented artist Gregg Davies was available to do the layout. So, it was back to the drawing board. With my printer repaired and the internet restored, everything was falling back into place. Phew!

What a journey! The time offered by South Africa's lockdown ultimately proved to be a Divine gift. Inspired to continue writing once this awesome publication is in the can, I plan to get on with the other four books anxiously waiting in the wings. In the meantime, I am learning to take each day as it comes with an enormous amount of gratitude, knowing that everything happens for a reason.

I do hope that you enjoy this publication as much, if not more than I have enjoyed creating and sharing the charts.

TAKE THE NEXT STEP - 3

UNDER-STAND-ING THE CHARTS

Everybody sees something different in these charts, drawing attention to whatever is meaningful to THEM. The general write-up accompanying each chart gives you the opportunity to devise your own impressions and story. It is by observing patterns within personal experiences that the significance of life is realised. This is particularly powerful in evoking new perspectives when encountering something unfamiliar.

'E-motions' are constantly felt, yet the true impact of what occurred can take aeons to sink it in. There are so many different layers, each with their own separate meanings. Contemplating and refining these life events helps to add richness and texture to life.

Feet offer the most profound 'under-standing', with them being 'UNDER' the body and the body 'STANDING' on them. As the body's roots, feet are ideally positioned to provide a firm, stable and mobile platform for ongoing growth and development. Constantly taking it upon themselves to reflect life impressions through their ever-changing characteristics, feet have earned the reputation of being the 'Soul's messenger'.

Here is a brief outline of the meanings behind each chart.

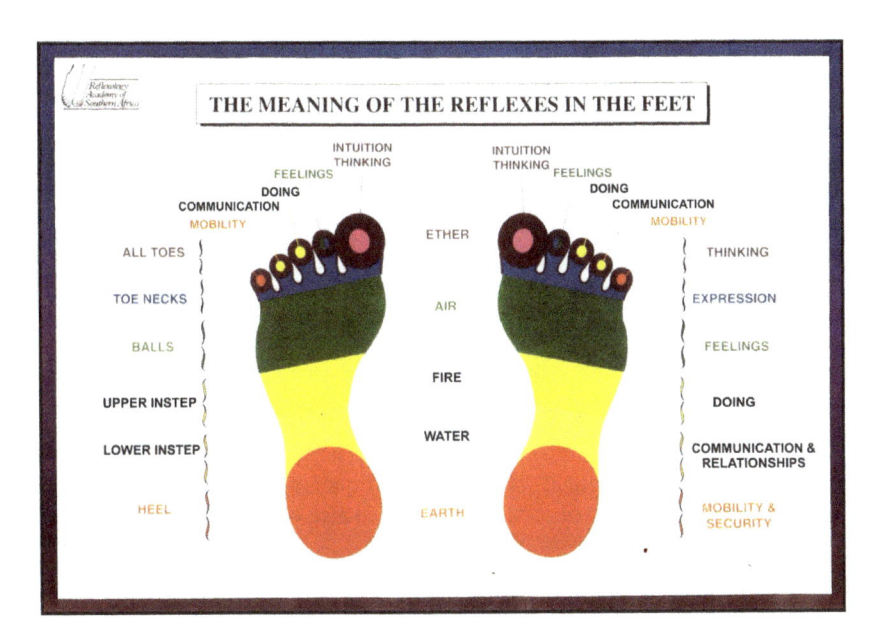

THE MEANING OF THE REFLEXES IN THE FEET

Left foot labels:
- INTUITION
- THINKING
- FEELINGS
- DOING
- COMMUNICATION
- MOBILITY
- ALL TOES
- TOE NECKS
- BALLS
- UPPER INSTEP
- LOWER INSTEP
- HEEL

Centre:
- ETHER
- AIR
- FIRE
- WATER
- EARTH

Right foot labels:
- INTUITION
- THINKING
- FEELINGS
- DOING
- COMMUNICATION
- MOBILITY
- THINKING
- EXPRESSION
- FEELINGS
- DOING
- COMMUNICATION & RELATIONSHIPS
- MOBILITY & SECURITY

All toes reflect the impact of thoughts on the mind. Being multi-dimensional thinkers, each toe is representative of different aspects of the various philosophies, all of which are derived from memories, that then form beliefs.

Meaning Filled Feet
by Chris Stormer

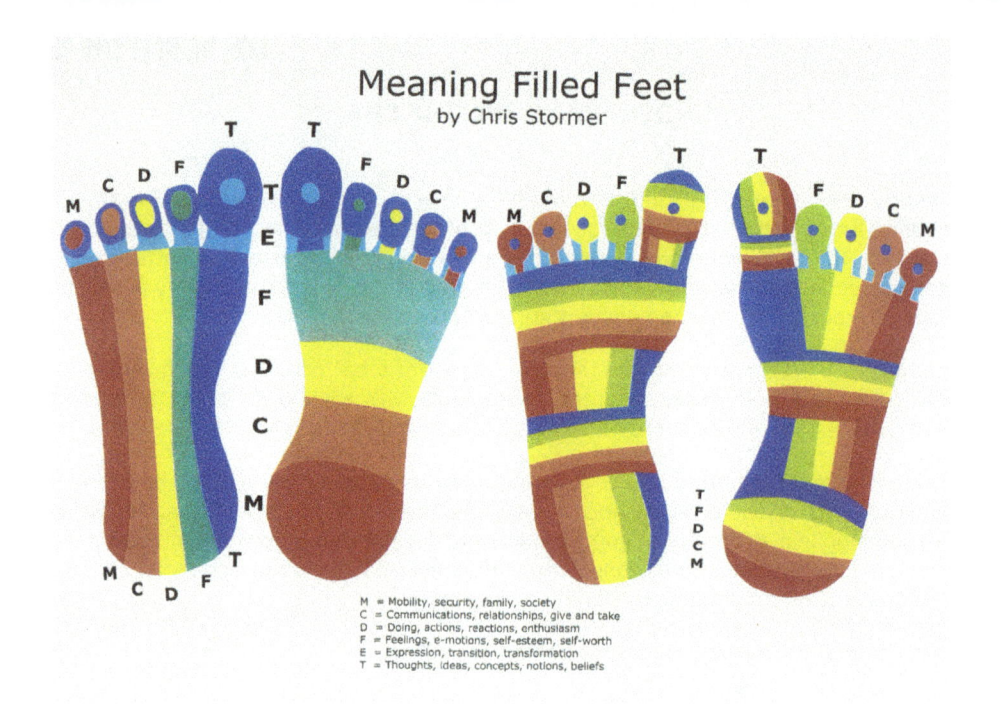

M = Mobility, security, family, society
C = Communications, relationships, give and take
D = Doing, actions, reactions, enthusiasm
F = Feelings, e-motions, self-esteem, self-worth
E = Expression, transition, transformation
T = Thoughts, ideas, concepts, notions, beliefs

The quality of the ideas running through the body from head to toe impacts different groups of organs, with the varying effects reflected onto the soles.

SIGNIFICANCE OF WORDS

Words are one of the body's most powerful tools. Specific vibrations within words carry energies that give language weight and power. The potential to heal or hurt. To be destructive or constructive. Disempowering or empowering. Two of the shortest words in the English language, 'Yes' and 'No', often require a lot more thought before being said.

Constantly plagued by negative self-talk, many Souls fill their minds with notions of being doomed to fail, not being good enough, or not worthy of love – and yet are astonished when these become their reality.

The subconscious mind accepts critical statements as the absolute truth. As such, positive affirmations (once within the realm of consciousness) can also enter the subconscious mind with the power to change the quality of life.

Certain letters 'fix-ed' before the stem of a word are referred to as a 'prefix'. An 'affix' (also known as a 'performative') changes the energy of a word to mean the opposite, or something quite different.

When surveying the charts, do keep the following prefixes and affixes in mind.

A- or **an-** meaning not, without, absent, e.g. a-pathetic and an-aemia. **Alter-** other, change, modifies, adjust, amend, revise, correct – e.g. alter-native. **Anti-** opposite or against, e.g. anti-body. **Auto-** by itself, e.g. auto-immune. **Dis-** negative or remove, e.g. dis-ease. **Down-** reduce low sad unhappy, e.g. down-hearted. **Dys-** negative badly wrongly, e.g. Dyspnoea. **Epi-** upon, addition, above, on, over, near, at, before, after, e.g. Epi-dural. **Extra-** to a greater extent, beyond, additional, more ultra, e.g. Extra-ordinary. **Fore-** before, front, e.g. Forehead. **Hemi-** half, e.g. Hemi-plegia. **Hyper-** over, excessive, exaggerated, beyond, hyped-up, e.g. Hyper-active. **Hypo-** under, too little, not enough, e.g. Hypo-active. **Ill-** unkind, unfriendly, hostile, harsh, mean, cruel, unpleasant, bad, harmful, injurious, destructive, detrimental, hurtful, e.g. ill-logical. **Im-** I am, e.g. impossible. **In-** inside on not, e.g. Intuition. **Infra-** above or penetrating, e.g. Infra-red. **Inter-** between or connecting, e.g. inter-leading. **Intra-** within toward marginal or not, e.g. Intra-cellular. **Ir-** within, toward, marginal or not e.g.ir-regular. **Macro-** large scale or exceptionally prominent, e.g. Macro-scopic. **Mal-** bad, unpleasant, not, undesirable impact, faulty or inadequate, e.g. Mal-function. **Meso-** middle, intermediate, halfway, e.g. Mesoblast. **Meta-** self-referral e.g. Meta-data. **Micro-** on a small scale, e.g. Micro-organism. **Mid-** in the middle, e.g. Mid-line. **Mini-** smaller version, diminutive, tiny, e.g. Mini-scule. **Mis-** incorrect, bad, wrong, e.g. Mis-demeanour. **Mono-** one, e.g. Mono-tonous. **Multi-** many, more than one, e.g. Multi-ply. **Non-** no, not, e.g. Non-entity. **Over-** excessive, too much, on top, e.g. Over-expressive. **Pan-** all, e.g. Pan-demic. **Para-** beside, beyond, related to, altered, e.g. Para-medic. **Per-** through, throughout, e.g. Per-cutaneous. **Peri-** around, e.g. Peri-cardium. **Poly-** many, e.g. Poly-gamous. **Post-** after e.g. Post-operative. **Pre-** before, already, e.g. Pre-assembled. **Pro-** on behalf of, before, e.g. Pro-fessional. **Proto-** first, primitive, precursor, e.g. Proto-col. **Pseudo-** false, quasi, virtual, mock, fake, artificial, pretend, simulated, imitation, poser, fraud, e.g. Pseudo-intellectual. **Quasi-** somewhat, pseudo, would-be, wannabe, e.g. Quasi-particulate. **Re-** again, e.g. Re-establish. **Semi-** partial, somewhat, half, e.g. Semi-circle. **Sub-** below, deputise, represent, substitute, stand-in, associate, junior, e.g. Sub-ordinate. **Super-** superior, better, above, more than, great, top-notch, e.g. Super-intendant. **Supra-** above, e.g. Supra-orbital. **Trans-** across, connecting, e.g. Trans-verse. **Ultra-** beyond, extremely, particularly, mega, especially, e.g. Ultra-violet. **Un-** not, remove, opposite, e.g. Un-easy.

Also, be mindful of letters at the end of a word such as **-able-** capable, confident, proficient, adept, e.g. Ador-able. **-ate-** cause or make the outcome of what has been taken in, be it thought, feelings, food, conversation e.g. appreci-ate. **-ion-** an atom or group of atoms either charged positively or negatively. **-dous-** 'do to us' – there are only four words with this at the end: tremendous, horrendous, stupendous, hazardous. **-eat-** there are so many 'eat' words all requiring extra energy to digest. e.g. B-eat, h-eat, m-eat, s-eat, etc. Also, in the middle as in cr-eat-e, w-eat-her, f-eat-her.

Becoming more conscious of the meaning of words, recognising that they are a powerful source of feeling, deepens our relationship with them. Carefully listening to others before speaking gives words more integrity. As intelligent messengers of healing and light, words can transmit deep and positive feelings. It is a good idea to always keep words soft and palatable, just in case you need to eat them.

Words hold great sway over the kind of life created!

FOOTNOTE

When asked: 'What one thing about humanity surprises you the most?' the Dalai Lama answered: "Man. Because he sacrifices his health in order to make money. Then he sacrifices money to recuperate his health. And then he is so anxious about the future that he does not enjoy the present; the result being that he does not live in the present or the future; he lives as if he is never going to die, and then dies having never really lived."

What we are is the Universe's gift to us what we become is our gift to the Universe

6 - CHRISTINE LYNNE STORMER-FRYER

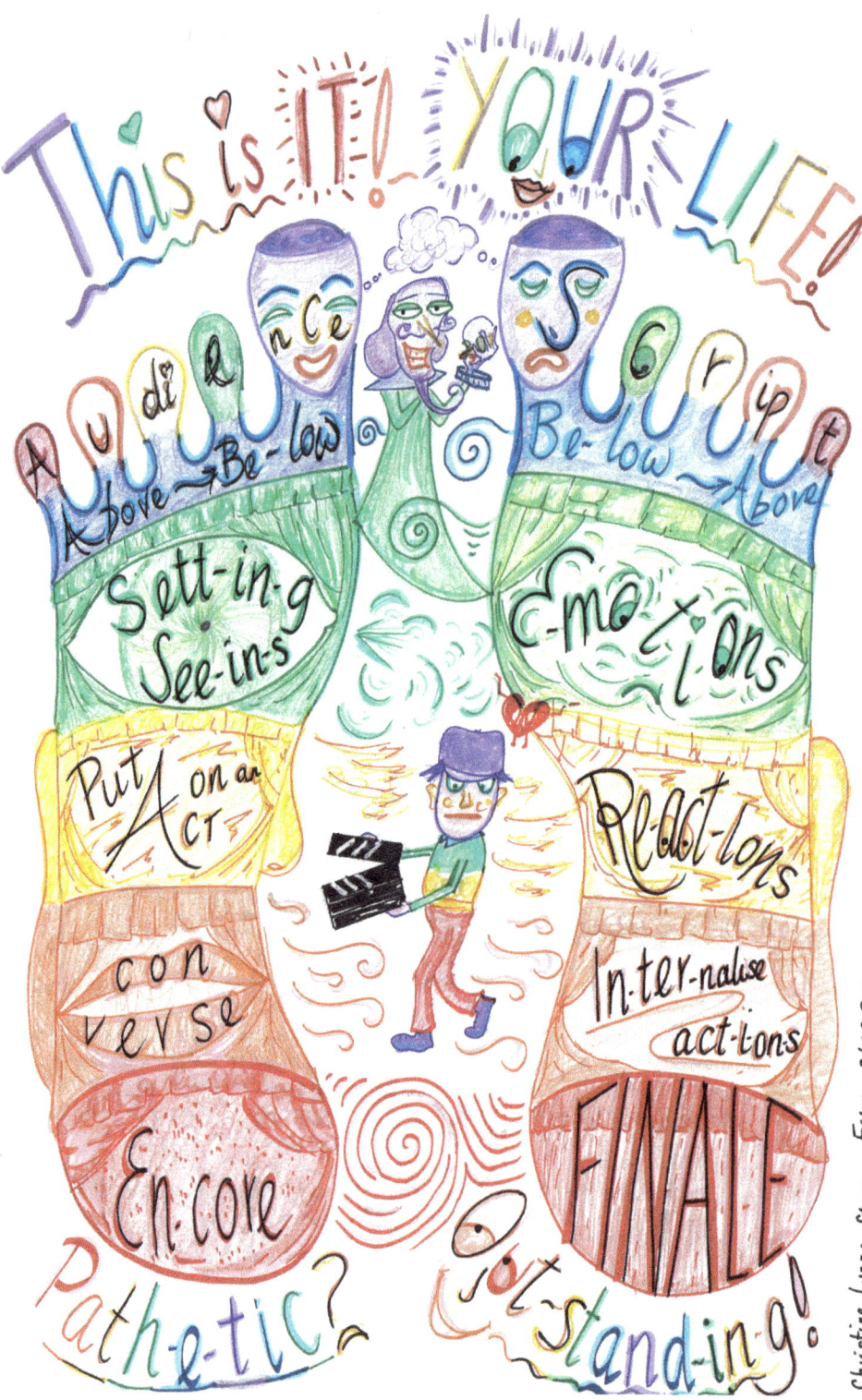

THIS IS IT – YOUR LIFE! PATHETIC OR OUTSTANDING?

Accelerating at such a rapid rate, Universal energy is throwing many into a flat spin. Forced to let go of old worn-out ideas, set routines, and anybody or anything getting in the way, there is now a chance to start afresh and openly and lovingly embrace the next stage in human evolution.

Every body is a Universal production, and each Soul is in charge of its own performance. Selecting the most suit-able mind and body, the best roles are chosen to achieve its sole purpose on earth – the opportunity of a lifetime for the Soul.

The Spirit required for each stage of life is determined well in advance, along with the appropriate costumes, make-up and props, apt scenes and locations, as well as the required back-ups and resources. Each co-star, performer, crew member and assistant is individually hand-picked to match the required parts.

With everything seen in the mind's eye long before physically appearing, the script is made up well in advance. Cues from oscillating e-motions set the scene, frequently dramatised by personal perceptions and points of view. The apparatus used for forming opinions are constantly adjusted since the eyes only 'see what they believe but do not always believe what they see'.

The body's cells, the ever-patient audience, have differing reactions to the various scenarios and roles played throughout life. Conversing among themselves, they continually set the tone.

Bored by the same time-worn spectacles, cells love to be entertained by exciting, innovative acts that keep them alert and 'on their toes'. The more passion injected, the better! Being filled with zest and confidence makes it so much easier to internalise and be enthralled, all the better for producing the best possible performances.

Choosing a family with the same genetic coding makes it easier to work through similar Soul issues that still need to be worked out of the chromosomal system. Repeating the 'same old, same old' acts, generation after generation, gets monotonous and hardly ever provides a worthwhile solution.

What is required is up-to-date insights and unusual ideas to inspire new, light-hearted and outstanding performances. Much-needed evolution engenders exciting reproductions craved by the audience to 'wipe the mud off the feet', to make mind-blowing progress, and to be the star of the show.

When it comes to the 'Final Curtain', will the reaction be "How absolutely pathetic – they could have done SO much more with their life", or will it be "Brilliant! Fabulous performance! Encore!"?

Everybody is the author of their own story, free to create a masterpiece!

8 - CHRISTINE LYNNE STORMER-FRYER

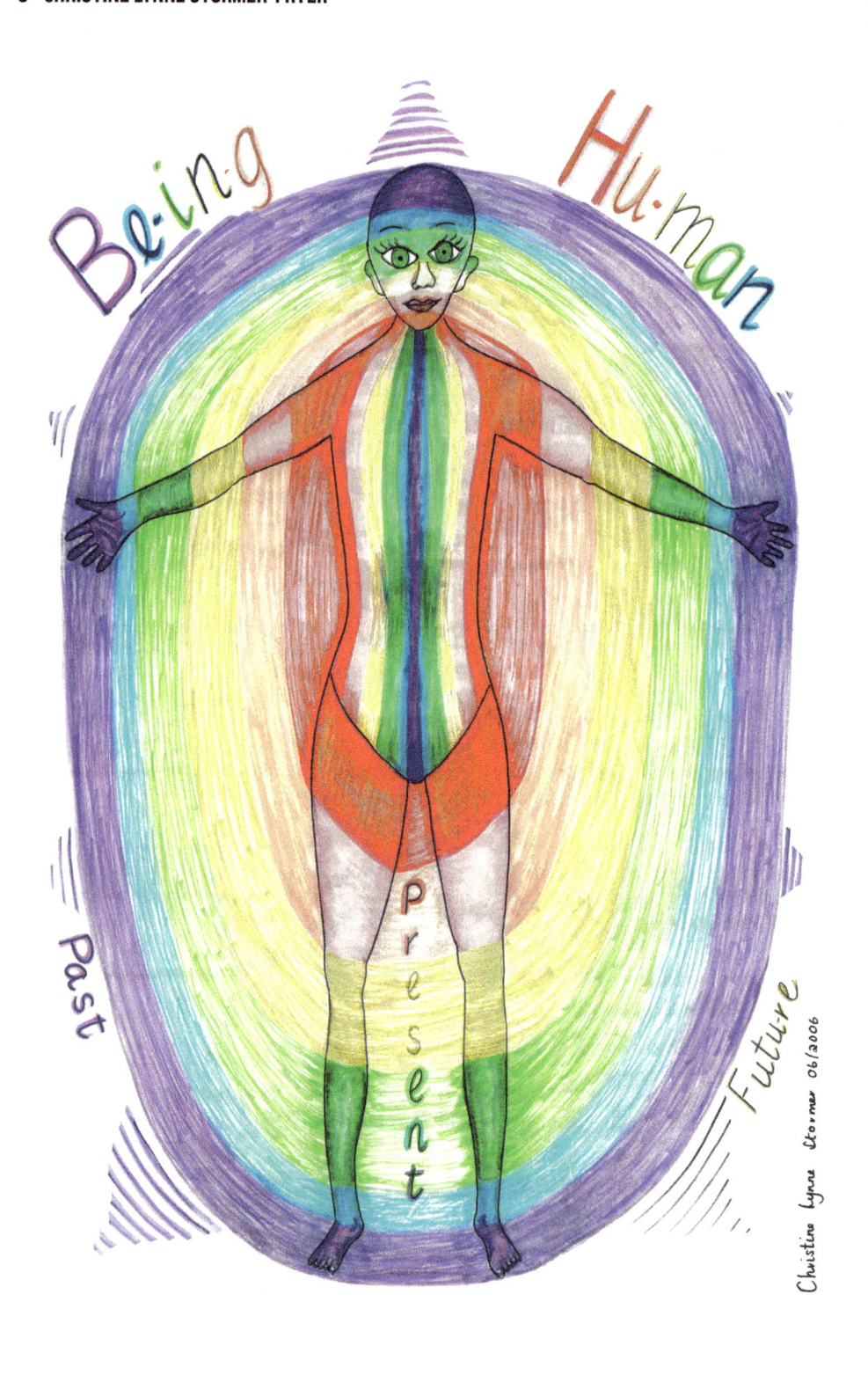

BE-ING HU-MAN

'**Being Hu-man**', the '**Man**'-ifestation of colour (**Hu-**) coming into **Being**, is to be a creation of energy full of chakra colours. Cosmic and earth energies mingle in these vortex points, known as 'power centres', with distinct energy patterns holding consciousness in the physical body. Bringing the colours to life is input from the mind inoculating the body with enthusiasm, passion and vibrancy.

Constantly living in the **past** wastes time and energy, consistently draining the whole of these vital lifeforces. This scenario is detected by the **right** side of the head and body, as well as the **right** arm and **right** foot. All are '**dead right**' about everything. 'Letting go' of any stumbling blocks that prevent progress is heaven-sent.

The **pre-sen**t, a **gift** ordered in advance by Spirit, is ideal for manifesting dreams. Resonating at the very core of being human, whatever happens in the now influences **future** possibilities. The resultant energy is picked up by the **left** side of the head and body, along with the **left** arm and **left** foot, since 'all that is **left** is the **present.**'

Inspired by **indigo/violet,** the **brain** generates **thoughts.** Ethereal Universal energies are detected and absorbed by the body's antennae, its hairs. Bashing personal concepts tends to turn the skin into an indignant **purple** hue. **Hands** handle and engineer individual ideas, while **feet** get them out there. Both are essential tools for participating in the journey of life.

Transforming non-physical energies into physical energies (and vice versa) is **blue,** the colour that connects the sky to the sea. Blue is linked to the **expressive** parts of the body with functions relying on openness and flexibility, the **forehead, neck, shoulders, wrists** and **ankles**. Being given a 'cold shoulder' for instance, is enough to turn the skin blue.

The predominance of **green** in nature, surrounded by **air**, resonates in the **chest** and **breasts**. Opinions and perceptions formed by what the **eyes** take in influence the breath, moving contained energy into **e-motions**. These, in turn, stir various deep-seated **feelings** with a noticeable bearing on the **lower halves** of the **forearms** and **shins**.

The **fiery** qualities of **Yell-Ow**, yell '**ow**' if you don't like it – are provoked by all that happens or does not happen. Yellow is initiated by what is heard via the ears and smelt through the nose, along with responses to impudence provided by the cheeks. Subsequent **actions** and **reactions** profoundly impact the **upper digestive tract**, as well as the **upper halves** of the **forearms** and **shins.**

'**O the Range**' of relationships instigated by **orange** enthuse life with gushes of lively conversations, balancing bodies of **water**. Taking this effusiveness on board is the **lower digestive tract.** Its ability to give and take with ease has an impact on the **lower halves** of the **upper arms** and **thighs**.

Earth, with its **reddish** tones, represents **family, society, stability**, and **mobility**. Innate resources to 'stand on one's own two feet' and be '**B-One**' of a kind come from solidarity within the **skeleton**. Closely related are the inherently lenient **muscles**, with more than enough flexibility for personal expansion and progression. Meanwhile, the **excretory** organs flush out and eliminate the 'old' to make space to **reproduce** and keep the bloodline going.

Living life to the full makes for a colourful, healthy personality.

To be humane is to be benevolent and compassionate!

10 - CHRISTINE LYNNE STORMER-FRYER

I-N-C-L-IN-AT-I-ON

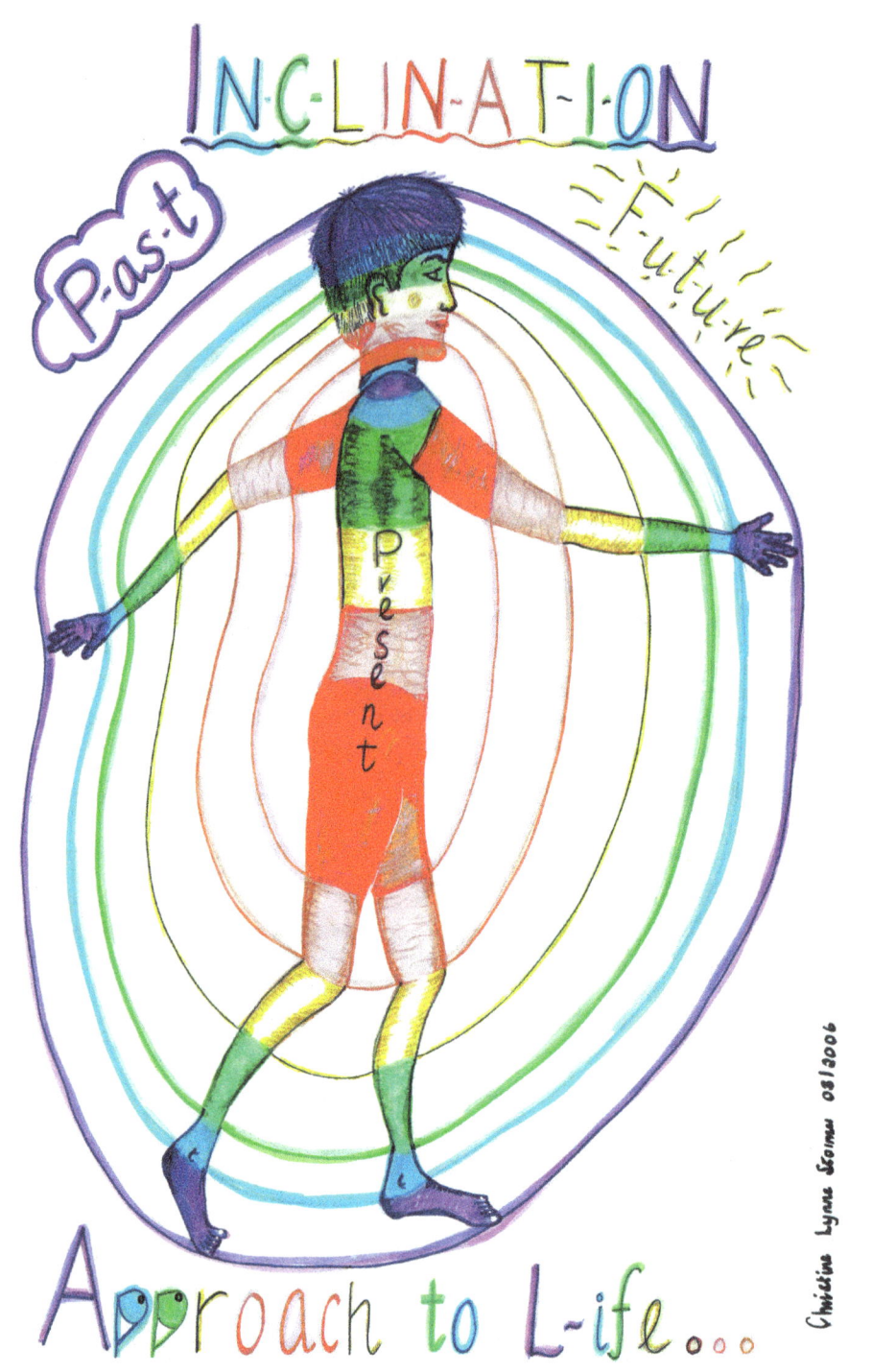

P-ast · F-u-t-u-re

Present

A-p-p-roach to L-ife...

Christine Lynne Stormer 08/2006

INCLINATION – THE APPROACH TO LIFE

The fastest and most dramatic progress ever in evolutionary history is intentionally 'knocking humanity off its feet'. The natural and innate tendency to keep moving a-head is being tested. Ultimately, it is the inclination to do so that makes all the difference. With all movement being transitional, challenges encountered along the way are meant to engender innovative ways to live and continue existing in a perpetual state of creativity.

When moving on, if past events or non-events are not 'left behind' and linger menacingly at the back of the body, the situation can become problematic – especially when unable to provide the torso with its much-needed back-up. Selecting the best from previous life experiences builds a firm, solid and strong backbone to keep the body upright. Positioned completely in the present, the mysterious future can then be confidently con-fronted.

Once 'on the go', limbs effortlessly swing 'to and fro' between past and future, briefly encountering the present in between until coming to a standstill. The leg that has just 'set foot' in the past is always the last to leave it behind, while the alternate arm simultaneously reaches forward into the future to 'get a feel' for whatever lies a-head. At the same time, the counterpart leg 'sets foot' on the virgin territory of the future, while the alternate hand moves on from the past – unless it is gripping on too tightly for fear of letting go.

Taking a step back to observe the bigger picture is one thing, but without 'eyes in the back of the head', constantly moving backwards is futile. Fear is the ruling force when it comes to having 'cold feet', making it exceptionally difficult to make any form of progress. Terrified muscles recoil and stiffen as the body becomes increasingly defensive, closing itself off to all possibilities.

Times like this require a positive approach to life, the courage to bravely step away from the comfort of the known into the possible discomfort and uncertainty of the unknown, even if it is with a forced 'smile on the dial' to convince oneself and fool others. It certainly takes guts with a head held high to explore and discover the untapped potential within and set it free.

Making time to get away from daily concerns and stepping away to reconsider all options helps in working out the best approach to inevitable challenges. Challenges are nothing more than exciting stumbling blocks encountered along the way to forcefully change the mind.

With every move influenced by thoughts, ongoing positivity helps the body orchestrate its movement in such a way that every step becomes increasingly worthwhile. Having moved forward, there is no going back. Fortunately, the human body is generally inclined to keep moving a-head, especially when sparked by exciting new prospects of ongoing innovations.

Acquiring wisdom, knowledge and never-ending experiences all take place when progressing onto the next stage of life. Endless encouragement comes from the Spiritual movement as it opens mass consciousness, nudging it to extend from dimensions of illusion into dimensions of awareness.

The best angle to approach any challenge is the 'try-angle!'

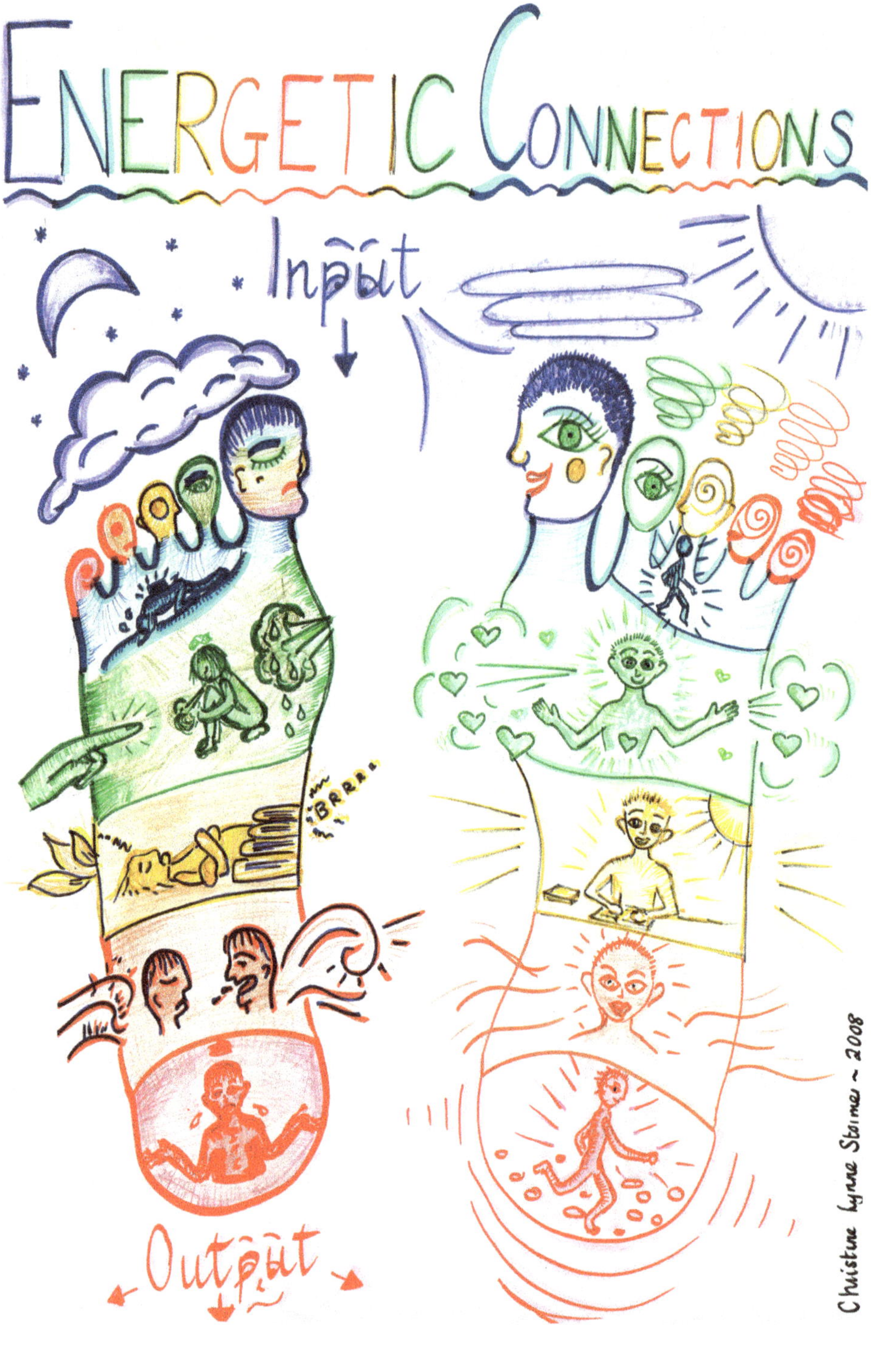
ENERGETIC CONNECTIONS
Input
BRRR
Output
Christine Lynne Stormer ~ 2008

ENERGETIC CONNECTIONS

Energy flows are the very essence of life – the life-sustaining force that infiltrates every atom of the body, giving it life and keeping it alive, vibrant and energised. It is the very essence of vitality, emanating from the core, that shapes personality and physical characteristics.

During times of health, the body harmoniously vibrates to different frequencies, all beautifully intermingled. Feet absorb the solid, grounding, stable energies from Mother Earth to energise and rejuvenate cells. Bounced back to the feet, the reflected energy accurately reflects what is going on inside mind and body.

A tremendous amount of precious life force energy is wasted through the build-up of tension. Depression dulls, dims and narrows the energy beam retracting the aura towards the body. Fearful, threatening thoughts and perceptions immediately restrict and inhibit the energy flow. In contrast, an artificial, unfulfilling experience depletes the amount of energy absorbed and utilised – draining the mind, body and Soul of vibrancy and enthusiasm.

The right side of the body and the right foot resonate more to electric, outgoing and giving male energies of the past, while the left side of the body and the left foot are more magnetic, receptive and receiving, reverberating to a more creative, emotional and sensitive female energy. Aligned vertically through the centre of the body near the spine is an electro-magnetic system, a series of vortex points or power centres known as chakras – the doorways between the ethereal and physical realms.

Whatever is put into thought is where energy known as the "ego" is Connected with the Universe, when 'thinking off the top of the head', the crown chakra relates to Spiritual understanding and trust in life's purpose. Purple and ether offer the incentive to play with ideas, while violet from the third eye provides intuition and clarity. Blue from the throat centre opens everything to self-expression.

Personal development relies on self-love emanating from the heart chakra. Combined with air and the colour green, there is plenty of space to breathe and share that love. Tapping into the heart's passion, the wisdom of life's lessons is discovered.

Every action and reaction shift the energy, either constructively or destructively, with a vibrational match to whatever is put out there. The sunshine yellow and fire emanating from the naval chakra excites the energy into meeting challenges, in the hope of having a favourable impact on the world.

Within every body is a unique life force, a mixture of positive and negative energies that balances the whole. Related to creativity and sexuality, the sacral chakra provides the opportunity for joy through orange, as well as fluidity through the element of water.

As the body's energy emanates outwards, it touches everything and everybody, meeting at a midway point. The down-to-earth root chakra uses family and society to ground Universal energy through various hues of red.

Each chakra energy relates to a theme of nature, which determines the output. Moving energy is the best. It is a healthy energy.

Energy flows where energy goes!

14 - CHRISTINE LYNNE STORMER-FRYER

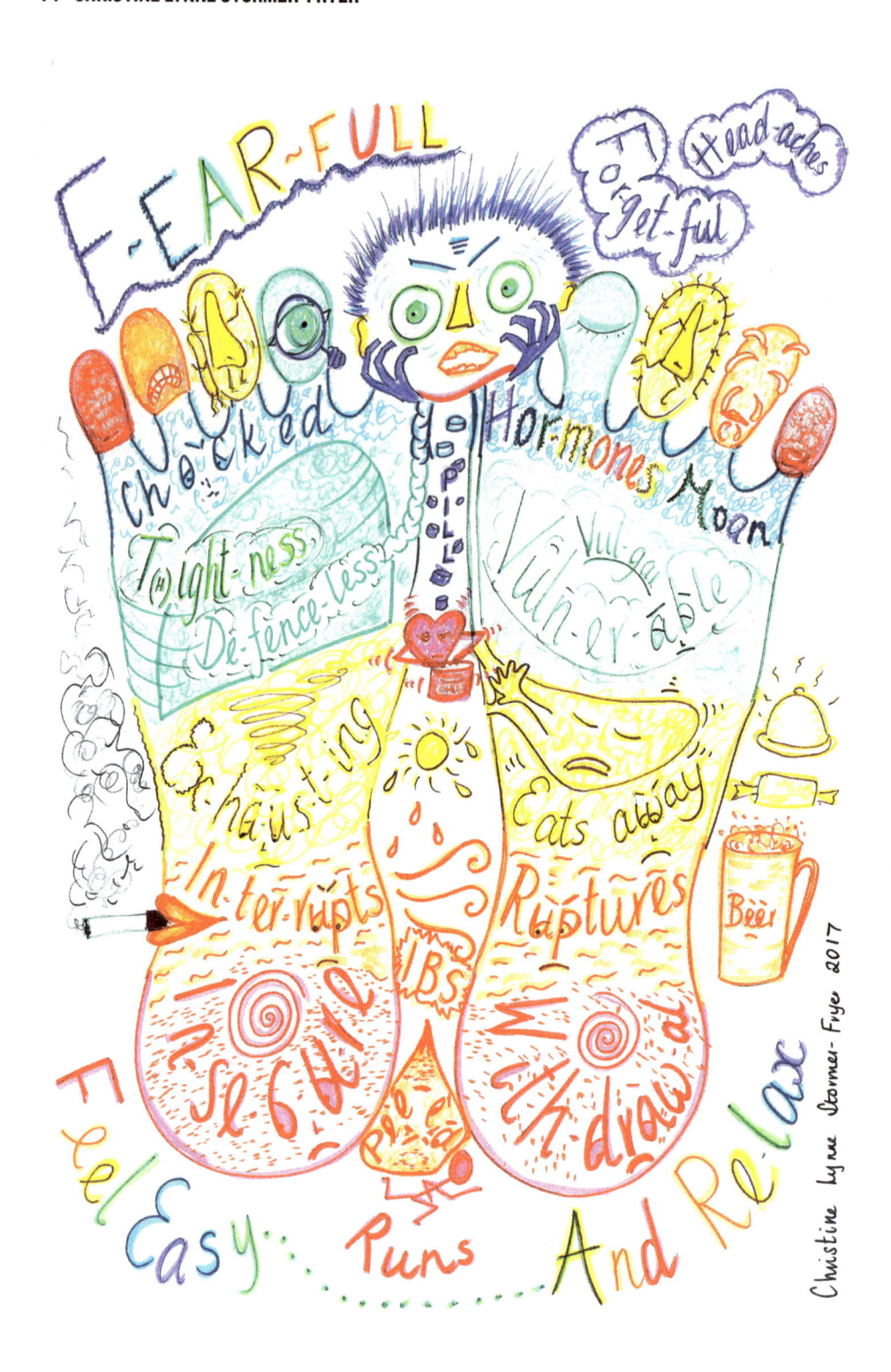

FEARFUL

Fear is an innate form of protection and a natural part of being human. Being fearful can be so utterly ungrounding. Unfounded fears are the worst, engendering feelings of uncertainty and insecurity, and throwing everything completely off balance.

Ultimately, fear is a state of mind. The creation of fearful thoughts is an illusion that goes only as deep as the mind allows it to. Gulps of fear choke the body. It is far too 'hard to swallow' all the deceit and mistruths, along with all the swallowed tears.

With hormones moaning mercilessly and constantly feeling under threat, it is impossible to give peak performances.

As the chest tightens, the breath is relentlessly squeezed out of the defenceless body. Extreme vulnerability is unnerving, especially when perceived to be disadvantageous. Yet letting the guard down is a chance to be free of having to pretend that all is well. Revealing the authentic self is surprisingly empowering, and the key to genuine happiness.

Caught up in collective terror, fear has become rampant within the human heart. A consciousness of victimisation, poverty, lust (and so on) is but a choice.

The other option is to face the fears. Overcome inner obstacles by changing the mind, and move into new life-enhancing territories, inside and out.

There is always an element of fear attached to anything worth doing. It is a way of questioning whether the inevitable changes are welcome or not. Trying to integrate fearful energies is exhausting. Overloading energetically with anxiety can eventually end up eating away at the innards.

Resorting to eating sweets to compensate highlights other issues. Believed to lead to tooth decay and bone deterioration, sugar draws attention to 'rotten' decisions made over 'bones of contention', leaving the body without 'a leg to stand on'.

Highly annoying fear-induced interruptions irritate the bowels, compounded by the pressure to perform under unreasonably high expectations. Turning to alcohol for comfort only brings temporary relief, with the notorious 'beer gut' not only subconsciously concealing the fear but also a punching bag.

Strained communications that rupture relationships pull related parts of the body apart. 'Pee-ed' off with everybody and wishing to run away engenders the temptation to retract and 'curl up and die'.

Yet fear is not meant to be discouraging. Its role is to create an awareness of being on the edge of a comfort zone poised between an old life and a new one. It is the harbinger of transformation.

Instead of acting from fear-based past experiences, allow spontaneous thoughts and actions to establish a firm, confident base that cannot be swayed by the scepticism and the fear of those still entertaining the mistruths of the old world. There is nothing to fear but fear itself.

'Feel Easy And Relax!' Conquering fear is the first step towards wisdom!

16 - CHRISTINE LYNNE STORMER-FRYER

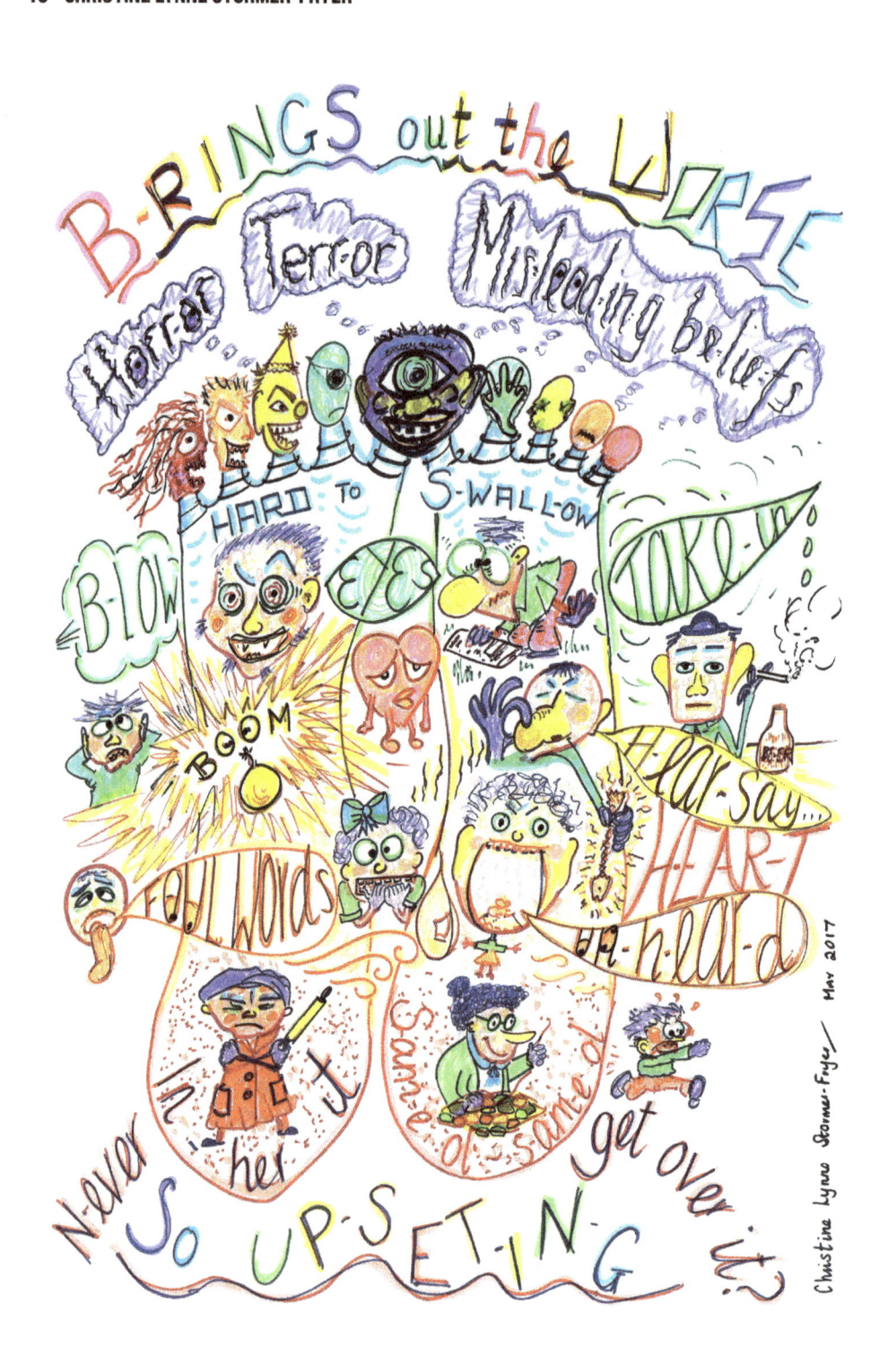

BRINGS OUT THE WORST – SO UPSETTING

Fear is the greatest cause of dis-ease. Fed by the horror and terror of misleading beliefs, it is constantly intensified and re-enforced through the media and modern technology.

Consequently, society has become overly achievement-orientated, greedy, selfish, aggressive and materialistic. So much so that that mounting confusion, pressure and tension have become inevitable.

An innate subconscious desire to feel comfortable, well, and healthy soon becomes a 'pipe dream' when fearful thoughts topple the distressed mind. Terrified and in a state of panic, the body contracts, perturbing the already-perplexed Soul 'at its wit's end'. It just cannot understand how living off other people's dramas helps address the fear of facing one's personal crises. It is too bizarre for words.

Acting as a pause button, fear, when invited in, is more than capable of bringing life to a complete standstill. Coming from an overdose of negativity, it ends up consuming copious amounts of vital life force energy. The dis-empowered ego feels so weakened that it is a hard blow for it to swallow.

Taking in distorted points of view and horrifying opinions is enough to terrify the 'living daylights' out of anybody. In absolute panic, energy is withdrawn. Feeling vulnerable opens the body to hostile attacks usually fabricated by the mind.

When focused on fear, fearful energies that live off fear for sustenance are constantly attracted, keeping the fear quotient dangerously high. Fear feeds off fear, seeking out more fear to grow.

Spread by false 'hearsay', anxiety is a thin stream of fear trickling through the mind, eventually cutting a deeper and wider channel to suck in even more negativity.

Pesky notions persistently 'getting up the nose' become a bugbear. Having a 'short fuse' in such an unstable, volatile environment is an invitation for an explosion to happen whenever a 'bomb is dropped'.

Previously unheard foul words escape through gnashing teeth, ricocheting straight through the pounding heart already panicked by fear.

Distressing beliefs that life is filled with endless stress and strain upsets and hardens the body further in a desperate attempt to avoid feeling the pain of confrontation, and having to go through any further 'e-motional' upset. Locked in the lower astral plane, fear fuels the collective poverty consciousness, limiting the ability to live freely.

So much more is passed on than just material belongings when inheriting an inheritance. The 'same old' fearful beliefs handed down from one generation to another pass on sickening perceptions of inherent misfortune and uneasiness. Until one brave family member 'steps out of line' and refuses to take on all the worn-out BS, Belief Systems.

Thinking that something is impossible to get over is **F**alse **E**vidence **A**ppearing **R**eal – fear only goes away when released.

Those who fear limit themselves at times that faith is needed the most!

18 - CHRISTINE LYNNE STORMER-FRYER

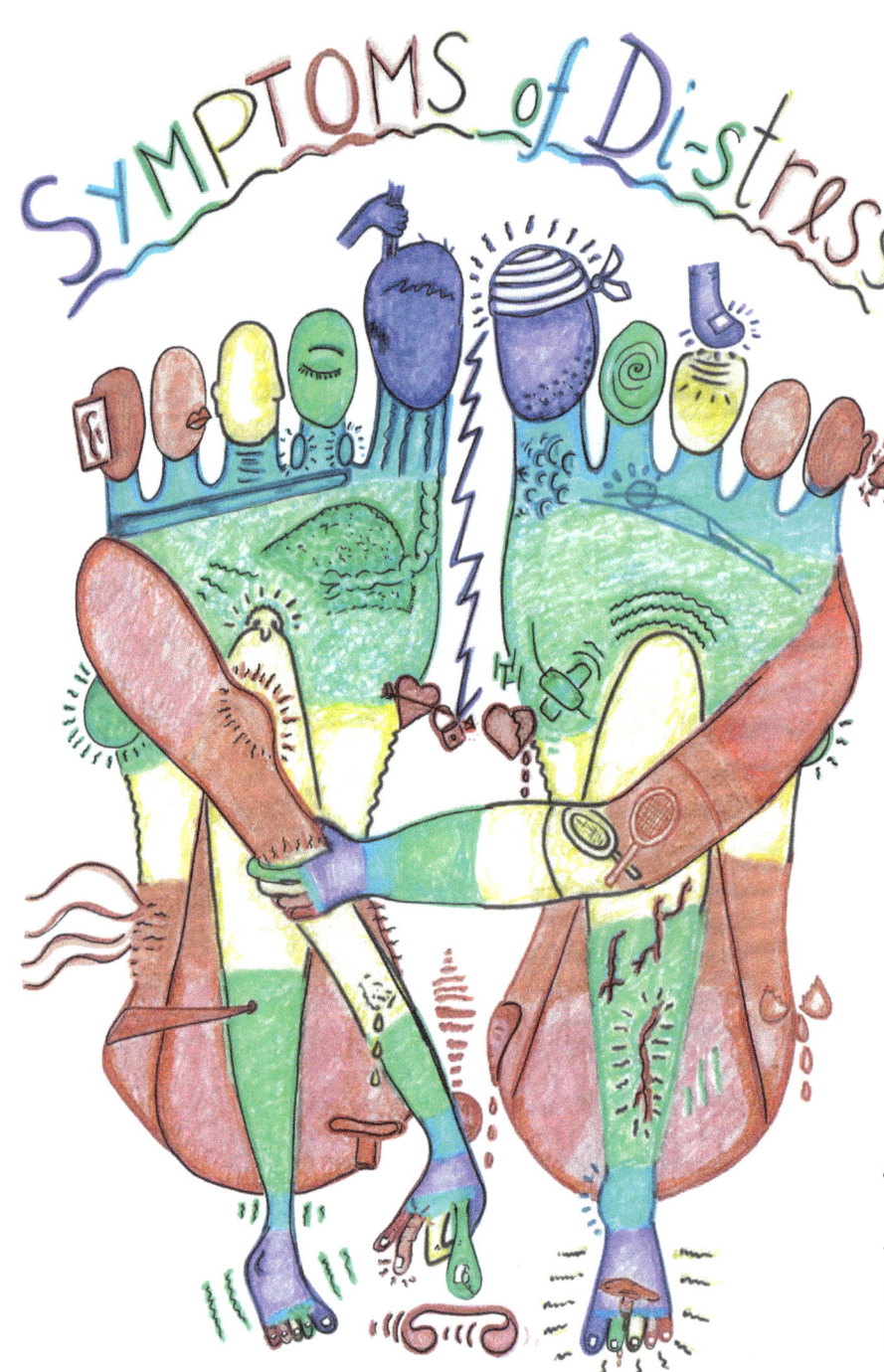

SYMPTOMS OF DISTRESS

Symptoms are the body's way of expressing despair at pertinent feelings being ignored or shoved into the background. Never an isolated event, every symptom has its own story, with the gist being that something unacceptable, even alien, is going on.

Going back seven generations or more, nobody is to blame. Ancestors unable to remedy outstanding issues at the time pass them onto future generations in the hope that sufficient advancements have been made to solve the issue for once and for all – a solution for all inherent uneasiness.

Symptoms of dis-ease provide insight into how to become a better, more authentic being. Uneasiness happens when circumstances begin to matter, thereby affecting the matter – in other words, the body.

Tipping the balance is too much or too little of anything. Too much or too little sensitivity. Too much or too little tolerance. Withdrawing or holding back when too much, or going over the top to compensate when too little. The 'issue' shows up in the 'tissue' to highlight 'the issue'.

If symptoms of 'dis-comfort', 'dis-turbance', 'dis-order', 'dis-location', 'dis-association' (and so on) are a sub-conscious concern, it can ultimately lead to 'dis-ease'. The right side of the body, empathising with the past, is influenced by men and anybody older. This energy is passed onto the receptive left side, more affected by females and those younger.

From memories, beliefs of good and bad are formed. Should these beliefs entangle mind, body and Spirit, the panic makes things go haywire with the ability or inability to cope being the ultimate test. With the state of mind determining the state of health, constantly 'aching' to 'get ahead' 'makes the head ache'. Racking the nerves are control issues and constant internal battles, making nerves quiver with dread, shake with frustration, go numb when traumatised, or become paralysed with fear.

Social restraints and restrictions strangle and stifle creative expressions. All the 'shoulds' and 'shouldn'ts' weigh heavily on the 'should'ers. Choked with e-motion, swallowed words often get 'stuck in the throat'. No day passes without feelings. Within seconds, a disturbing thought or distressing e-motion makes the body go from ease to a state of turbulent chaos.

Physical restraints produce the urge to rebel. When anger and frustration become motivating forces, the built-up inner fury raises temperatures, with affected parts becoming inflamed about what was done or not done. 'Hard to digest', such intensity upsets the upper digestive tract, causing dis-orders.

Inappropriate, misleading or inadequate communication, misunderstandings and estrangements, no information or co-operation, and staying in a relationship out of fear are all unacceptable to the lower digestive tract. Any form of insecurity 'rocks the boat', disintegrating the very structure and foundation of the body.

Symptoms, therefore, are the perfect opportunity to make vital changes and improvements.

Pain makes a person think. Thinking makes people wise. Wisdom is the appreciation of life!

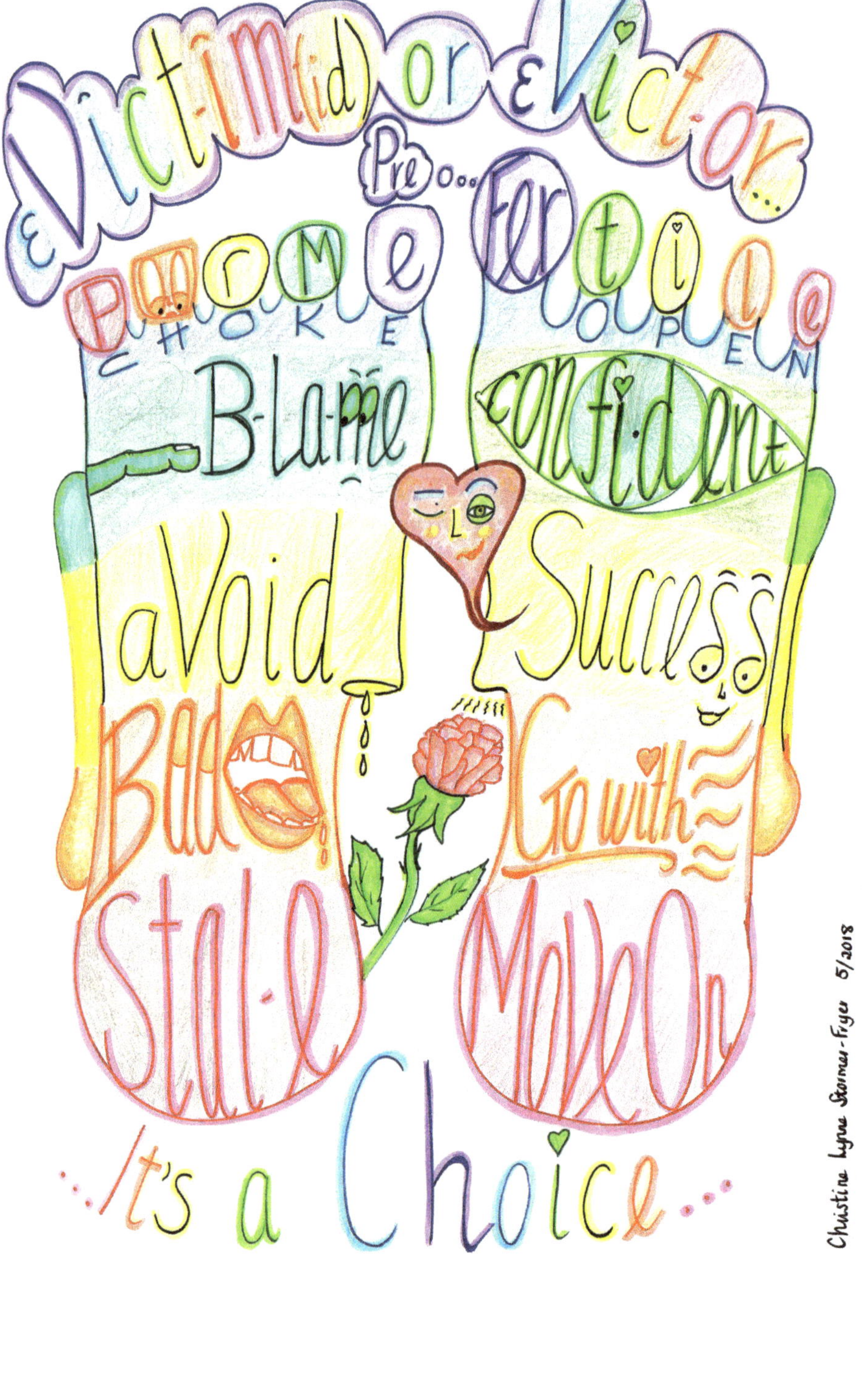
Vict-im(id) or Vict-or...
Pre... Fer
CHOKE
OPEN
B-La-me
con-fi-dent
aVoid
Success
Bad
Go with
Stal-e
Move On
...It's a Choice...
Christine Lynne Stormer-Fryer 5/2018

VICTIM OR VICTOR – IT'S A CHOICE

Those who continue to fall victim to past conditioning hang on relentlessly to stale memories and outdated and detrimental beliefs. Whether self-denial, lack of confidence, guilt, envy, shame, anger, poverty consciousness or lust, victims come from a place of powerlessness. Quick to blame childhood situations, pathetic 'poor me' sagas abound amid wails of 'why me?'

Choosing to be a victim serves in many ways, especially when craving sympathy and attention. Terrified of being proactive, a deep-down fear of failure curses these unhappy Souls, preventing them from taking responsibility for their actions.

As life passes rapidly by the drawback of wallowing in victim consciousness is the constant feeding of heavy despondency compounded by growing negativity filled with doom and gloom. Self-deprivation of 'happiness' is a choice.

Unwilling to spontaneously allow and make things 'happen', victims are invariably surprised to be swimming upstream against the current, giving further ammunition to bemoan the ongoing unfairness of life – albeit self-inflicted.

Blame avoids delving into one's deep-seated fears. 'A-void-ing' issues and filling the 'void' with further piles of self-pity only makes matters worse, as does 'bad-mouthing', speaking critically or disloyally, all of which foul the breath with halitosis.

'Choking' on untrue words or 'gagging' on overwhelming e-motions, society frequently finds truth too strong a medicine to take undiluted. Rather than abiding by counterfeit notions construed in the mind, abiding by authenticity borne in the Soul eliminates dark shadows of pretence, illuminated by rays of enlightenment.

Victims fail to realise that change is essential for humanity to evolve. Every exciting new phase comes with an exhilarating, albeit turbulent and chaotic, beginning. Only then can appropriate adjustments be made to embrace the unknown. Personal growth and development are all part of the process that comes in handy when venturing out on the ever-expansive journey ahead.

Victims with no hope can be transformed into victors with everything going for them. By being openly authentic and confident enough to 'step up to the plate' and accepting accountability without any complaints, constant alterations, modifications and adjustments ensure ongoing progress.

Even when shunned, ignored or banished for being perceived as a threat to society, victors proudly continue to express their individuality and just keep going. With fertile imaginations open to receiving Universal Insights, the self-assured victor has the wherewithal to go with the flow, constantly moving beyond social limitations.

Victims attract victims; victors attract victors!

22 - CHRISTINE LYNNE STORMER-FRYER

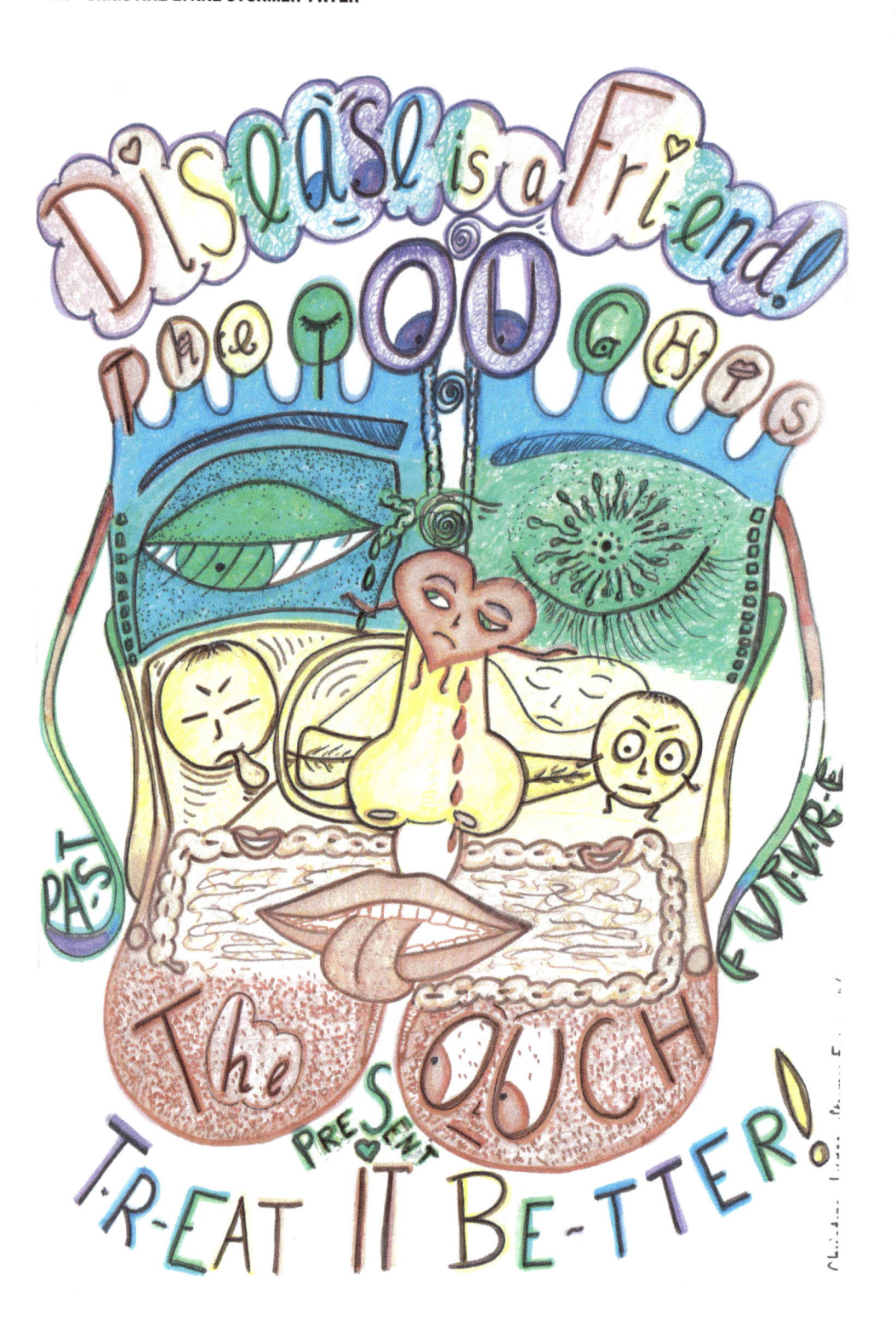

DIS-EASE IS A FRI-END – TREAT IT BETTER

Relentlessly plagued by intense distress and extreme discomfort, there is more disease and neurotic anxiety on this planet today than ever before. An over-whelming desire to fit into a desperately confused and insecure society, along with trying to meet unrealistic expectations of outdated family and social belief systems, soon shows signs of huge strain.

General fatigue and lack of energy from living an artificial, unfulfilling existence wastes a tremendous amount of precious life force energy, drained further by the inevitable build-up of inner tension and ongoing anxiety. Trying to master the visible outer world ignores the strength and power within.

Words used when dealing with dis-ease have a profound impact. 'Struggling' with a dis-ease intensifies the skirmish within. The clashing energy of 'battling' or 'fighting' an illness only makes matters worse. 'Suffering' from an ailment immediately creates a conflict situation, with the complaint perceived to be the over-ruling force. Disempowering words distract from the actual cause of uneasiness.

Detrimental circumstances taint 'thoughts', with all '**THe OUGHTS**' blemishing beliefs – circumstances that could otherwise be transformed by a changed mind and a more positive attitude. Ultimately, 'dis-ease' uneasiness within is purely and solely corrective, with every dis-eased person being a potentially healthy person temporarily imbalanced and out of sync with Universal life forces.

Despite trying to hide behind masks, eyes are the real give-aways. Unable to conceal deep feelings of discontent about the Spirit not being sufficiently nurtured, through failing to keep 'a-breast' of innermost needs. Unacceptable situations 'getting up the nose' make all the ridiculous hearsay 'hard to digest'. Being conscious of the 'e-motion' behind the uneasiness eases the transition from a state of extreme distress to one of inner harmony.

'Words put into the mouth', and stuff shoved 'down the throat' is enough to make any body puke. Mastering the mouth prevents becoming a slave to words that would otherwise 'get under the skin' when a sensitive issue is 'touched upon'. With touch being so fundamental to life, without it, feelings of being unwanted and insecure inevitably arise. Yet many still prefer to dwell on '**The OUCH**' of the past instead of appreciating 'touching incidents' in the present.

Regardless of the dis-ease's severity, intensity, frequency, or duration, self-acceptance and pure love, along with regular doses of warm-hearted belly laughs, are proven to be the best medicine. Love is well-known for 'healing all'. The purer the love, the better. With its marvellous recuperative abilities, the body, when fully appreciated, is more than capable of regaining its equilibrium and homeostasis.

Embracing 'dis-ease' as a friend, thanking it for drawing attention to 'the issue' within, is a giant step in healing. Treating dis-ease with respect, taking care of the affected tissue, and accepting the lessons on offer is to value the situation as a means of getting better at being oneself, trusting that the strength required to do so will be provided. As each Soul discovers the true meaning of life, world conditions will heal and change, and there will no longer be any place for dis-ease.

Optimists proclaim we live in the best possible world. Pessimists fear that this may be true!

24 - CHRISTINE LYNNE STORMER-FRYER

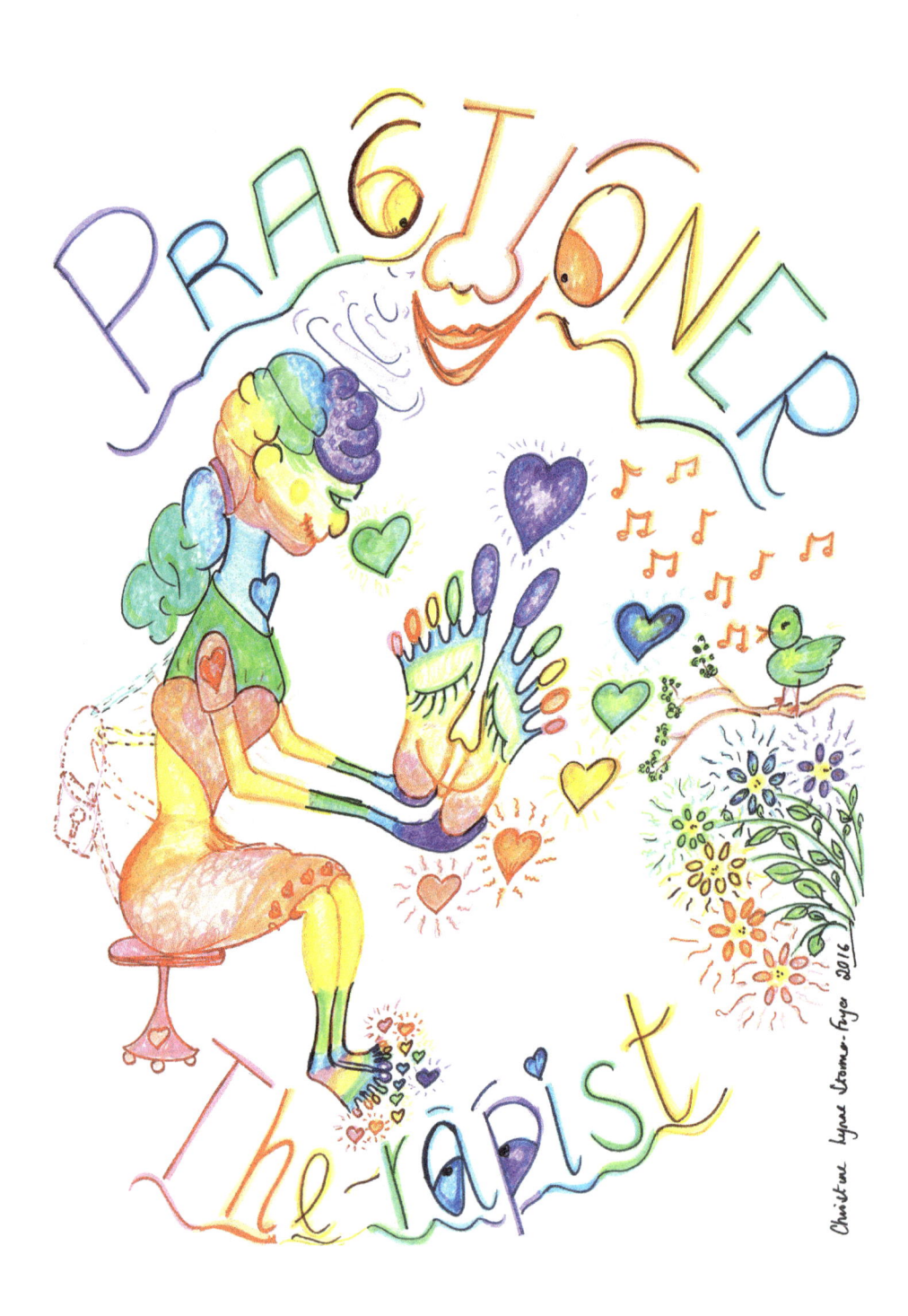

HEALTH PRACTITIONER

Everybody is a healer. Able to heal and feel better about oneself is an innate Universal gift bestowed upon everyone. It is an honour and privilege to encourage others to do the same by touching their Soul through their soles and being entrusted with connecting to innermost thoughts, dreams, hopes and fears.

Within every Soul dwells unlimited Universal energies waiting to be released on all levels. When offering 'Rei-flexology' (or any other healing modality), it is essential to ask for Soul permission. By connecting with the Higher Source, the practitioner becomes a more effective conduit for Universal energy. As life force energies are benevolently guided, it is up to the client to decide how best to use them.

As with any profession, the occupation chosen is ideal for 'working out' inherent Soul issues handed down from previous generations. In the health profession, those in need of curative measures are those administering them. With like attracting like, specific clients are magnetically and energetically attracted to reflect outstanding issues that require attention. Under-standing how to 'work out' personal issues while assisting others in the process is an absolute gift.

From time to time, certain clients may test the practitioner's patience and, in so doing, offer valuable and worthwhile lessons. Also insightful is the facilitator's decision to exclude specific individuals. For instance, choosing to 'treat' only females could reveal deeply entrenched issues of being taken advantage of by men. Those rejecting homosexuals, prostitutes, other races (and so on), are being shown the 'red light' of discrimination within their own family. When clients constantly present with similar complaints, it is time to look more deeply within to reveal what is really going on beneath the surface.

Health practitioners can only heal themselves by intuitively tapping into life force energies all from the same Universal source. It is the practitioner's demeanour that makes all the difference in gaining the client's trust and creating space for them to help themselves move towards improved health.

Many Souls have lost touch with their true Spirit and meaning of life. Having distanced themselves from one another, touch is essential (and vital) for healing the gaps. Made unique by the personal touch, miraculous responses occur when the energy is generated from a place of love and compassion.

As the body activates its own healing power, latent contents are unleashed and 'e-motional' congestion eased. Being considered a failure when symptoms get worse is a misconception. Instead, it is a good sign of the body bringing issues to a head, to be dealt with in their own way.

Understanding the client's story and their Spiritual hi-story assists in adjusting treatments to suit individual needs. Taking credit for another's recovery places the health practitioner in an uncompromising position. It immediately changes the energies, leaving them surprisingly powerless – especially when the client chooses *not* to improve.

With each health practitioner offering a unique and individual approach to reflexology and natural health, clients have a wonderful choice of which practitioner and what technique suits them best. Ultimately, it is up to the health practitioner to inspire and encourage others to help themselves to a better way of life.

Healing is a Divine energy available to all!

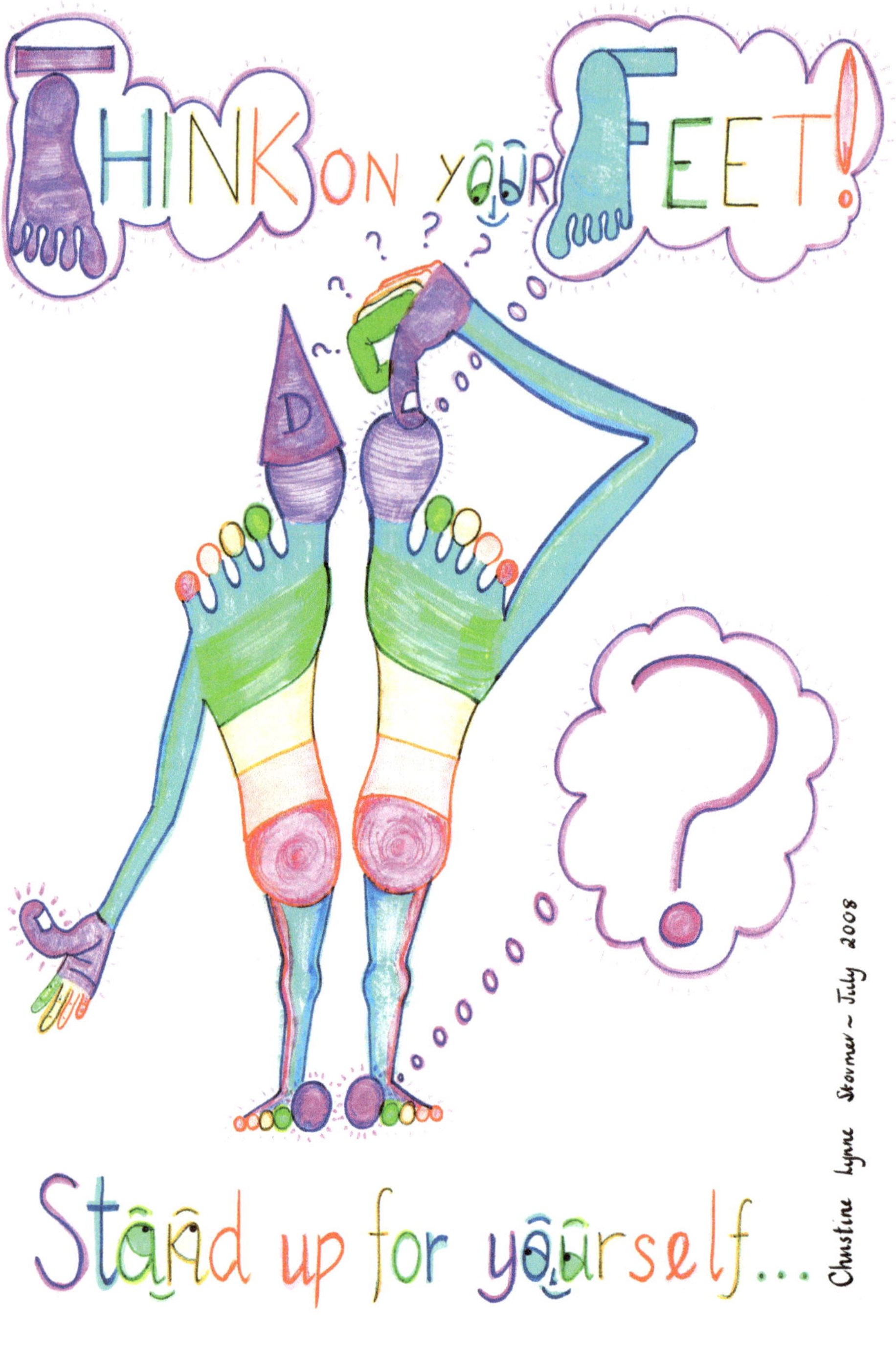
THINK ON YOUR FEET!
Stand up for yourself...
Christine Lynne Stormer ~ July 2008

THINK ON YOUR FEET – STAND UP FOR YOURSELF

Thinking is humanity's greatest tool of creativity – an energy that evolves as the human race becomes increasingly advanced and enlightened.

Ultimately it is all '**THe OUGHTS**' that determine the type of impact on each miniscule cell. As ideas run from head to toe, the vibration jogs memories, evoking 'e-motion' – 'energy in motion'. Subsequent feelings act as stimuli, determining what to do or not do next, thereby affecting relationships. Once 'on the go', feeling secure is the motivating force to making progress.

'Putting on the thinking cap' requires planting seeds of energy in the mind to create reality. Based on personal perceptions of life, the outcome is determined by the quality of these concepts and the intention behind them.

Sowing old seeds way past their 'sell-by date' and expecting healthy plants is a non-starter, as is planting worn-out beliefs and time-worn notions – it is detrimental to personal wellbeing.

Whether conscious, subconscious or unconscious, every thought generates its own kind of energy – either constructive or destructive, significant or insignificant. Either way, the chemical and physical composition and characteristics of individual cells are altered, influencing the ever-changing characteristics of feet.

The mind keeps dwelling on the circumstances that it has created. Programmed in the elusive sub-conscious mind, continuous modes of thought yield certain types of behavioural patterns, postures, eases and dis-eases. Concentrated thoughts, like a powerful magnifying glass, have the greatest impact.

Hovering overhead are 'en masse' thoughts – purposefully distorted through misleading patterns of belief at a sub-conscious level, for mass control and manipulation by a self-elected minority. Exceeding boundaries of popular thinking can have significant, albeit exciting, life-changing consequences, offering other ways to 'make up the mind'.

No thought is an original thought. Each one is drawn from the Universal Library of Thoughts and has been thought through zillions of times before. To claim certain thoughts as one's own and to copyright them is to 'have another think coming' since it interferes with their free flow.

To assist in raising consciousness is the Universal spotlight of enlightening UV ultra-violet, ultra-Divine rays, pouring through the hole in the ozone layer. Misconstrued fear is intentional, preventing THE light from showing the way.

Nothing is 'impossible' when 'I'm possible'. If it can be imagined, it is possible. It is impossible to stop thinking, except during meditation, but it *is* possible to change thoughts. Becoming aware of the ability 'to think on the feet' and 'stand up' for oneself makes it possible to control thoughts and 'think for oneself'.

It is time to 'think for a change' and allow resplendent thoughts to influence worldwide conditions. Once stretched by new ideas, knowledge, and wisdom, the mind never goes back to its original dimensions. Thank goodness!

Be daring! Think of what to change!

28 - CHRISTINE LYNNE STORMER-FRYER

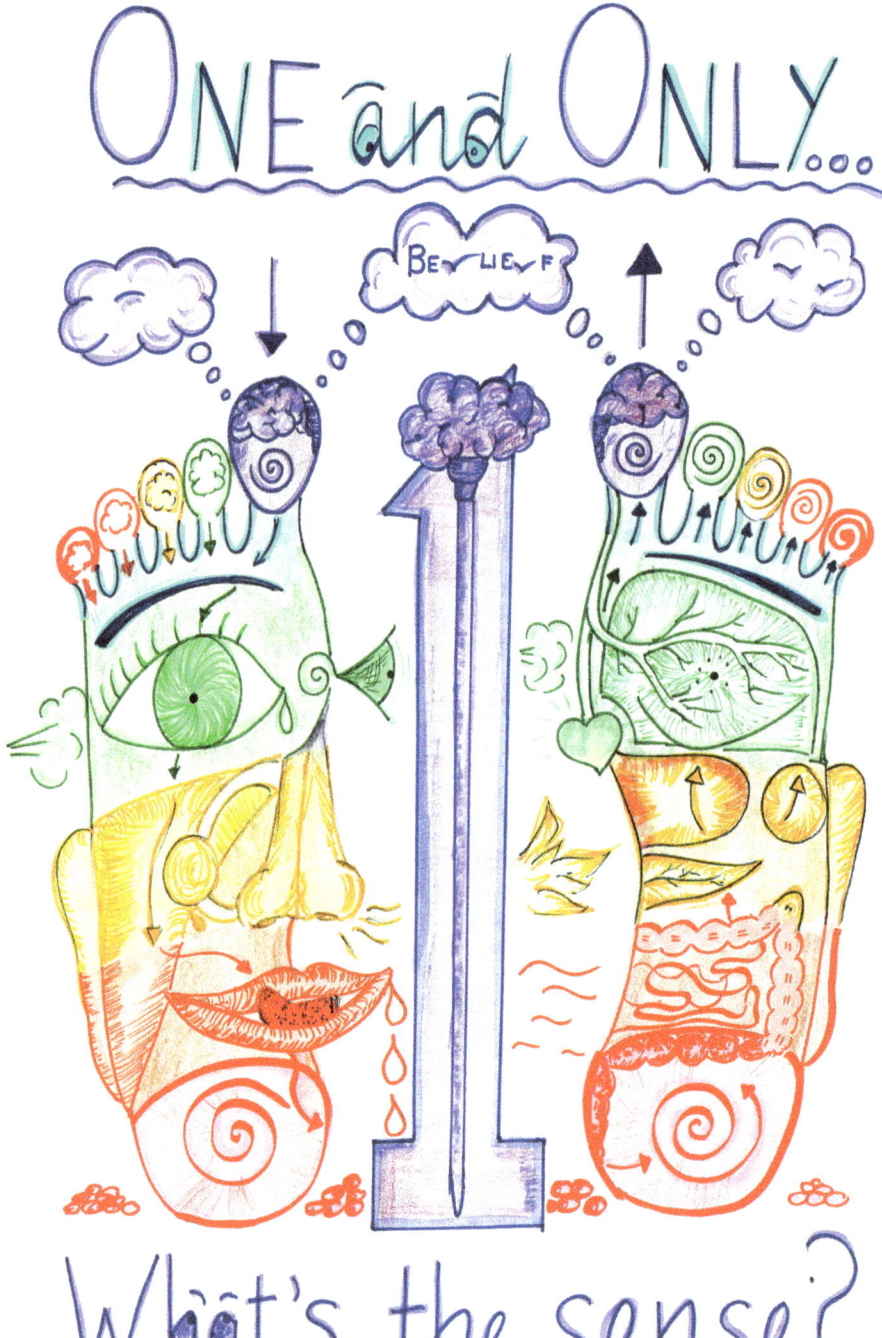

ONE AND ONLY – WHAT'S THE SENSE

'What's the sense' of being the 'one and only' 'one of a kind' standing out from the crowd being noticed for being the same but different? Linked to the ethereal realm of thought, this is the role of the big toes.

Perfectly straight like an arrow, 'one' is a strong, assertive symbol of individuality, making the beginning of self-discovery and self-empowerment. The Spiritual essence of singularity, 'one' seeks and reaches out, exploring ways to define the self.

The aim of 'one' is to be at 'one' with the Higher Self, by getting reacquainted with the power residing within 'one'. Knowing 'one's' personal potential, 'one' can then generate new projects, completely changing course in life. 'One', being creatively confident, is always on the look-out for new adventures.

Putting out feelers, the big toes lead and point the way towards the next step, making the most of the many 'one and only opportunities of a lifetime'. Standing proud and tall and being unique is their forte.

Generally larger than all the other toes, big toes are in the perfect position to embrace all the sensory vibrations that come their way. The greater the sensitivity, the greater the imagination. Meanwhile, each of the smaller toes picks up and resonate to a specific sensational aspect.

For the second toes, it is sight; third toes prefer sounds and smells; fourth take on taste, while little toes are the 'touchier' 'feely' 'ones'. The energetic commonality between all the toes unites them as 'one'.

When 'one' feels uncomfortable about standing out, the tendency is to 'pull back', but when 'one' wishes to 'get a point across' or 'be in another's face', the toe pad sticks out and leans forward.

Sensitive about being separated from the crowd but not wishing 'to close the gap', a space is often found between the big toes and the neighbouring second toes, invariably as a sign of enhanced Spiritual awareness.

Preferable to 'one-upmanship' (trying to outdo or be more successful, admired, or respected than someone else) is to move beyond comparisons. It makes it so much easier for 'one' to accept being a 'one and only'. Embracing personal values defines 'one's' unique identity, keeping relationships on a more 'even keel'.

'One's' Soul choice is to achieve great things on Earth by manifesting 'one's' innovative ideas. Individuality sets 'one' apart, yet 'one' still relies on the contribution of others to ensure the continuing evolution of humanity.

Even though every 'one' is 'al-one' on 'one's' own unique journey, every 'one' is 'all-one', connected by humanness – every 'one' an extension of the Creator's Spirit; the 'one' energy that unites all of creation by permeating everything, uniting all atoms in the Universe.

Mind, Body and Soul are one, present throughout the journey through life!

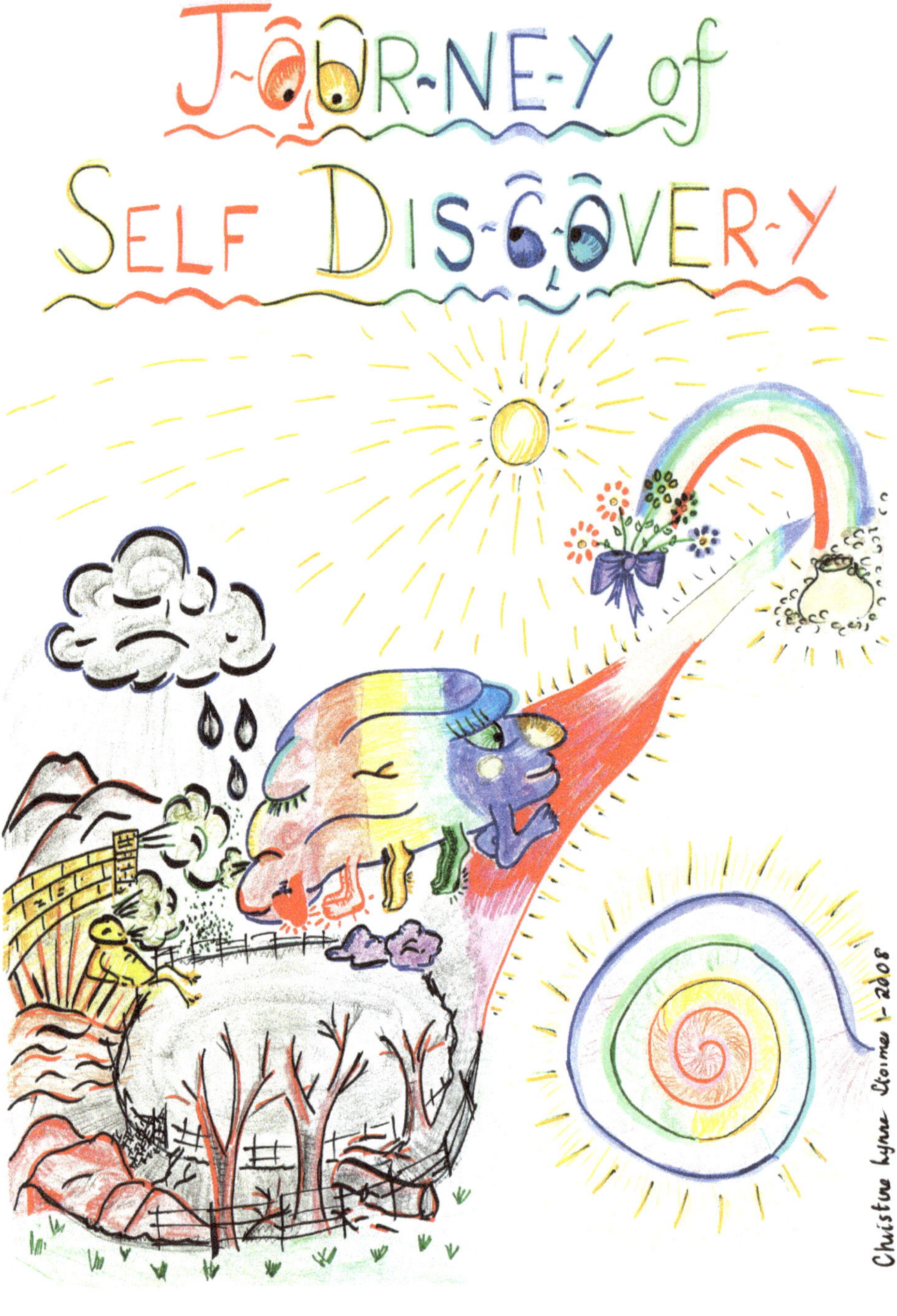
J~OUR~NE~Y of
SELF DIS~COVER~Y
Christine Lynne Stormer 1-2008

JOURNEY OF SELF-DISCOVERY

Life is an adventure of the mind making the impossible possible, a journey of self-discovery opening the Soul to endless possibilities through countless experiences, thanks to the body's ability to move. No wonder life is such an intriguing mystery!

Being courageous enough to enter the human race is to discover many exciting approaches and enthralling ways to follow the route of the Soul. Ultimately, it is choice not chance that determines our destiny. Never before have there been so many exciting destinations with the power to change reality by instantaneously transforming the mind, instead of struggling with current conditions.

Getting wrapped up in repetitive thoughts 'going round and round in circles' makes it impossible to concentrate on the gifts of the present. Fearful Souls are often too frightened to venture out into the elusive unknown.

Rebellious Souls are frequently tempted to veer off track, invariably losing their way. With the mind digging up endless doom and gloom, depression sets in and deepens into a large abyss of nothingness, making it seem impossible to function or even be understood. This is only an 'ill'-usion.

Pre-occupation with instant physical, intellectual and material gratification puts the more intuitive aspects of being human on the back burner, depriving the Soul of its true essence. The natural balance of life-generating forces is easily upset until the treasure chest of talent and wisdom is discovered within and utilised for ongoing success.

Blessed with the gift of a creative mind, life's journey is all about visualisation, purposefully creating all life experiences. Being 'out of the mind' is a great time-saver. Without having to review, analyse or criticise past encounters and events, decisions are instantly reached, and choices rapidly activated, a delightful way of getting back in touch with the senses.

Being mindful of what is being projected is the first step in reclaiming authentic power. As the 'one and only' maker of the mind, filling it with well-meaning productive thoughts leaves no room for detrimental, harmful ones. What happens is not nearly as important as the response and reaction.

It is not good enough to have a good mind. The main thing is to *use* it well, a matter of 'mind over matter', with the body being the 'matter'. When things are 'made to matter', it 'affects the matter'. When it 'doesn't matter', there is no difference.

'In many minds', the 'conscious mind' oversees the physical body. The 'subconscious mind' cares for the 'e-motional' body. The 'unconscious mind' governs the mental body. Spirit administers the 'superconscious mind'.

As the Soul creates, so the mind reacts. The Spirit understands what the mind cannot begin to conceive, while the body follows the mind wherever it goes. Even when the 'mind is made up', changes will always be required along the way.

Never be in two minds – be in many minds!

32 - CHRISTINE LYNNE STORMER-FRYER

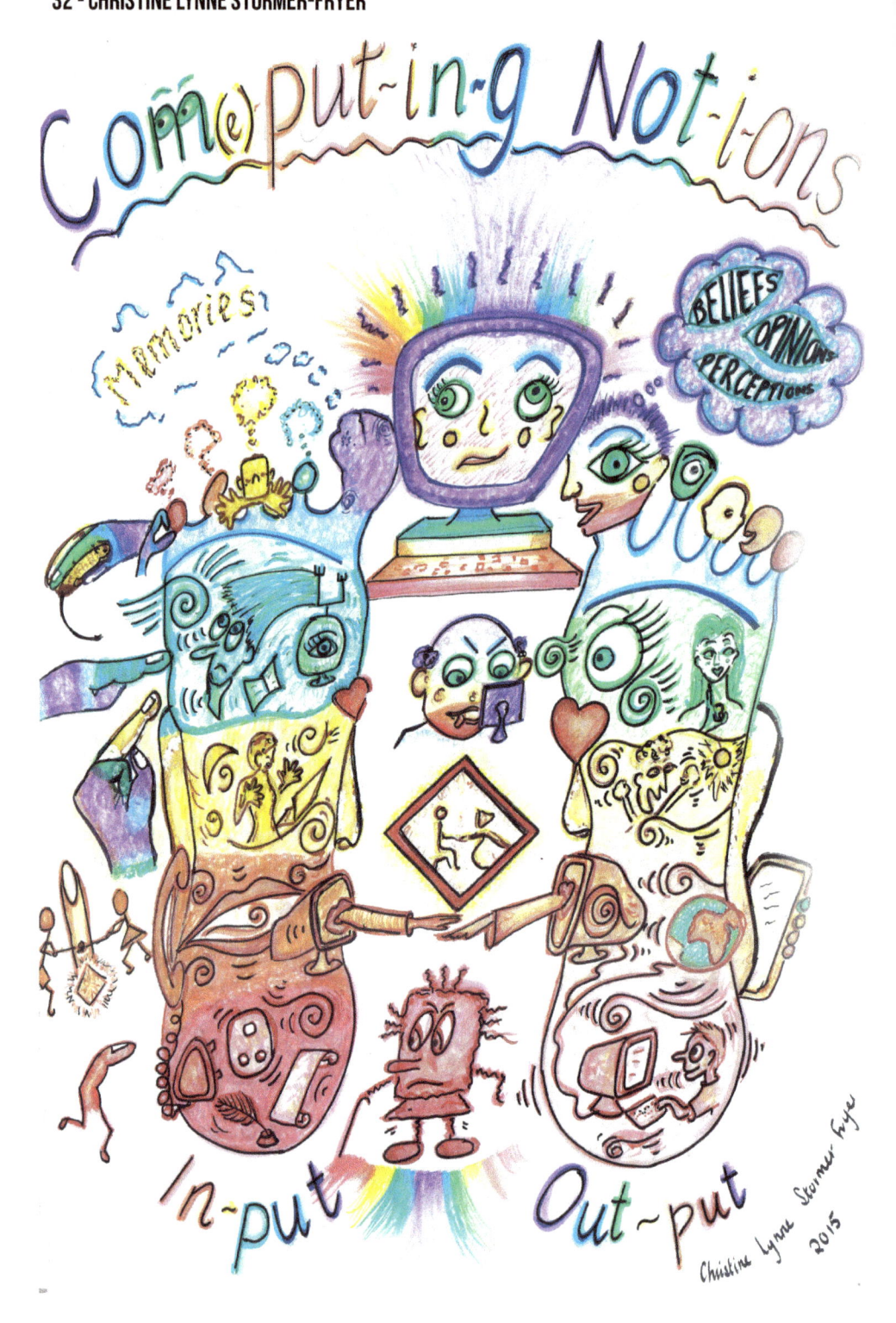

COMPUTING NOTIONS

The brain is the world's most complex computer. Sub-consciously fed and programmed by belief systems, values, and stored memories, all perceptions become reality. Consulting a bank of zillions of memories, a decision is reached within a split-second after having analysed an onslaught of incoming information. Pertinent messages are then relayed to appropriate parts of the body for action.

The generation known as 'BBC', 'Born Before Computers', believed computers to be a way-out science fiction concept only seen on television. A 'window' was something to look through. A 'ram', the father of a goat. 'Meg', a girl's name. A 'gig', a night-time job. 'Cursors', a form of profanity. 'To compress' was to zip an over-packed suitcase. A 'mouse pad', a rodent's home. 'Logging on' was to add more wood to the fire. A 'hard drive' was a difficult journey. Interesting snippets were 'cut and pasted' into scrapbooks. A 'virus' was the flu. A man with a 'three-inch floppy' was nothing to be bragged about, and openly 'unzipping' was a public offence.

Highly evolved minds get IT, and invariably have jobs in the computer industry to invent further advancements in processing and dealing with life. The functioning of the brain's grey-white matter depends on how well it is treated and appreciated. The mind's way of dealing with 'factual input' has a powerful influence on the computer's performance.

The network is a mishmash of 'webs' – some 'webs of lies', others 'webs of truth' – that capture the imagination to draw in like-minded Souls. 'Sources' of information can either be deceitfully enticing to trap unsuspecting mentalities or 'openly honest', offering gems of wisdom. Either way, extensions of the working of individual minds impact actions on a daily basis.

Dislike of computers due to the belief that 'they never work properly' is likely to be a reflection of the regular rejection of personal concepts 'not working out'. So much so that an overload of conflicting notions befuddles the mind, often causing the whole system to 'crash', requiring periodic rebooting.

'Troublesome thoughts' are asking for 'trouble', necessitating constant 'troubleshooting' to sort things out. The problem with 'troubleshooting' is that 'trouble often shoots back'. Information-related crises require a deep analysis of the conflict. It takes a brain and heart to restore any sense of orderly comprehension of what to do next.

Men and women compute incoming information very differently. Females are the only ones to understand the internal logic and language used to communicate with same-gender computers. A 'bad command or file name' is as about as informative as 'If you don't know why I'm so mad at you, I am certainly not going to tell you!'. Even the smallest mistakes are stored in the long-term memory bank for later retrieval.

Meanwhile, male computers are convinced that, had they only waited a bit longer before committing, a better (and more attractive) model would have come along.

Beneficial choices made today make for worthwhile ones tomorrow!

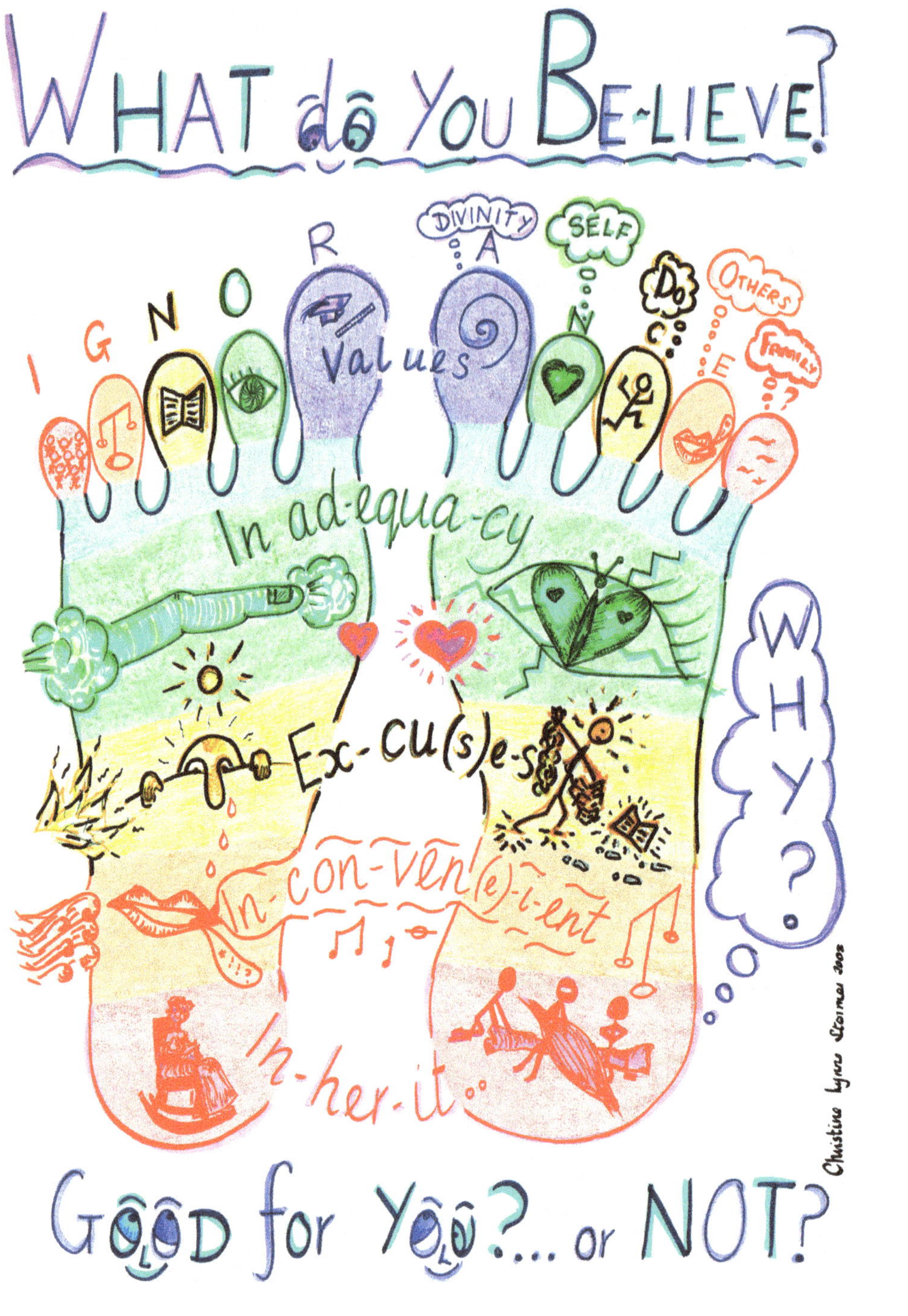
WHAT do YOU BE-LIEVE?
I G N O R A N C E
DIVINITY
SELF
DO
OTHERS
FAMILY
Values
In ad-equa-cy
WHY?
Ex-cu(s)e-s
In-con-ven(e)-i-ent
In-her-it..
GOOD for YOU?... or NOT?

WHAT DO YOU BELIEVE? GOOD FOR YOU OR NOT?

Beliefs are a load of 'BS', '**B**elief **S**ystems'. Whether inherited, hearsay, or derived from the memory banks of personal experience, a belief holds great power. Ultimately, beliefs are the basis of all perception and concepts.

Beliefs change expectations. Accepted as true or real without proof, being absolutely certain or convinced about the existence of something, personal beliefs contribute their 'penny's worth' to the collective consciousness. All too often though, unquestioned beliefs settle deep in the unconscious mind, influencing the heart, mind and reality.

Many beliefs arise from ignorance. The more the truth is denied, the greater the ignorance. Ignoring divinity, oneself, personal talents, others, family (and so on) is to recklessly entrap the mind, holding it prisoner within the dense vibrations of lower consciousness. Furthermore, 'buying into' limiting beliefs stifles inner potential, thereby limiting personal expectations.

A belief is not an idea possessed – it is an idea that takes over. Experiences do not determine beliefs. Beliefs of what to expect determine the experience. Despite playing a key role in being convinced and getting behind something, beliefs do not always serve as reliable guides.

'Entertaining' inner beliefs of 'inadequacy' and 'not being good enough' eventually evolve into the body's personal trademark. Highly protective of these misconceptions are the ribs and chest. The right lung favours principles laid down by Father and society, while the left lung resonates with the more intuitive and Spiritual beliefs of Mother and the Universe. Low self-esteem hampers the breath, preventing the heart and blood from circulating love and joy, both internally and externally.

Free to choose 'what to believe', the only limitations come from the 'self-restraining ones'. Most energy-sapping notions revolve around not having the talent or wherewithal to succeed. Personal identification becomes lost when taking 'other beliefs' on board, believing and conforming to all that is heard.

'Ex-cuses' are just not good enough. Whether used to lessen pain, justify a fault or an offence, or conceal the truth, using these over-used 'ex-cuses' as 'props' is a real 'cop-out'. A pathetic attempt to try and buy more time, an excuse eventually becomes a 'crippling disease' of the failure to 'step up to the plate'. Worst of all, deep down, everybody knows it.

Heavy childhood baggage sabotages a multitude of amazing opportunities. A deep-seated conviction that suffering and sacrifice have to be endured in order to succeed is hugely debilitating. While this may have been the experience of an ancestor, it is no longer the case. Poverty conscious beliefs undermine self-worth and are at the root of never being able to manifest abundance, even when well-deserved.

No two people have the same beliefs. What is deemed 'inconvenient' by one is not always believed to be the situation for the other. Each has their own specific belief system, programmed by life, with many being 'in-her-it-ed'. Releasing negative beliefs opens floodgates of energy, offering endless opportunities to be sensational. It may mean 'going against the grain', but trusting personal instincts and going with the heart's desire – regardless of prevailing opinions – is the 'way to go'.

Beliefs are decisions and choices actively creating reality!

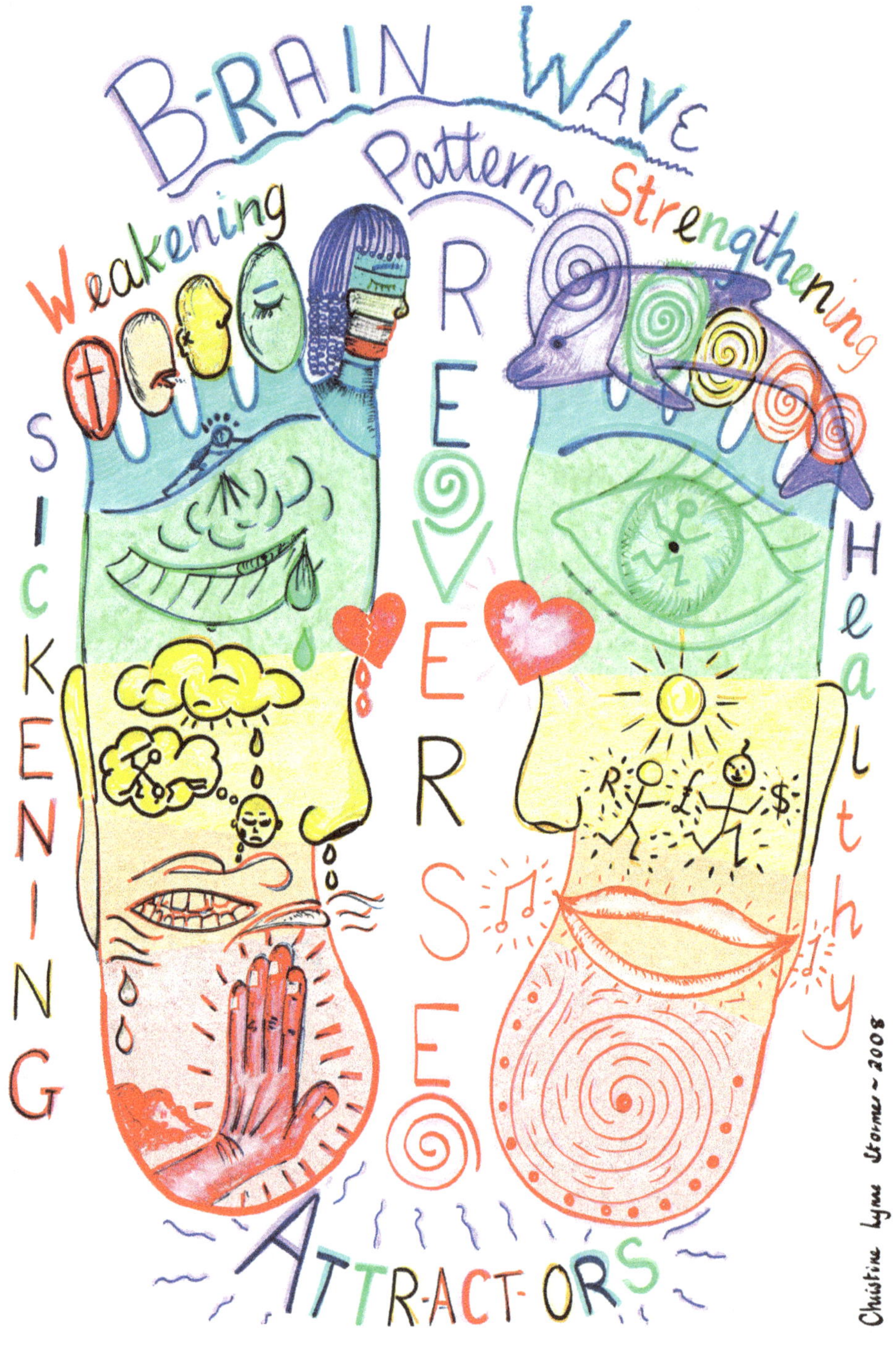
B-RAIN WAVE
Patterns
Weakening
Strengthening
SICKENING
REVERSE
Healthy
R £ $
ATTR-ACT-ORS
Christine Lynne Stormer ~ 2008

BRAIN WAVE - ATTRACTORS

Waves of force, passion and understanding ripple continuously from the brain throughout the body, bringing insight and exciting concepts to the fore. Being on the 'same wavelength' as the Universe ensures a smooth transmission of internal and external messages along nerve fibres, triggering highly beneficial impulsive responses. Vibrating on 'alien wavelengths' distorts reality and creates confusion – enough to want to 'throw a fit'.

Every thought 'pattern', 'e-motional' response and behavioural display attracts a series of synchronised electrical pulsations from masses of neurons, all collaborating with one another to either 'weaken' or 'strengthen' the brain waves. This continuous spectrum of consciousness is determined by bandwidths, from slow, loud and functional to fast, subtle and complex.

Low-frequency waves, much like a drumbeat, are profoundly strong. The more elusive higher waves are akin to the sound of a high-pitched flute. Joined together through harmonics, these 'patterns' change in line with one's perceptions and beliefs.

When tired or dreamy, slower brainwaves become predominant, slowing the body down and often making it feel drowsy and sluggish. To prevent persistent 'weakening' thoughts from 'sickening' the body, a positive input is required to 'reverse' the situation, revving up frequencies and generating a 'healthy' outlook. Going to either extreme makes the body jumpy, or turns one into an over-stimulated hyper-active 'live wire'.

Deep meditation and dreamless sleep lower the frequency of brainwaves, with deeply penetrating 'delta waves' suspending all external awareness, ideal for ongoing rejuvenation.

Fleetingly experienced when drifting in and out of sleep, the twilight 'theta waves' are gateways to a vivid imagination and enhanced intuition, way beyond normal conscious awareness. As senses become oblivious to the external world, so the focus goes within.

Quietly flowing 'alpha waves' relax brain activity to induce mental co-ordination, serenity and enhanced sensory awareness. The exquisite state of 'being' experienced during 'Rei-flexology' creates the ideal space for the Soul to rejuvenate itself.

Dominant during the normal waking state, 'beta waves' focus on mental activity and the outside world. High-frequency waves are quick to participate in cognitive tasks, decision making and problem-solving, but continual processing at such a hectic rate takes an enormous amount of energy, not a particularly efficient way to run any brain.

For information to be passed quickly and quietly, the brain needs to be silent to access the high frequency 'gamma' brainwaves, the fastest of them all. This 'pattern' of neural oscillation correlates to a widespread brain network that is amplified through meditation. These wave patterns are drastically altered when functioning on 'alternate wavelengths', as in Alzheimer's dis-ease, epilepsy and schizophrenia.

By simultaneously processing information from different brain areas, consciousness is elevated. With an increasing awareness of Spirit, a sudden 'brainwave' engenders innovative concepts, raising humanity to a completely different, and exciting, level of consciousness.

As perceptions change, so too do brainwaves!

38 - CHRISTINE LYNNE STORMER-FRYER

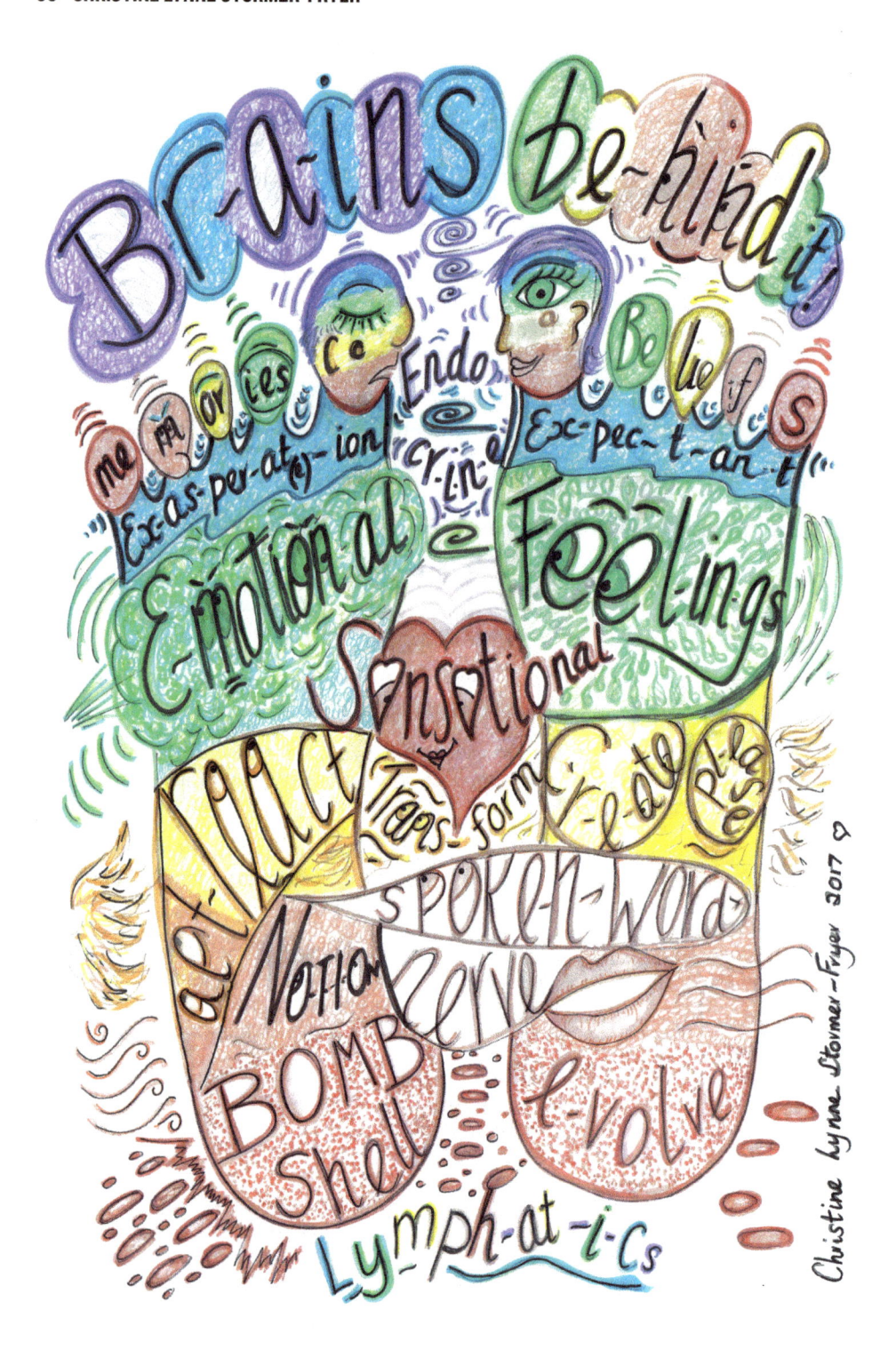

BRAINS BEHIND IT

At any one time, millions of messages course through the brain, providing ongoing stimulation and knowledge. Much more than a centre of intellectual activity, the brain can either ascend to the ethereal realm to attain Universal wisdom and Spiritual awareness or stretch both inwards and outwards to explore the magnificent creativity of the Soul.

The 'brains behind it all' are highly intellectual, extremely imaginative, and incredibly intuitive. Thanks to them, the potential for natural talent and unbelievable aptitude is enormous. Endless decisions are based on thoughts, memories and beliefs constantly 'entertained'. Whether destructive or constructive, each has its own consequences.

From the brain (and the brain alone) arises 'exasperation', sorrows, pain, grief and fears, as well as 'expectations', pleasures, joys, laughter and jests. All 'sensational feelings' that have a profound impact on the flow of lymph. Devouring the input of thoughts fed to it, brain cells react by retrieving and selecting meaningful information. Anything that does not resonate with its belief network is rejected immediately, not even 'given a second thought'. Moulding all the stored data from previous experiences and remembered e-motions pre-determines the quality and events of life.

By choosing one's own thoughts, every body has complete control over deciding how best to 'act and react', ideally in a 'pleasing' manner, without having to resort to the 'dis-ease to please'. Initiating, monitoring, 'transforming' and controlling the performance of all organs and endocrine glands according to what is 'uppermost in the mind' is not only essential for survival but vital for determining personal wellbeing.

A mass of paired, inverted pyramids of nerve fibres run vertically down the centre of the brain, providing the 'nerve to speak up' and 'get a move on'. Innovative, exciting Universal concepts present the greatest impetus to magnify thoughts, inflating the mind to make a much-needed world of difference.

Ultimately, the brain offers a dwelling place of love. The 'spoken word' is a superb vehicle used by the super-conscious mind of the Higher Self. It helps to create consciousness of the self and the world – 'hand in hand' with unconscious awareness, creativity, and everything human.

Even with a 'bombshell' coming its way, the brain is subconsciously capable of determining a multitude of life-saving bodily functions by objectively obeying conscious choices.

The only way the body can respond to the outside world is to 'evolve' through the activity of the 'brains behind it'. Great importance is attached to hands and feet to get its brilliant ideas and magnificent concepts 'out there'.

The brain minds the matter while the matter shows how much the mind cares about the matter!

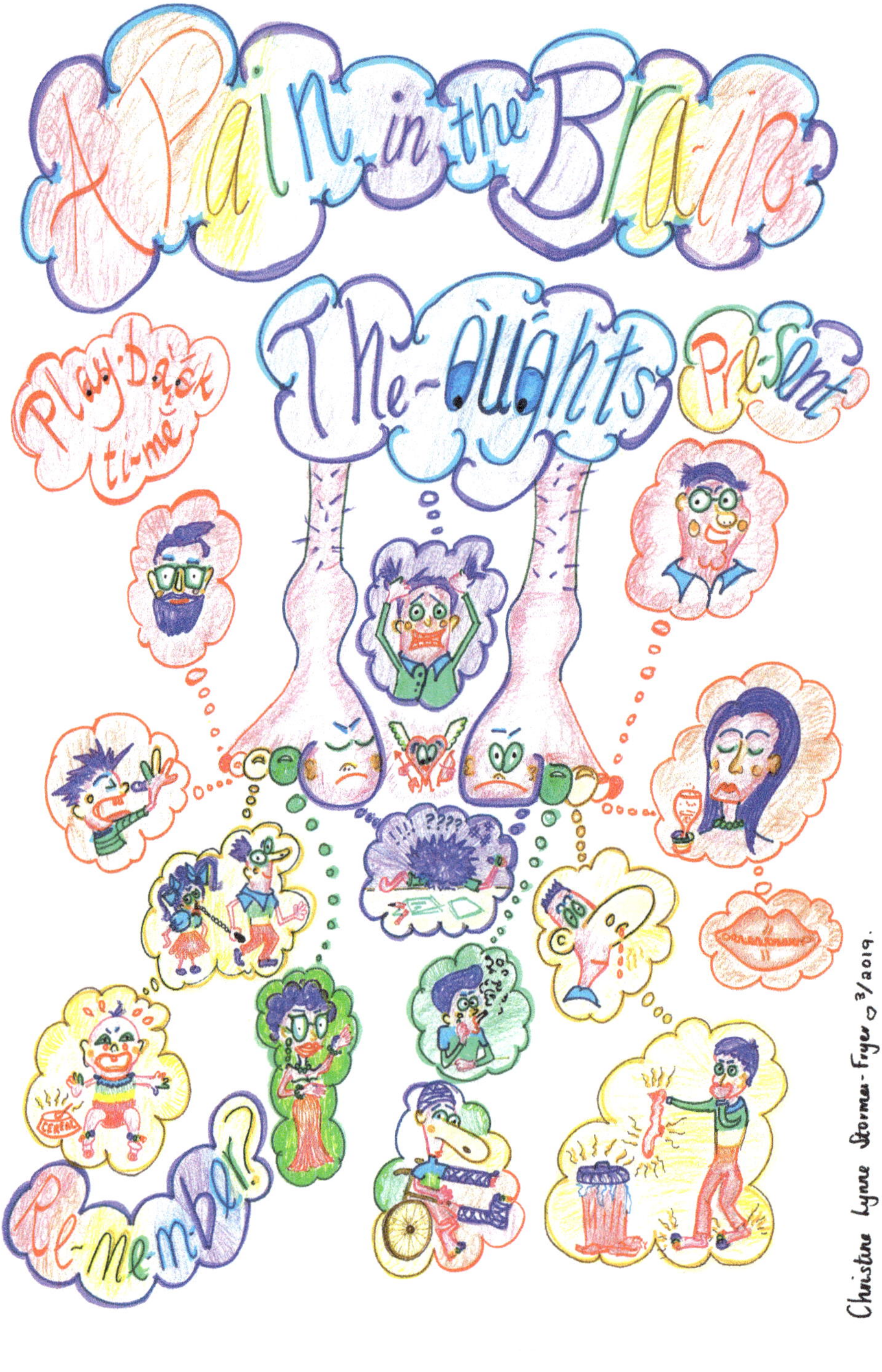
A Pain in the Brain
The-oughts
Play-back ti-me
Pre-sent
CEREAL
Re-me-mber?
Christine Lynne Stormer-Fryer 3/2019.

A PAIN IN THE BRAIN

A head crammed full of hectic memories, outdated beliefs, frantic fears, and feverish anxiety is a real pain in the brain. Being dulled by all '**th**-e **ought**s' makes for a sluggish body more susceptible to uneasiness, and eventually dis-ease, with endless whims of possible disaster tipping the balance.

Dwelling in the past, with constant repetition and 'playback' of obsolete memories and archaic beliefs, irritates the brain and 'gets on its nerves'. 'Banging the head', 'pulling the hair out' in utter frustration, or 'throwing a tantrum' when totally 'out of control' is 'just the pits'.

'Dis-turbed' by deceit and dishonesty from 'bearding the lion', overthinking invariably proves useless. Even though 'bad' attitudes are rarely tolerated in others, the brain is forced to put up with ceaseless critical mind chatter. Dis-gusted by the stream of self-limiting, condemning thoughts makes it want to 'put its head in the sand' as moods and outlook become increasingly dismal.

Dis-comfort arising from 'smokescreens' used to conceal its abhorrence at being forced to accommodate stale e-motions and old hurts, goes straight to the chest. The lack of authenticity injures its pride. Always 'looking back' or continually 'looking ahead' is exceptionally unsettling, making it impossible to focus on the present. Having made such 'spectacle' of itself means that eventually 'spectacles' are required to see what is 'right under its nose'.

'Getting on its wick' is to be reluctantly 'led by the nose' and obliged to do something despicable. Being jeered at and snubbed by those with their 'nose in the air' is hurtful and pains the brain. On the other hand, trying to be a perfectionist is highly irritating, 'getting up its nose' and making it drip mercilessly.

Another 'pet hate' is being force-fed with repugnant ideas. Memories of having cereal, non-sense that 'goes against the grain', shovelled down the oesophagus and then told to 'zip the mouth' makes the brain want to 'blow its top'. Dis-appointment and dis-trust in those who adversely force the brain to question its values undermines its self-assurance. Turning to drink to lighten its head and 'drown its sorrows' is not the solution of choice, especially when left with a 'hangover' of note.

'Dis-turbed' at being 'rubbed up the wrong way', becoming incapacitated and stopped in its tracks, really puts the brain to the test. It knows that accidents, the 'act-I -see- indent' me, occur when 'going headlong' into life in search of a 'break' from rigidity. A less drastic way of showing difficulty in meeting social expectations is to cover up the true self with a double chin – being two-faced to please others and oneself.

The brain is more than capable of rising above all the pettiness and regaining complete control. All its healing centre requires is a change of mind.

A positive attitude begets positive health benefits!

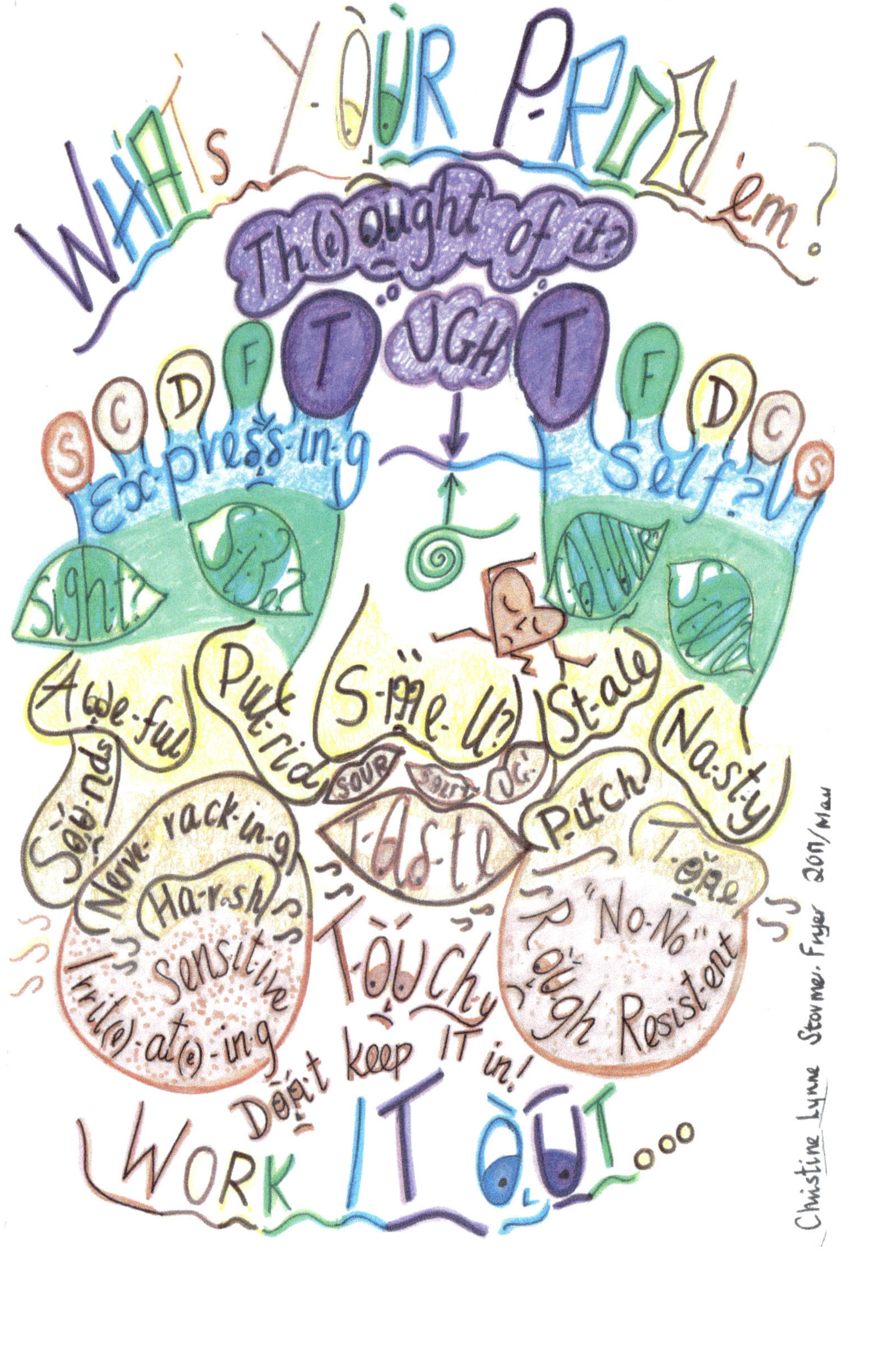
WHAT's YOUR PROBL'em?
Th(e)ought of it?
T UGH T
Ex-press-in-g
Self?
Sight?
Awe-ful
Put-rid
S-me-ll?
St-ale
Nasty
SOUR
SALTY
Pitch
Taste
Sounds
Nerve-rack-in-g
Ha-r-sh
Sensit-ive
Irrit(e)-at(e)-ing
Touchy
Tone
"No-No"
Rough
Resist-ent
Don't keep IT in!
WORK IT OUT...
Christine Lynne Stormer-Fryer 2017

WHAT'S YOUR PROBLEM?

The problem with problems is that they pose a problem, often perceived as mentally insurmountable with an overwhelming feeling of defeatism before a solution is sought.

Invariably, the unresolved issue is tucked well 'out of sight' 'at the back of the mind' in the hope that it will go away. Yet trying to 'run away' from it is of no help whatsoever. The problem relentlessly tags along, its tenacious presence 'eating away' at the mind until it eventually targets the body and develops into an ulcer, eroding bodily tissue.

The location of the ulcer reveals the problematic source. If in the mouth, it could be rummaging over festering words gnawing away from not 'speaking up'. In the stomach, annoyingly plagued by excessive anxiety about what to do or not do. In the duodenum, an all-consuming worry about what happened or did not happen. In the colon, fretting over an ongoing concern about the inability to meet unreasonable expectations. On the skin, persistently annoyed by irritating 'kin'. The list goes on.

Deep-seated beliefs from disquieting memories engender some of the most problematic reactions. Based mainly on assumptions, history has a profound hand in shaping life events. The senses help in getting to the root of and 'under-standing' the experiences responsible, thereby unravelling and resolving the mystery.

So, 'what is your problem?' Is it the 'thought' 'th'e 'ought' of somebody or something that is so maddening it 'gets on the nerves? Or is it the exasperation of being 'under another's thumb' and told (in no uncertain terms) what to do and how to do it, regardless of better options?

Or not being authentic and 'speaking up'? Is finding 'unsavoury' words 'shoved down the throat' 'hard to swallow' becoming 'a pain in the neck'?

Perhaps it is the burden of all the 'shoulds' and 'should nots' dumped on the shoulders?

Maybe the 'Sight', 'Size', 'Colour 'or 'Scenes' serve as a painful reminder of being made a 'spectacle' of, evoking injurious e-motions, lowering self-esteem, and 'taking the breath away'?

Possibly 'nerve-wracking', 'harsh' sounds along with certain 'pitches' or 'tones' being too nasty and sickening for words? Or even the lack of 'sound advice'?

Perhaps a foul 'taste' left in the mouth, serving as a disgusting reminder of unsavoury relationships? Either too 'sour' and bitter or too 'salty' and needy? Ugh!'

Then there are the 'rough', 'irritating 'types of 'touch' constantly 'getting under the skin'. 'T'he **ouch** of a 'no-no' 'touch' generating a defensive resistance to either protect or cover up highly 'sensitive' family issues 'not to be touched upon'. Conditioned into being told 'to keep things hidden' so as not to upset others prevents the relief of 'working things out'.

Solutions are only be found on a level higher than the one on which the problem was created. Embracing it as a 'challenge' rather than a 'problem' alters the energy, making it far more manageable. Once a workable solution is found and successfully applied, the benefits derived can be phenomenal.

So-called 'problems' hide the most unbelievable opportunities!

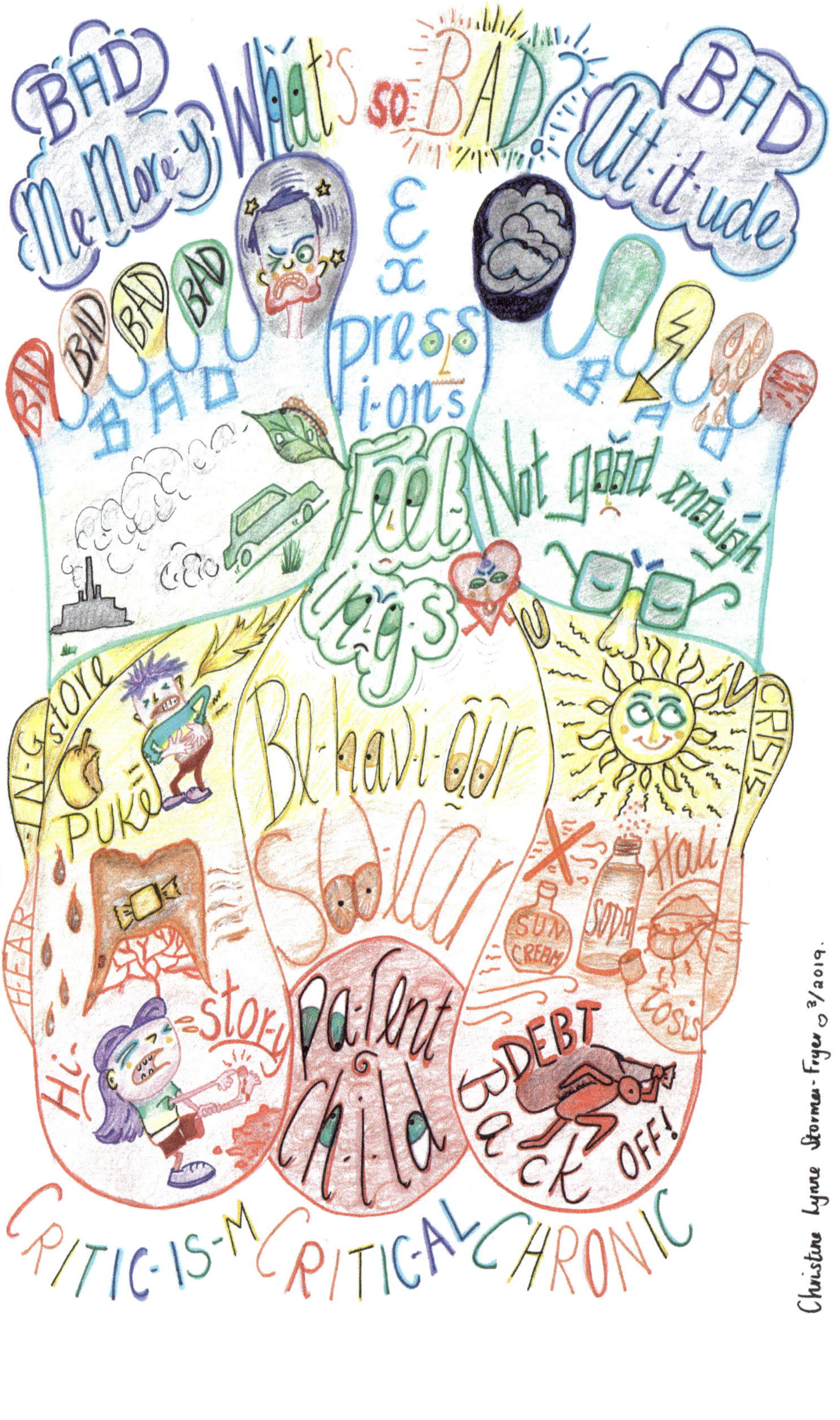
BAD
Me-More-y
What's so BAD?
BAD
Att-it-ude
BAD
BAD
BAD
BAD
BAD
B A D
Ex
press
i-on's
B A D
Feel-ing-s
Not good enough
IN-G store
PUKE
Be-havi-our
CRISIS
Hali-tosis
SUN CREAM
SODA
HEAR
Hi-story
Pa-rent
Child
DEBT
Buck OFF!
CRITIC-IS-M CRITIC-AL CHRONIC
Christine Lynne Stormer-Fryer 3/2019.

WHAT'S SO BAD?

Many centuries ago, Shakespeare wisely proclaimed that nothing is 'good' or 'bad', but only 'thinking makes it so'. With nothing being 'all good' or 'all bad' everything is a complex mix of challenges and gifts.

The tendency to be hard on oneself and others either overtly or subtly is a key component of human consciousness. It is easy to get into a 'bad' mood, making things get steadily worse. Also having a 'bad' attitude along with 'wanting something real 'bad'. That just compounds matters.

Those complaining of a 'bad memory', otherwise known as Craft's disease ('Can't Remember A Flipping Thing'), are using a perfect excuse for the mind constantly wandering into the past, or venturing aimlessly into the elusive future. There is either little or no interest in the 'now', or a profound fear of facing the present.

'Bad' notions plaguing the mind are injurious to the cells. Blaming 'bad weather' is just one reason for feeling 'bad' – little realising that 'clouded points of view' and miserable thoughts are responsible for 'making heavy weather'. As are unhealthy e-motions hanging gloomily in the air, polluting the atmosphere. Going straight to the chest, many complain of 'feeling under the weather'.

Extreme criticism adds to this critical situation. Food critics provide 'fuel for thought', with 'bad food' taking the brunt. Neither 'good' nor 'bad', once food is contaminated by beliefs 'past their sell-by date', its energy changes. Stored resentment has a hand in stirring and making the body puke when exposed to the same old despicable behaviour.

'Bad news' spreads like wildfire in a desperate attempt to replace the monotony and lack of excitement in certain lives. News is generally a negative medium, creating more of what is not needed. Highlighting corrupt prejudicial relationships not only 'rocks the boat' but is intentionally damaging.

'Bad governments' are continually held responsible for the ensuing chaos voted in by people little realising that going to the polls is a complete mockery. The results are always determined well in advance, based on who would make the best 'bad choices' to rile significant sectors of the masses.

A life overwhelmed with challenges, grief and pain is perceived to be 'bad'. Far less is achieved on a 'bad day', when the tendency is to be nasty.

Ironically, 'bad' and 'good' are 'opposames', two extremes sharing the same energy, with everybody and everything being the 'neutral' point on the spectrum, before injected perceptions 'tip the balance'.

Making the best of a 'bad situation' is to start a 'new trail' that has the ability to transform with a shift of perspective and a positive attitude.

Focusing on 'good' and all that accompanies it highlights its qualities resonating to the 'God' within. Any doubt is replaced by sympathetic tolerance, with a noticeable energetic shift.

'Bad' thoughts and' bad' actions or reactions rarely, if ever, bring about 'good' results!

46 - CHRISTINE LYNNE STORMER-FRYER

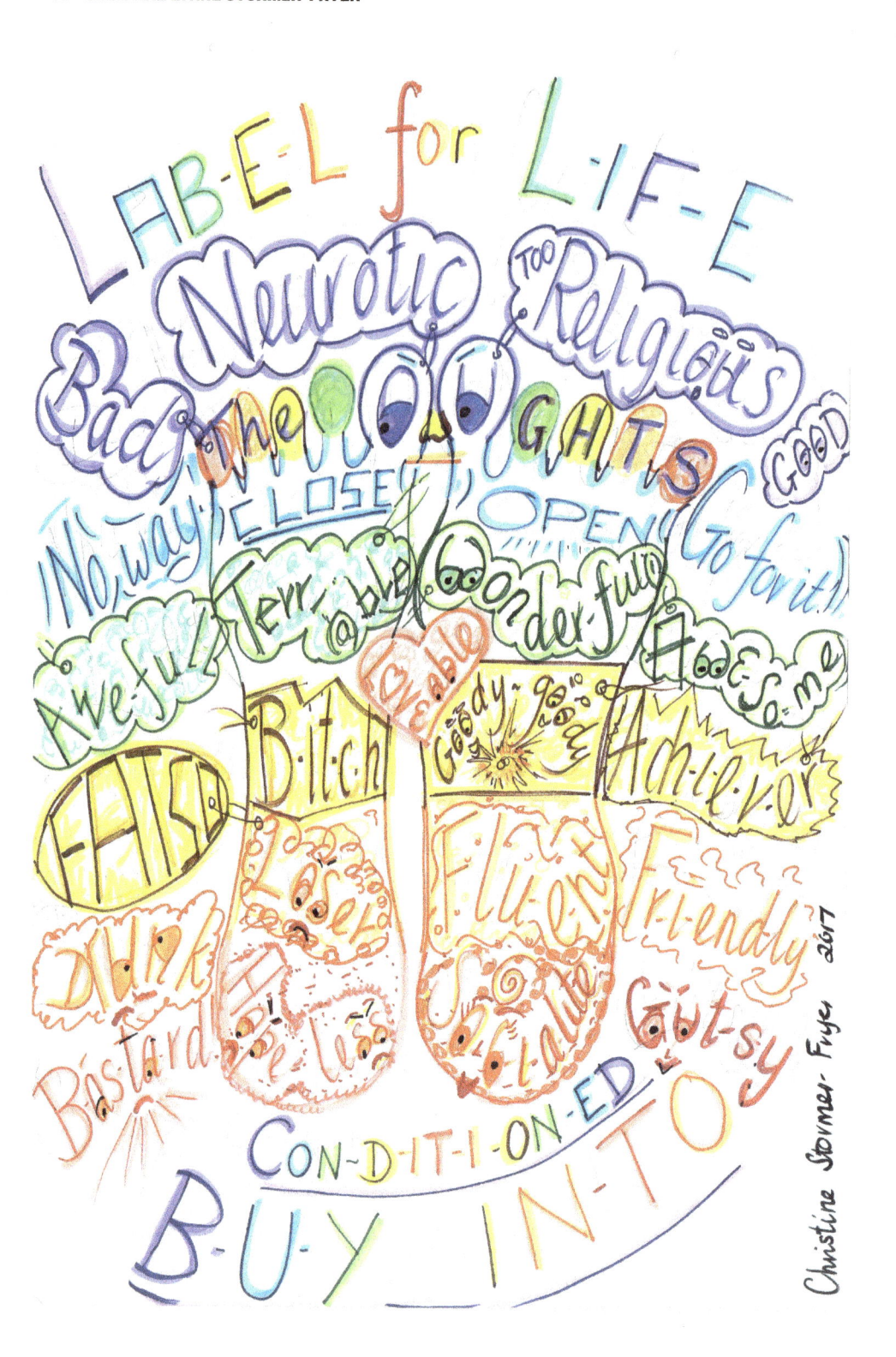

LABELLED FOR LIFE

A 'label' does not capture the essence of whatever or whomever is being named. It generally only captures a specific quality, but only if aptly applied.

Misleading 'labels' can become self-fulfilling prophecies, often accompanied by a trail of disaster.

Youngsters frequently grow into detrimental labels bestowed during childhood, often remaining oblivious to their true potential. Being 'labelled' as 'bad' places a lot of responsibility on small shoulders, precluding the ability to respond appropriately.

A tag of 'shyness' may conceal an adventurous Spirit. Instead of being daring, fear eliminates the chances of taking risks.

Meanwhile, a rebellious 'label' is 'asking for trouble'. Yet, beneath the defiant attitude, there could be a co-operative and understanding Spirit.

'Labels' need to be worn lightly. Accepting them is a choice, knowing that a 'label' is not the 'truth'. A wayward attempt to under-stand the world and its people, a 'label' generally falls short of its desired goal.

'Neurotic' when dealing with intensely disturbing circumstances may be true, but once the situation passes and things settle down, the behaviour often changes. To be lumbered with an 'irrational' label is highly irritating.

The words 'awe-ful' (full of dread) and 'terrible' (able to terrorise) are in themselves frightfully off-putting and morally deflating. In contrast, 'wonder-ful' (full of wonder) and 'awe-some' (filled with awe at the possibilities) are far more effective in boosting self-esteem.

The fiasco of being tagged a 'fatso' is that it is so hurtful, derogatory, and exceptionally depressing. Taken on board, added to the excessive weight of hefty e-motions, this label can escalate into extreme unhappiness.

'Beyond one's tether', going from being an 'angel' to a 'bitch' in three seconds flat, is easy enough, although its lifespan is generally limited.

'Drunk' with happiness is one thing. Being considered a 'loser' and a downright 'drunkard' though is enough to 'drive anyone to drink' and 'drown deep sorrows in alcohol'. These 'highly evolved Souls' are completely misjudged by an exceptionally critical two-faced 'goody-two-shoed' society, also known to freely imbibe 'behind closed doors'.

Being 'too religious' with a 'holier than thou' attitude is of no earthly good to anybody. Being horrified and prejudiced towards 'bastards' simply for being 'born on the wrong side of the blanket' is another form of hypocrisy.

It is likely to be more advantageous to 'go with the flow' by befriending strangers, mirroring the stranger part of oneself.

Labels belong to the labellers, not the labelled!

48 - CHRISTINE LYNNE STORMER-FRYER

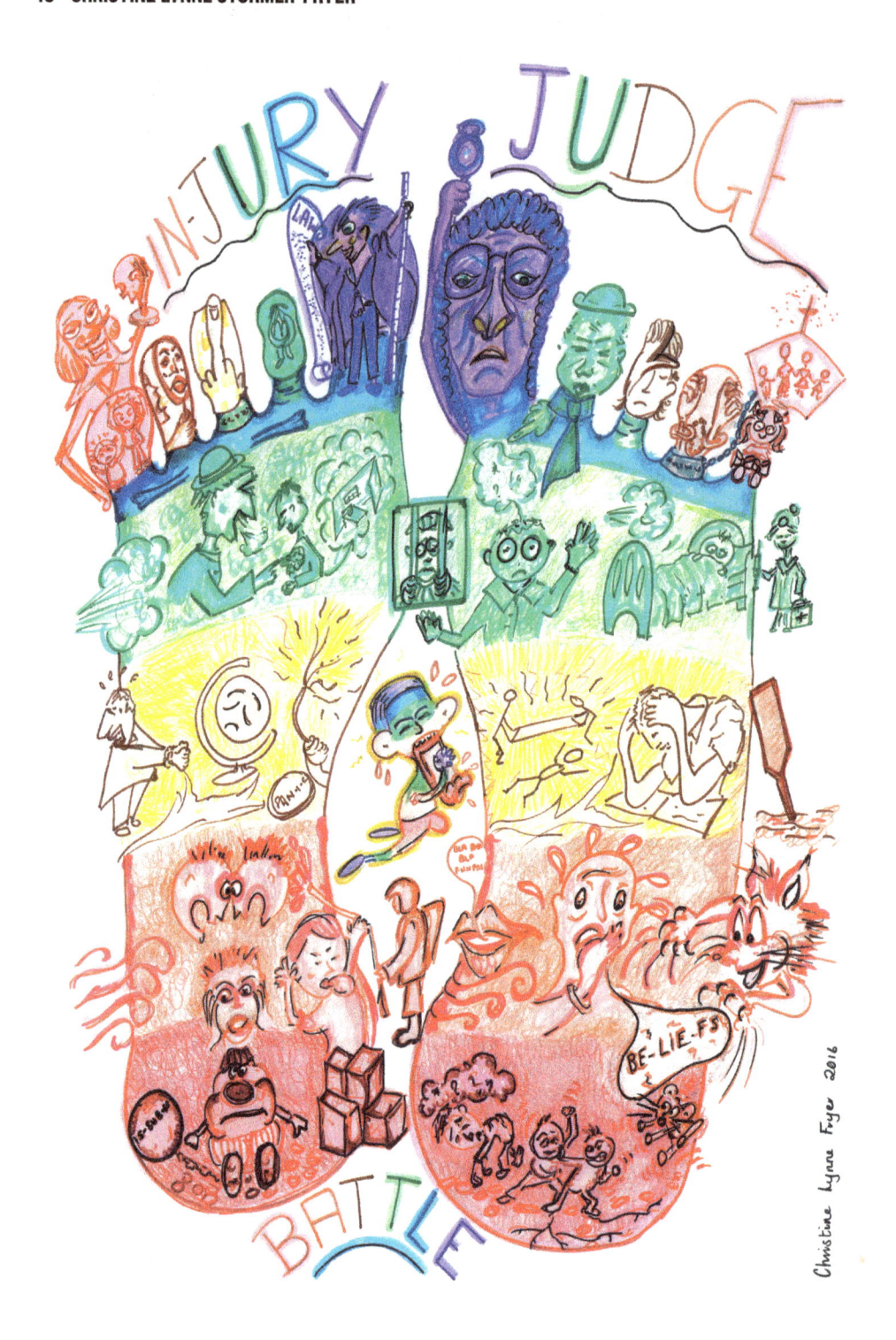

IN-JURY - JUDGE

It is human to evaluate people based on first impressions. Yet, at the heart of it, this categorising and criticising is insecurity, a desperate need to be set apart from what is internally feared the most.

Once 'judgment' is made, all conversations, considerations and debates come to an end – and the torment begins. It is then extremely difficult for mind and body to perform well.

To 'judge' others is to judge oneself. It is a form of inner torture, a negative 'e-motional' experience that does more harm than good, highlighting what is being repressed or rejected.

'Judged' to be unfit and unworthy creates an incredibly low frequency of entrapment and helplessness. Playing the role of the body's 'judge' is the relentless mind, quick to pick up on undesirable traits and pass a ruling without taking anything into further consideration. Its final verdict is echoed in the big toes.

As for the jury, the body's cells, it is difficult for them to remain impartial when taking the brunt of the so-called wrongdoing. The ruling is inevitable, punishment by pain, creatively and Spiritually paralysing. Crime, anger and animosity are evidence that pain has won the battle.

Conflicting e-motions, divided by an eclectic assortment of life's experiences, is confusing. The phrase 'rule of thumb', associated with domestic abuse, was discouraged owing to its perceivably false origin. Meanwhile 'Peter Pointer', the condemning index finger, has continued to reinforce this puzzling behaviour conducted by a so-called loved one, be it a partner or parent.

Trapped by an act of violence and unable to fight back- or run away is scary. It makes the victim believe that violence is the only means to get one's way and keep others compliant, a notion continually perpetuated through the media. Blame is pointless, since everybody has been brainwashed to a certain extent.

Wallowing in guilt is sickening. The fringe benefits to being ill are temporarily blotting out other issues, avoiding difficult situations, and evading responsibility. In other words, the 'poor me' mentality is a real cop-out.

With a war between hope and pain waging in the heart, all forms of conflict begin within. Motivated by unspoken needs 'head bashing' and 'fighting toe to toe' are to 'fight a losing battle', especially when caught up in the drama.

Adding insult to injury is intentionally wounding one who is already suffering. With injured pride and mounting anger, it becomes a struggle to trust and have faith in others. Trapped in the darkest, deepest place, the inherited instinct is to step into the stance of 'he said, she said' victimhood.

Being robbed and robbing others of the gift of life is the greatest crime. Yet with every 'break-in' comes the possibility of a 'break-through'.

Old rules no longer work. New developments need to take place outside rules and regulations for something extra-ordinary to be created. The Soul abides by the Spiritual laws of the Universe, based on the principles of pure love and seeing every new conflict as a chance to home in on empathy, compassion and tolerance.

It's a crime in life to never have tried!

50 - CHRISTINE LYNNE STORMER-FRYER

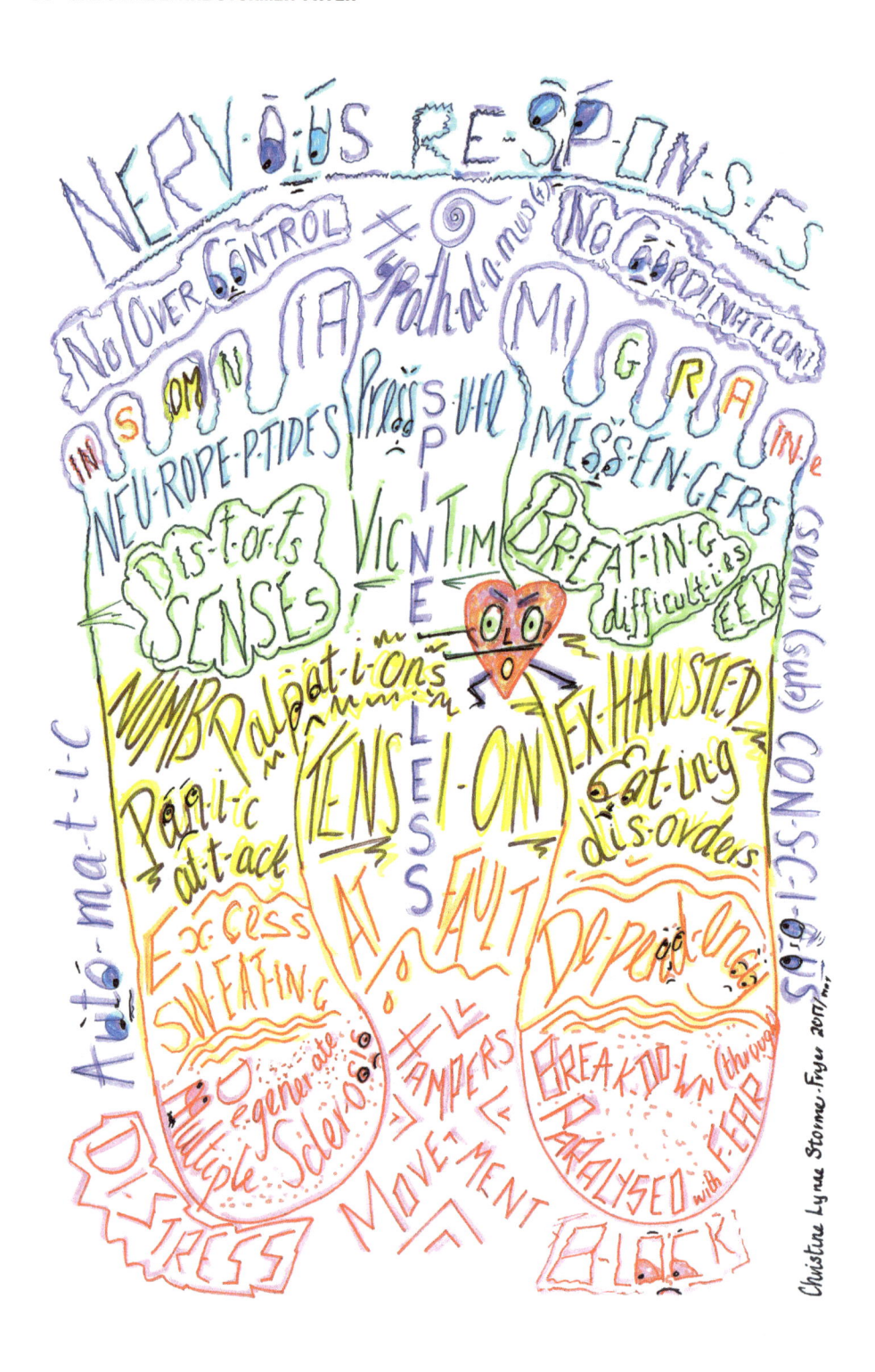

NERVOUS RESPONSES

Exerting control over mind and body is empowering. As nervous energy permeates the whole, it enlivens and thrills the Spirit for it to function in the physical world. A continual silent dialogue throughout the intriguing, intricate nervous network ensures that all cells stay up to date and well-informed of what is going on, internally and externally.

Constantly aware of the body's comfort or discomfort, the hypothalamus urges nerves to act and react accordingly. Distress and embarrassment about having no control (or lacking coordination) makes it tempting to want to control others. Even with the most honourable intentions, being bossy and 'knowing what's best' can 'go against me grain', causing 'migraines'. Utter frustration, bitterness and resentment keep the brain busy at night, resulting in insomnia.

Dictatorially dominating others or being arrogantly dominated can, in time, be enough to 'bang the head against a brick wall' and even 'throw a fit' as 'nerves are set on edge'. Constantly needing to manipulate and have the 'upper hand' makes the body shake with outrage, as it does with Parkinson's dis-ease.

At the root of all nervous issues is CONTROL, something humankind has struggled with for aeons. The ego battles to maintain an illusion of control, either trying to be too much in control, or feeling completely 'out of control'.

This puts pressure on the 'neuropeptides' the neurone messengers. Legs go weak at the knees, bringing the body to a standstill. Paralysed with extreme fear yet needing to gain 'strokes' leaves the mouth speechless, while the affected side of the body is immobilised.

Many things are 'beyond control'. As tension and anxiety block the way, mind and body become increasingly hampered. 'E-motional' uneasiness and distress distort the transmission of messages, hindering communication and making it difficult to breathe.

Being incapacitated and letting others 'get on with it' is how 'control freaks' manipulate others. Incredible things happen when 'letting go of the reins' and only controlling what is controllable.

Many hard knocks and trials in life shed light on the unconscious workings of the mind to deepen the experience of reality. Major happenings are meant to act as 'wake-up calls'. Resisting by 'numbing the pain' 'panics' the heart, making it palpitate with concern. Having 'exhausted all options', it is 'out of order' to even *consider* taking on board and digesting a new in-take, emphasised especially when plagued by 'digestive 'dis-orders.'

Never able to please others and constantly feeling at fault, the body breaks out 'into a cold sweat'. This excessive outpouring of anxiety increases dependency. With 'no leg to stand on' and everything appearing to be deteriorating, movement is hampered. In desperation, nerves are left with no choice but make an urgent plea for assistance through 'degenerate multiple sclerosis'.

Any nervous breakdown is actually an opportunity for a 'breakthrough'. Once in control of all that is humanly possible, it is time to relinquish control to the Universe. This requires trust but it is well worth it.

Trust is built by empowering one another!

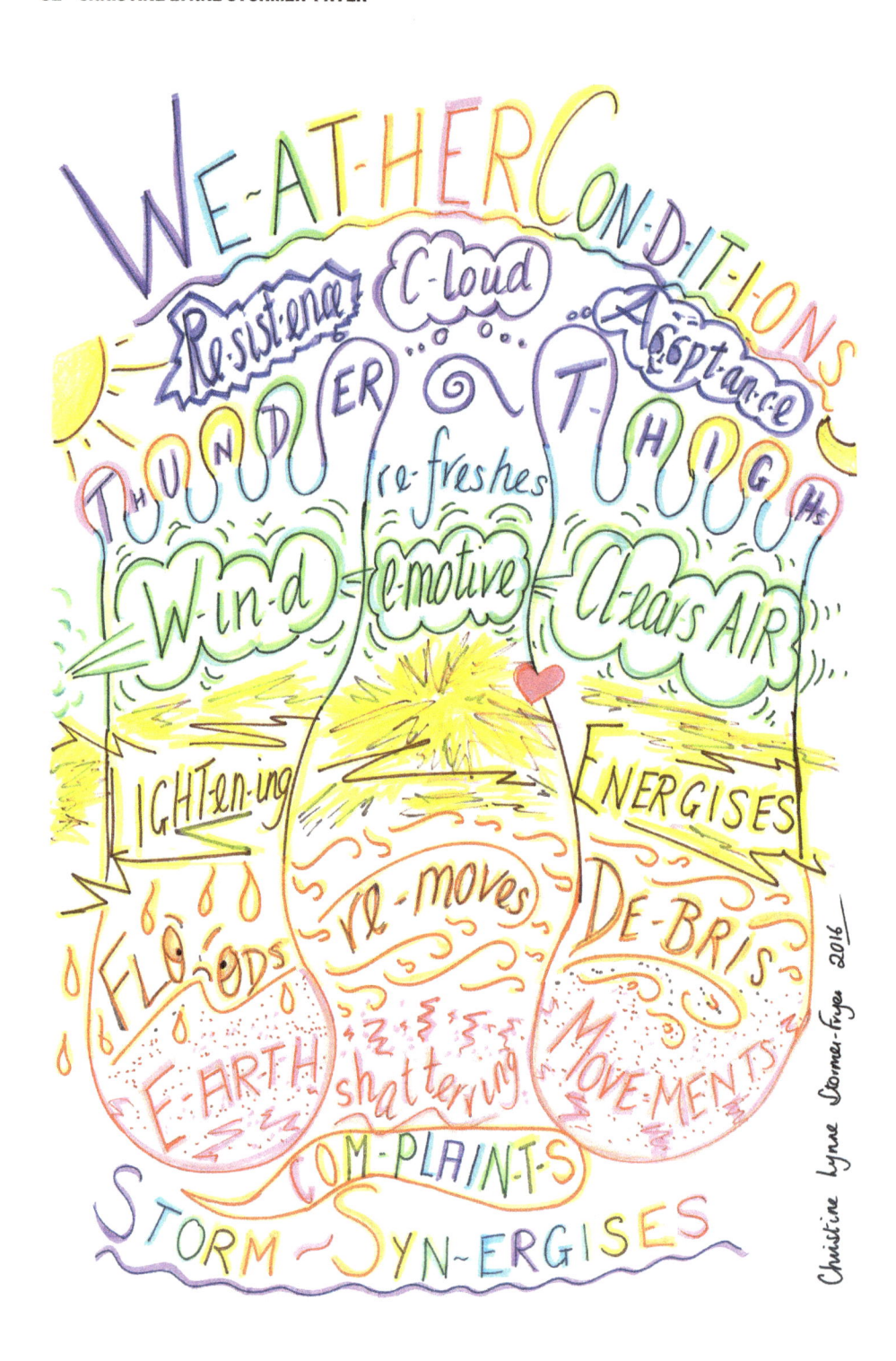

WEATHER CONDITIONS

- Resistance
- Cloud
- Acceptance
- THUNDER
- re-freshes
- THIGHs
- Wind
- e-motive
- Clears AIR
- LIGHTen-ing
- ENERGISES
- FLOODS
- re-moves
- DE-BRIS
- EARTH
- shattering
- MOVEMENTS
- COM-PLAINTS
- STORM ~ SYN-ERGISES

Christine Lynne Stormer-Fryer 2016

WEATHER CONDITIONS

Everything in life is connected, influencing and being influenced in unbelievable ways.

A thought bubble shares the same outline as the brain, clouds, trees, certain vegetables and so much more. Spelt out within each bubble is its inner content or dis-content. As ethereal thoughts formed in the mind are released and float into outer space, clouds form as all thoughts gather in the stratosphere.

Clouds provide welcome relief when others get overheated and 'let off steam'. From time to time, doubt 'clouds the issue', while doom and gloom contribute to the build-up of black clouds.

As disgruntled Souls 'storm off in a huff', stormy weather is a possibility. Getting 'hot under the collar' and 'blowing the top' thunderously, 'ranting and raving' and lashing out unexpectedly about anything and everything is extremely unsettling, creating a tense atmosphere.

With increasing humidity comes increasing 'humility' of those within 'striking distance', before spreading to the vicinity.

A 'clouded point of view' and not seeing further than the 'tip of the nose' 'clouds opinions', with ongoing deceit invariably leading to having to 'leave under a cloud', disgracefully dismissed for wrongdoing. Quite different from having one's 'head in the clouds'. With the mind residing on another planet, it brings back 'way out' ideas for human evolvement. Then there is the 'absent-minded' professor providing some light relief for everyone except this 'lost Soul'.

Happy, hopeful and optimistic dispositions 'clear the air', providing some space to breathe. Assisting the process is the sun, shining through to bring warmth and enlightenment. The sun is also there to highlight issues suppressed beneath the surface that flare up from time to time, through various skin issues, when mounting issues with 'kin' surface. Even when the sun is not shining, its warmth can always be felt in the heart.

Diverse cultural beliefs engender pockets of insecurity within individual societies. These insecurities are further compounded by localised turbulent and unstable conditions, areas of high and low-pressure, forcing the populace to conform. With ever-increasing stormy relationships comes the need for revenge.

Constant criticism engenders critical conditions worldwide, a build-up of impenetrable fronts, made up of an accumulation of mistaken beliefs. The elements are constantly held responsible for personal misfortune and dis-ease when, in fact, it is the other way around.

Current changes in global weather patterns and climatic conditions reflect mass uncertainty, the dilemma of 'whether' or not to 'buy into' the fear and panic. The truth of what is really going on is well concealed behind clouds of deceit, corruption, dishonesty and crime. Penetrating society on numerous levels, fraught volatile social climates periodically erupt, with hurricanes and torpedoes leaving a path of destruction in their wake.

Many are left in two minds, emphasising 'whether' they should or 'whether' they should not think for themselves to make a 'mass-ive' contribution to stabilising the changeable 'weather' conditions.

Behind the darkest, heaviest clouds, the sun still shines!

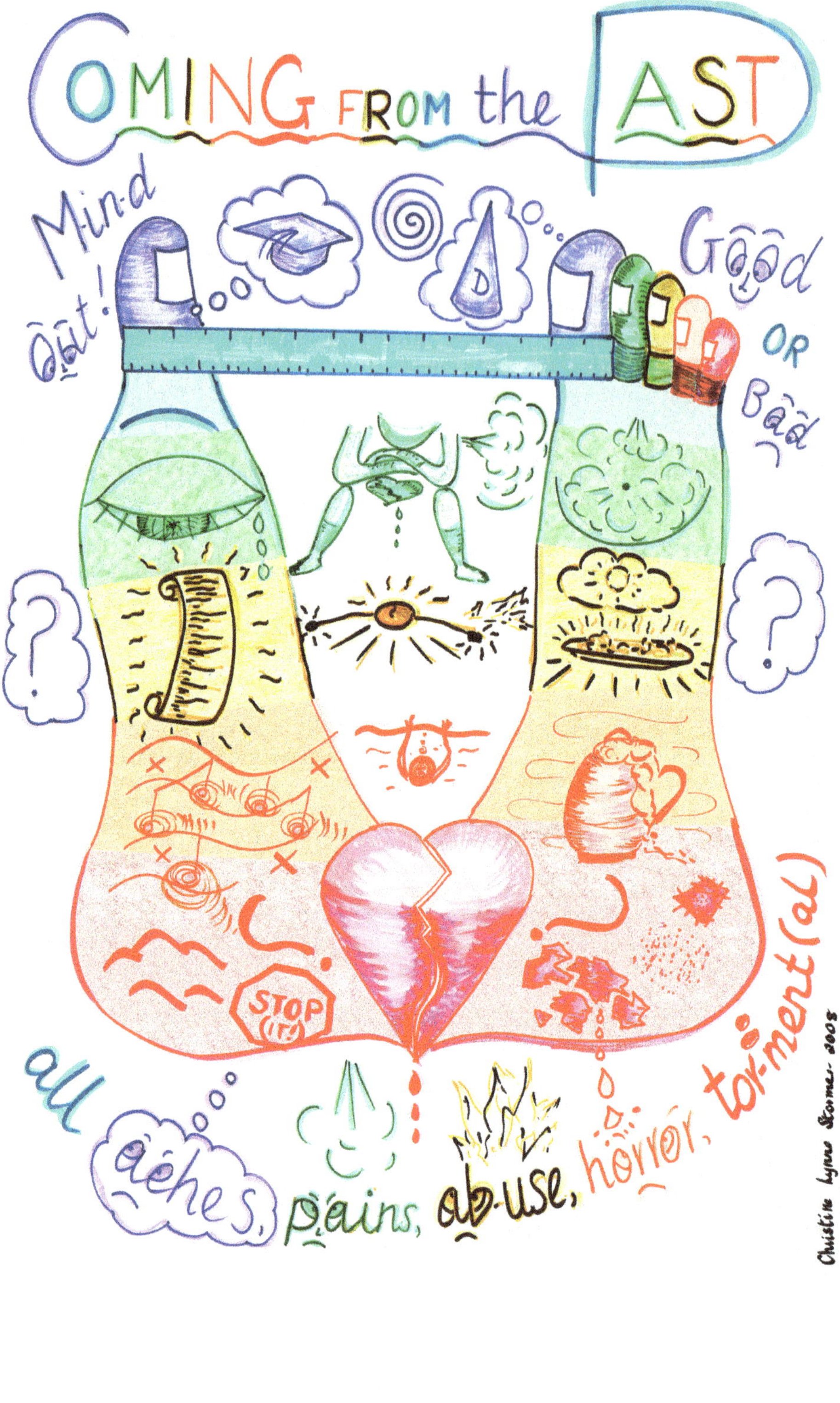
COMING FROM the PAST
Mind out!
Good OR Bad
STOP (IT)
all aches, pains, ab-use, horror, tor-ment(al)
Christine Lynne Stormer 2005

COMING FROM THE PAST

Mind out! There is so much stuff dumped backstage, behind the scenes and well out of sight so that the show can go on. All symbolic of what is going on 'behind the back'.

A backdrop is often used to conceal a whole host of undesirables that should have been dispensed with long ago. Until removed, the back becomes the dwelling place of numerous 'back issues'.

Niggling memories influence the script of life, with nerves having a massive role to play. Stockpiled at the back of the mind are all the 'aches', all the dreams ever longed for, and all the aspirations and ambitions still waiting to be fulfilled.

Hormones provide the undertones and overtones, taking their cue from the sensory organs. With every sensation being seen, heard or felt, the highly-tuned sensory organs alter the overall tone and tension level. Any issues are immediately amplified to draw attention to the problem.

With many backs turned on love because of pain, wounds stay wide open, improvising the moves of the respiratory, circulatory and lymphatic systems being compromised. The heart steps in to provide the passion and impetus to feel the love. Frequently, heartstrings are pulled to get a reaction.

'Ab-use', 'abnormal use', prevents things from working well. Every judgement, along with every criticism, is a form of self-abuse. Rejecting God-given talents is self-abuse. Doubt about personal capabilities is self-abuse. Ab-use manifests as self-deprivation. The refusal to participate and act the part.

Holding back in fear and trepidation and not having the courage to 'get out there' alarms the adrenal glands. 'Stepping out from the shadows' is scary. Lingering at the 'back of the mind' is the notion of struggling to 'perform well' and 'making a fool of oneself'. Even when a 'bag of nerves' once on stage, it is possible to 'calm down to a gentle panic'.

Meanwhile, stored in the liver is ample stock of ready-made items derived from previous experiences for ongoing performances. Prompts from the past jog the memory and serve as reminders of the plot, providing cues for the action or reaction required supported by the middle back.

Interacting with others involves taking on many different roles, each adapted to suit the 'e-motional' scene. Rather than risk having to compromise, old roles are fiercely hung onto, with the 'horrors' of in-house relationships soon 'getting out of hand'.

'Tormented' and being 'mentally torn apart' by family dramas can be agonising. At the root of instability is the general belief in insufficient financial backing and inadequate resources to 'get the show back on the road' – little realising that the most valuable resource is creativity, backed by the reproductive organs and supported by the lower back.

Remaining stoically in the background is the spine ultimately responsible for 'bearing the brunt' and providing overall support.

As each production comes to an end, everything must be cleared away to make space for the next performance. The break-up crew, in the form of the excretory system, is great at getting things moving, removing anything that is no longer required.

The Universe is always in the background providing back-up!

56 - CHRISTINE LYNNE STORMER-FRYER

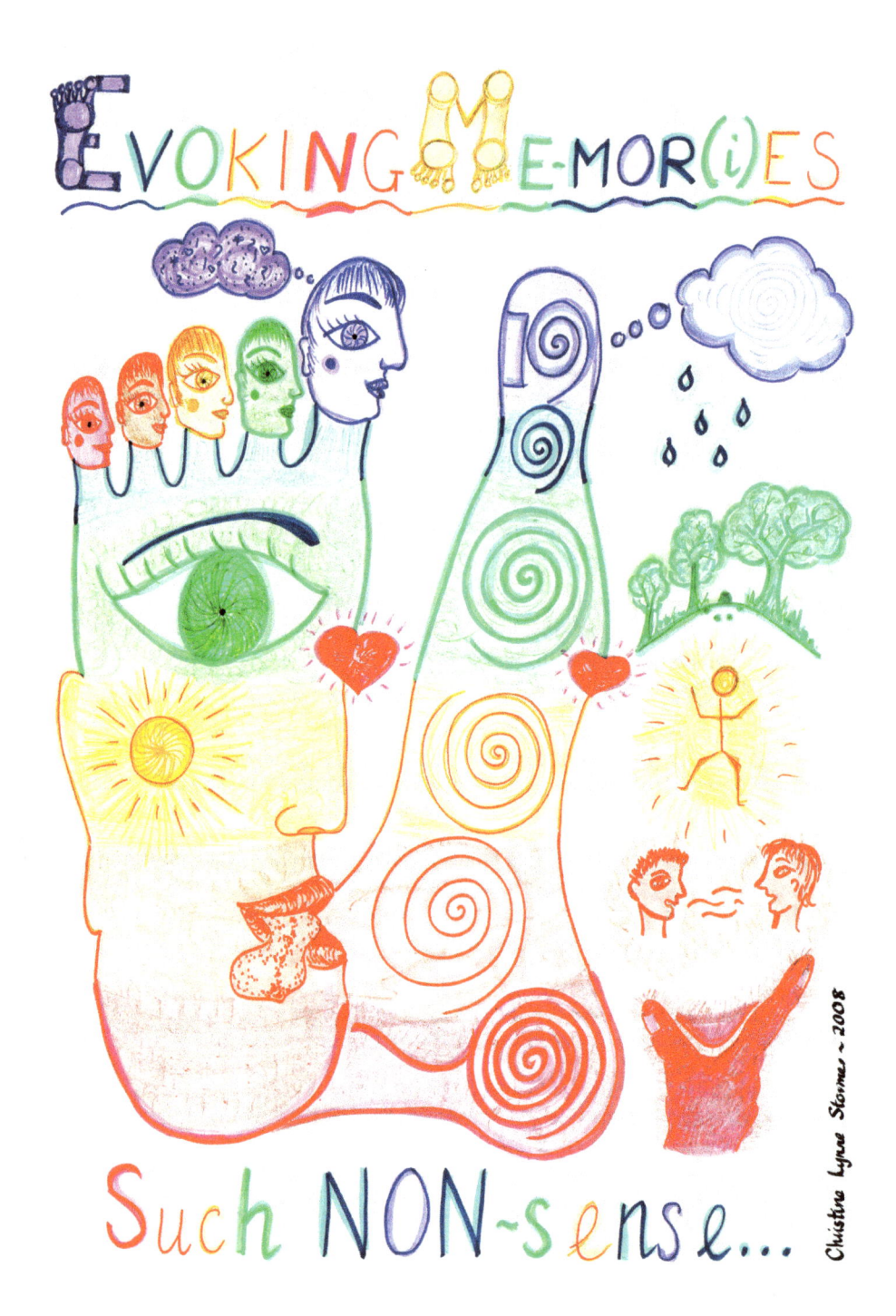

EVOKING MEMORIES – SUCH NON-SENSE

Long-lost memories residing at the back of the mind are sentimentally aroused by the highly evocative senses. Also casually dumped into the background and kept well out of sight is the energy of unresolved issues and unsettled feelings.

Despite all this, or possibly because of it, the resolute back continues to offer incredible strength and support, keeping the body upright and dignified. Representing the unconscious mind, the back has an enormously powerful communication system, with each spinal vertebra holding its own very specific library of information. Fear is the energy that holds it back.

Entrepreneurs and inventors spend most of their time 'out of the mind', breaking the bounds of conventional thoughts. Bringing back insights from the more psychic and intuitive realms of conception is by far the best way to get back in touch with the senses, particularly the sixth sense.

The mind sees what it believes, but it does not always believe what it sees. Looking back in 'hindsight' with 'eyes in the back of the head' evoke e-motions influencing the environment. The 'eye roll' performed unconsciously or consciously by rotating the eyes up and back down indicate incredulity, contempt, boredom, frustration or exasperation at all the scenes shoved to the 'back of the mind'.

Unhappy feelings tucked snuggly in the upper back are reflected onto the tops of the balls of the feet, revealed through the puffiness of unshed tears. Improved insight comes with viewing the past in a different light, especially when seen as a liability rather than an asset.

Too terrified to step out and 'put the best foot forward' and too fearful to sniff out valuable opportunities, the tendency is to 'bend over backwards' to please others. Hanging back, numbed by social conditioning and paralysed by panic, is utterly incapacitating and desensitising.

Smell, being the most evocative of all senses, is quick to conjure up memories and feelings of the past. Plagued by not being able to 'see beyond the tip of the nose', one's sense of smell is lost when way off track with the Soul's purpose.

Words emanating from the mouth create ripples in bodies of water, with vibrations of sound constantly running through the body to jog stored memories and arouse long-forgotten feelings. The deluge of unsound information received via the media and elsewhere has a significant role in undermining personal well-being.

'Picked up by the ears', adverse comments from the 'cutting edge' of the tongue stab the body and get it in the upper-middle back. Being 'fed up to the back teeth', with remarks made in 'bad taste', often evokes memories of unhealthy and possibly 'ab-usive' relationships.

Obsessing over misleading notions, entertaining the belief that material gain provides essential backing – is to be blind to the inner resources. Embroiled in such social 'non-sense' entraps and pains the lower back.

Common sense, it seems, is not so common after all. The knack of seeing things for what they are and doing things as they ought to be done is rare. Yet, despite all this, the greatest personal development is through sensational events, although it is actually when sensory input is reduced that creativity and insight come to the fore.

'Getting back to the senses' means getting back in touch with innermost feelings!

58 - CHRISTINE LYNNE STORMER-FRYER

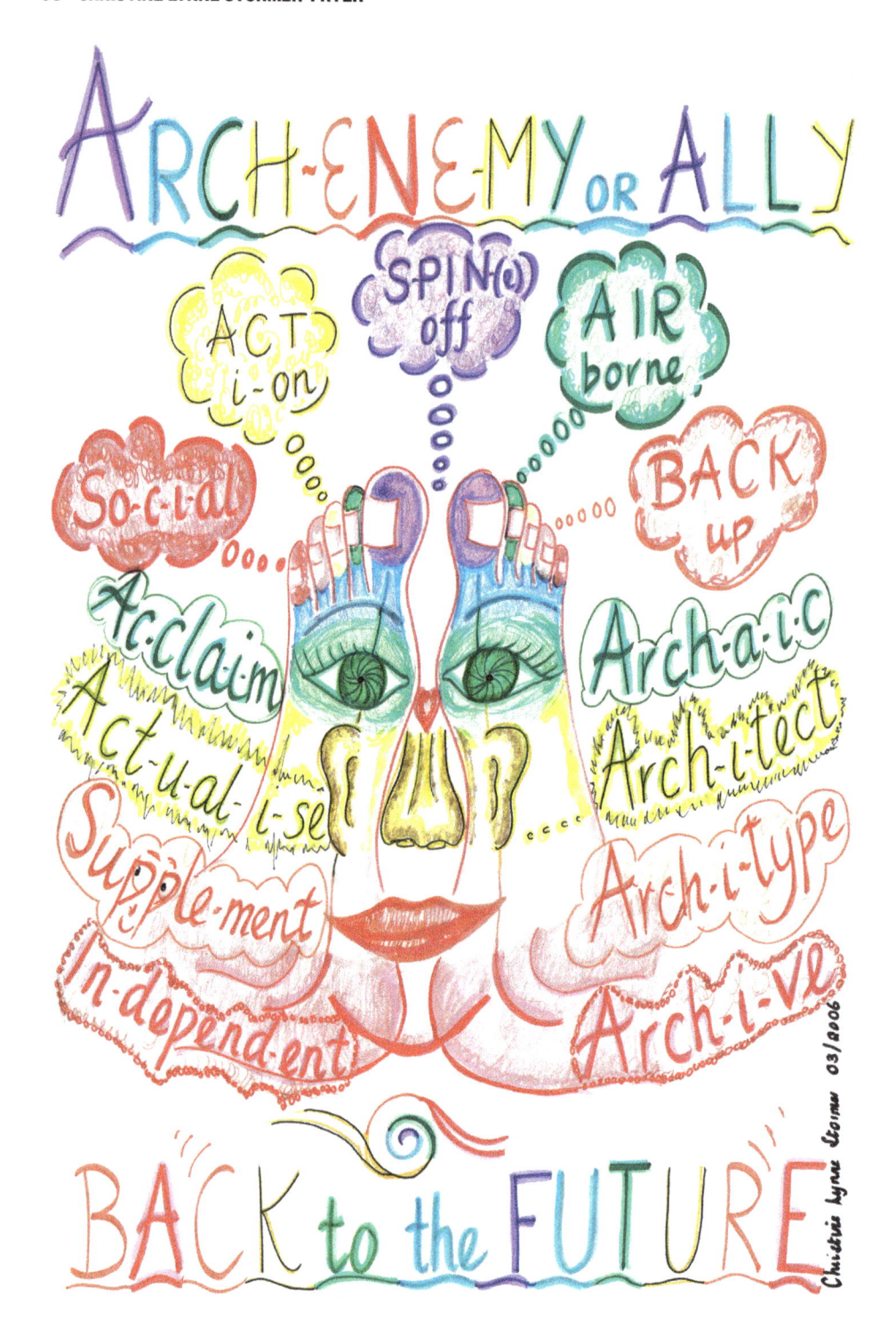

ARCH-ENE-MY OR ALLY – BACK TO THE FUTURE

When walking or jumping, the natural elastic spring of the foot takes place thanks to three arches in the feet. Two run lengthwise, while the third stretches crossways. Pressing the ground at the heel and the balls of the foot, the main arch makes sure that there is no jarring on the spinal cord.

Spinal reflexes, reflected along the bony ridges of both arches, represent the overall support system, providing backing for every thought, expression, feeling, action, reaction, relationship and movement. Entirely dependent on support from others, babies are generally born without arches, which only develop when capable of 'standing on their own two feet'.

As for 'arch-ene-my', 'my' arch 'ene'my, every body is ultimately their own worst 'enemy'. Just the 'th-ought' of it is enough to 'send shivers down the spine', evoking terrifying memories. Yet, it is the perceived perceptions which distort reality that are the enemies, inducing a stack of unfounded fear.

The fear of not having enough support or the fear of being incapable of supporting others often lurks gloomily in the background. A fabrication of the mind, it is easy enough to make *fear* an 'arch-ally'.

Springing into 'act-i-on' with the third toes derives many beneficial 'spin-offs' coming from the big toes. Once 'air-borne', with some light-heartedness from the second toes, the fourth toes provide the 'backup', along with the assistance of the 'social' small toes.

Replacing 'arch-aic' worn-out e-motions with 'acclaim' boosts the self-esteem. With commendation and praise puffing out the chest, the danger of the ego taking over often overly arches the back in haughtiness and superciliousness. It is important to remember that life is a happy balance of in-betweens.

Past 'arch-itects' set ideas in stone by building archways, providing the incentive for more modern designs on which to 'act-u-alise' and build a more realistic reality.

Midway along the curved arches a bony protrusion, affectionately known as the 'guilt bump', pops up when reaching out for additional support. It is mortified when help is not forthcoming. Not having the guts to support or stand up for oneself, and without a sufficient 'backbone', the arches flatten.

With 'arch-etypes' influencing subsequent behaviour, a fallen arch is generally indicative of the inherent tendency to feel 'rushed off the feet', without any of the required backing and support. Trying to 'supplement' what is missing becomes extremely exasperating and may just be too much for the arch to bear.

Over-extended arches become an issue when constantly overstretching the self to support others and be the 'backbone of society'.

Each ethnic tribe has its own 'arch-ival' experience. Highly evolved Spiritual Souls seen as a threat to society found themselves trodden underfoot. Being forced into submission left their Souls crushed and their feet flattened.

Regardless of the past, being 'independent', 'self-regulating' and liberated is the heart's desire for everybody.

Everybody needs to support and be supported to thrive in this world!

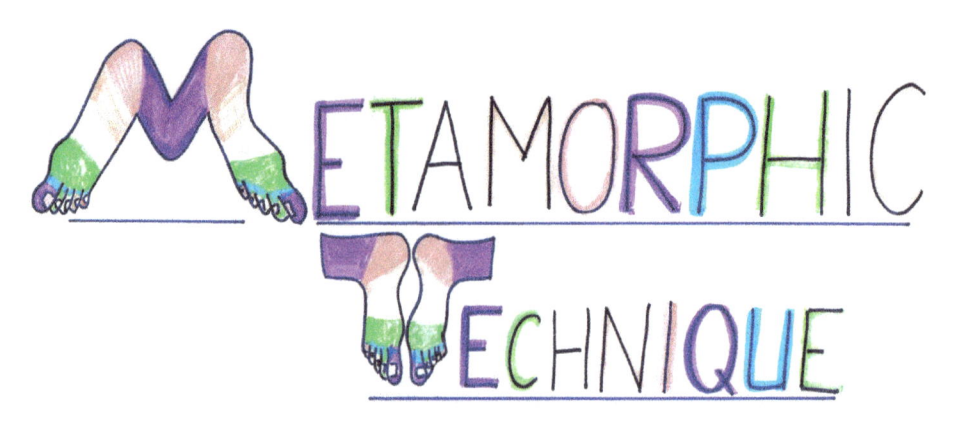

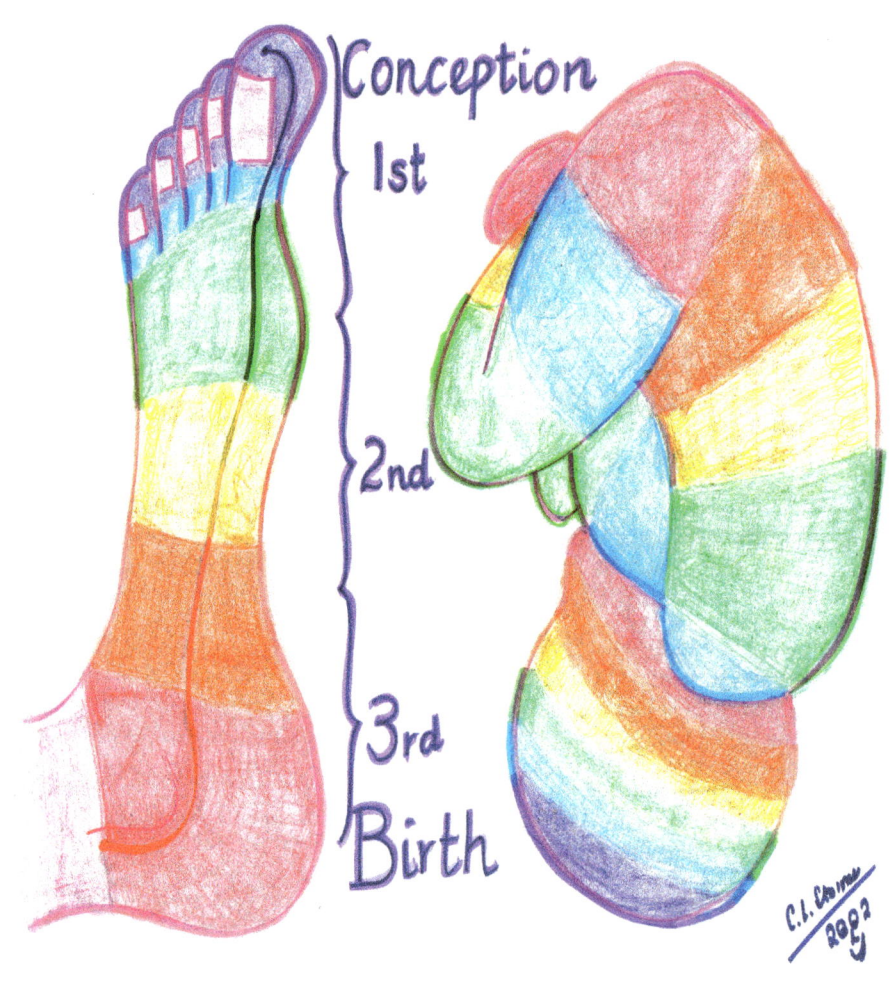

Metamorphic Technique

Conception
1st
2nd
3rd
Birth

METAMORPHIC TECHNIQUE

Going back many lifetimes, memories and impressions are stored in the sub-conscious mind with each vertebral disc containing the Spirit's divine plan. Meanwhile, the Soul's blueprint is cared for within the spinal fluid.

As the foetus physically and psychologically develops, its spine is in constant touch with the mother-to-be's ever-fluctuating thoughts and fluttering e-motions. Dominant memories that mattered during this time in the womb soon become embedded in the matrix of the foetus's backbone.

A dynamic technique, known as the 'metamorphic technique', is facilitated by a much greater intelligence than can be imaged. It lovingly weaves its magic from the inside out, encouraging a change of heart and a more understanding mind about experiences in the womb.

As Spiritual beings having a physical experience, the 'met-a-mor-ph-ic' technique is an invitation to enjoy and '**Me** *e* **t a more ph***ysical*' experience.

Reflexes on the tips of both big toes resonate with the time of conception. Intuitively resting any two digits on each reflex, while visualising 'white light and pure love', puts the circumstances around conception into a more loving context.

Continuing along the spinal reflexes, the three trimesters are equally represented.

The first trimester reflexes mirror the amount of 'e-motional' support required and received. When lacking, a bulging bunion reaches out in desperation for attention and affection – a craving passed onto future generations when unresolved, until the love is found within.

Second-trimester reflexes display personal convictions around the ability to cope. One's partner's actions and reactions have an overbearing impact.

Lower back dis-orders can be picked up in the third-trimester reflexes, revealing maternal issues going back many generations concerning the nature of the support provided within these relationships.

Just behind the inside ankles, at the very end of the spinal reflexes, are points representing the time of birth. Repeating the same procedure as that performed on the tips of the big toes assists in helping circumstances surrounding the delivery be more comprehensible.

Unusual spinal reflexes highlight back issues entertained in the background for far too long. Anything 'out of order' during the mother-to-be's pregnancy can sometimes show up as a back issue in the offspring.

The development of the nervous system and neck are predominantly influenced by male energies – rigidity and only 'seeing one point of view' being the main paternal principle reflected here.

Wielding greater influence over the digestive tract and lower spine are female energies more involved in birthing and nurturing new concepts.

Tremendous benefits can be derived from this technique by anybody and everybody, at any stage of life.

Expanding the mind accommodates new exciting concepts!

62 - CHRISTINE LYNNE STORMER-FRYER

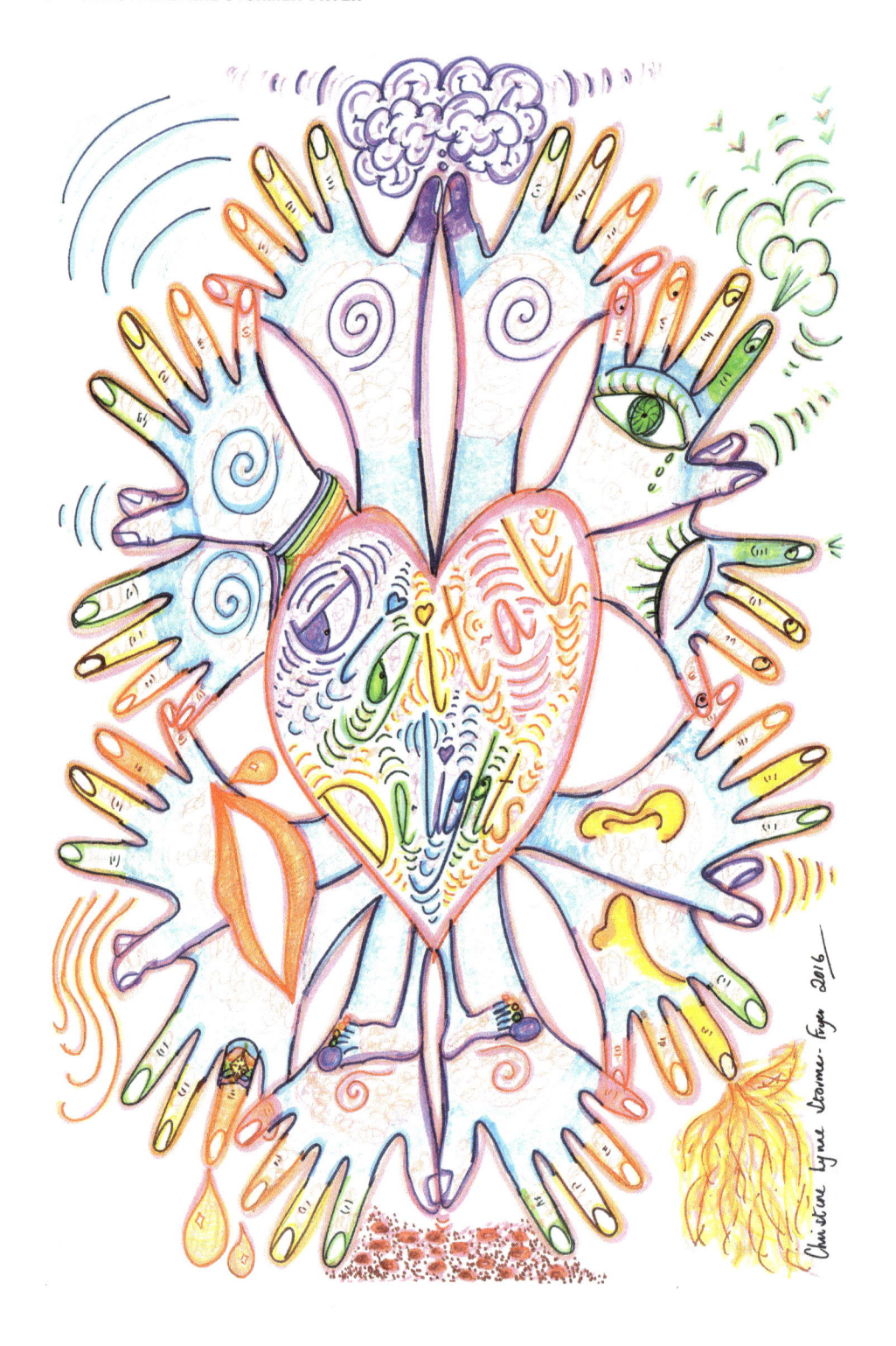

DIGITAL DE-LIGHTS

Activation of all bodily systems through healing touch helps in restoring equilibrium throughout. All sensory organs, particularly the skin, play a major role in this exhilarating process. As an acute awareness of both inner and outer environments is created, a happy medium can be found.

With the Universal approach to Reflexology incorporating Reiki, the importance of channelling of Universal energy, either through touch or intention, is recognised. Administered in a remarkably loving way, incredible sensations are transmitted from all the digits, rather than just the thumbs.

Each pair of digits has its own unique healing sensations.

Thumbs heighten Spirituality to strengthen the connection with the Higher Self. The nervous system, endocrine glands, sensory organs and lymphatics respond particularly well to this touch.

Index fingers soothe or agitate e-motions to boost self-confidence while providing the audacity to be authentic. A great benefit to the respiratory and cardiac systems, as well as the upper back.

Third fingers either calm or excite active and reactive energies, engendering the courage and 'guts' to put innovative ideas into practice with the upper digestive organs profiting.

Fourth digits balance the give and take within relationships, much to the delight of the lower digestive parts and lower back.

The wee little fingers provide a remarkable amount of stability, affording the confidence to stand tall within the family and society, thereby enhancing the skeletal structure along with muscular flexibility, while encouraging the excretory system to let go of the old, enabling the reproductive organs to generate new concepts.

The exceptionally light touch is intuitively adjusted throughout the session, according to individual physical, 'e-motional' and Spiritual requirements. Varying from hovering just above the skin's surface (to enhance healing energies) to being firm but gentle (to ground these Universal energies) is based on the same principle as homoeopathy, that being, 'less is more'.

The gentleness of this approach can initially be extremely irritating and annoying or incredibly soothing and reassuring.

Either way, there is the delight of becoming completely immersed in the loving sense of joy and wonder of being alive and enjoying all that life has to offer.

How beautiful a day when kindness touches it!

64 - CHRISTINE LYNNE STORMER-FRYER

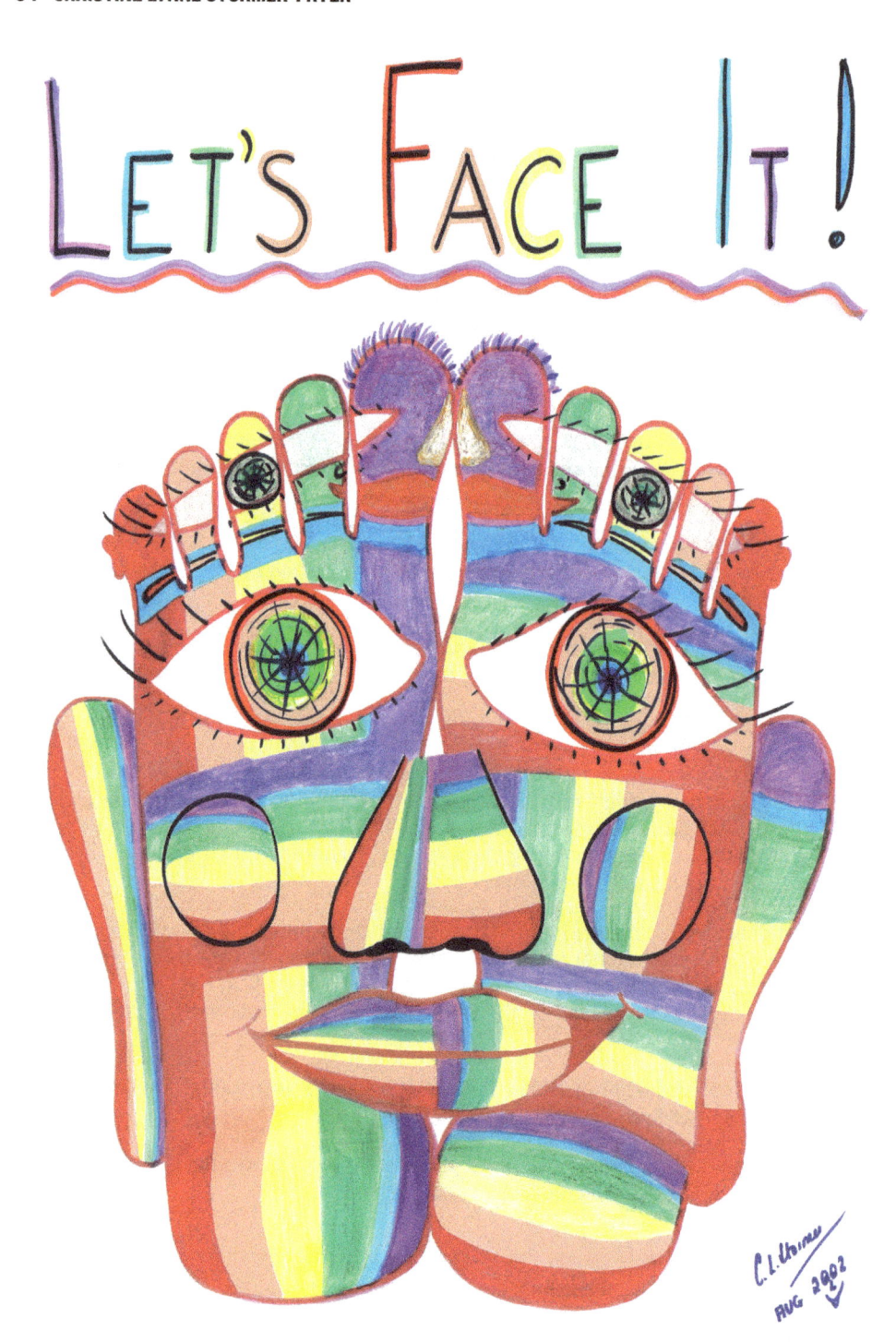

Let's Face It!

LET'S FACE IT

Concentrated in the face are highly tuned sensory organs, enabling the radar-like mind to pick up what is going on externally as well as internally.

Every sensory experience, whether seen, heard, smelt, tasted or felt, is detected and reflected in the toes, constantly altering the body's tone and tension level.

The right big toe reflects the right side of the face, and the left big toe the left side, each with the relevant sensory organs, together revealing how everybody faces life in their own way.

The eyes, being the 'windows to the Soul', radiate the true essence of the inner being, mirroring profound feelings. The sensitive second toes resonate to these 'e-motional' responses.

Triggered by sights, colours and images, the impressions of all that is seen goes straight to the heart to dwell in the chest. The essence of these 'e-motional' perceptions shows up on the balls of the feet.

Subconsciously aware of what is going on, the third toes get a 'sniff' of things to come, having picked up all that is heard by having the 'ears to the ground'. Ears are constantly in cahoots with the nose, which uses smell to keep mind and body on track. The talent of both the nose and ears processing and taking on board life events is reflected onto the upper halves of both insteps.

Initial sounds on either side of the head are influenced by family and society and mirrored on the little toes. Once deciphered by the middle ears, reflected mainly on the third toes, messages are passed onto the inner ears predominantly represented on the big toes. The brain can then 'make up its mind' as to what to do with the incoming information.

The mouth's shape indicates the ability to communicate and relate personal concepts and ideas openly and liberally. Whatever goes into or comes out of the mouth is detected by the fourth toes and relayed to the lower halves of both insteps.

Sensitive to touch is the skin, as related to the 'kin'. In other words, family and society. These sensations are related mainly to the little toes and heels.

Being the first port of entry into the mind, sensitive issues make the tissues of sensory organs react badly, depending on the type of issue. Irritated nerves agitate the already distressed body, erupting into a host of symptoms – not just on the face but also on related parts of the body, as well as in the feet.

Whatever is being faced encourages a shift from automatic conditioned robot-like responses to going with the flow and instinctively trusting the Universe.

Calmness within creates calmness without, affecting and enhancing environment conditions. Alerted to picking up meaningful universal messages, the senses are well-positioned to promote personal wellbeing through the accurate interpretation of external messages.

The Universe provides the strength to face life full-on!

66 - CHRISTINE LYNNE STORMER-FRYER

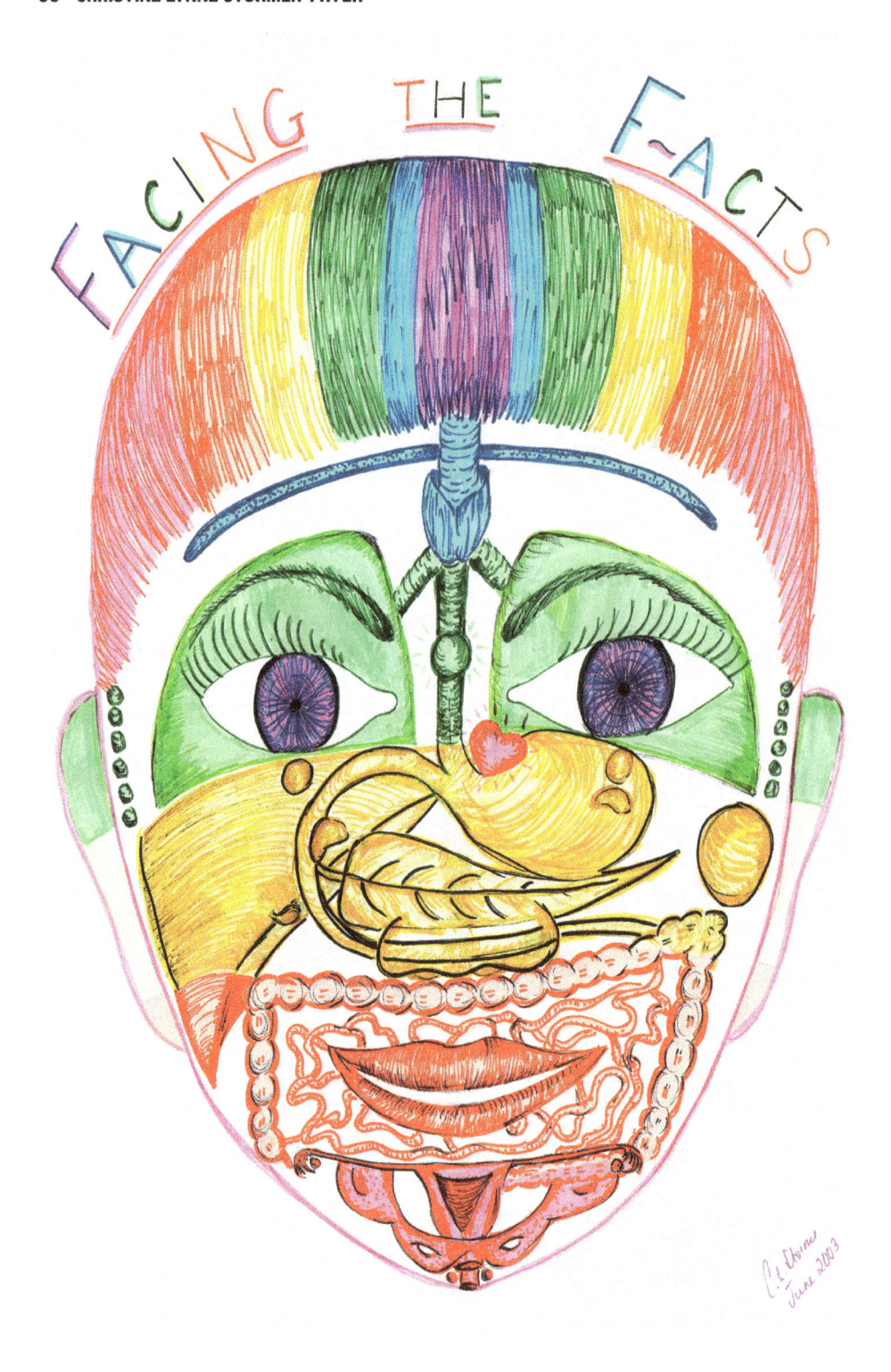

FACING THE F-ACTS

FACING THE FACTS

There can be no body without the senses, nor can there be any senses without the body. The two are inseparable and interdependent. It is only natural for the face to become the body's biography as it experiences life through all six senses. Its most noticeable aspects being its appearance and expressions.

'Thinking off the top of the head', hair acts as the body's antennae. Forever tuning into the Universal Library of Collective Thoughts, inspiration is drawn from the place where every concept is conceived, with the expression of these notions projected onto the neck and forehead.

Raised eyebrows show surprise in response to all the 'shoulds-but-don't-really-want-to' and 'should-nots-but-have-no-control' – although it is also a form of acknowledgement, affirmation or consent in certain parts of the world. These fringes of hair resonate to the energy of the shoulder clavicles.

Beliefs and memories play a massive role when it comes to perceptions of what is seen and not seen. As the windows of the Soul, eyes are completely in tune with heartfelt feelings. The elusive third eye between the two physical eyes has both the windpipe and oesophagus reflexes running through it, influencing everything entering and leaving the body. Mirroring the lungs, eyes openly display profound e-motions confined to the treasure chest of the body. When 'up to the eyes', dark 'bags' appear, giving them an ominous appearance. The heart of the matter soon makes its loving and empathetic presence known.

Then there is the 'sound of things' – whether 'sound' or not, heard or unheard, along with a whole lot of 'hearsay' – some reliable but generally misleading, all having an impact on the ribs, influencing what happens (or does not happen) next.

'Sticking the nose into other people's business' is irritating. Not recognising personal accomplishments is 'hard to stomach' and takes the pleasure out of life events, revealed by the pancreatic reflex over the nostrils.

With ears wide open and a 'nose to the ground,' the impact on the digestive tract shows up on the central panel of the face. The right cheek has the impudence to reflect the liver, while the left cheek has the audacity to mirror the spleen. Being different often leaves blemishes on the cheeks.

Whatever is taken in or spurted out of the mouth always sways relationships. Oscillations within the give and take are mimicked by the intestines showing up over the mouth. Meanwhile, the jaw reflects inner resourcefulness and personal stability within the family and society. It also displays stubbornness.

Holes made by piercings highlight significant gaps in life. In the nostril, it draws attention to an event that took away joy and happiness. A diamond stud is an attempt at bringing back some of the sparkle. A ring could indicate being 'led by the nose' or a situation involving a Taurean (the bull).

A stud in the lower lip emphasises the tendency to sulk or the desire to give lip. In the upper lip, it draws attention to nasty conversations that need to be stopped. A stud 'holding the tongue' makes it hard to 'speak up', despite wishing to do so.

Subtler than the body, the more life is experienced through all five senses, the greater the awareness of the sixth and higher senses.

Ignoring the facts does not change the facts!

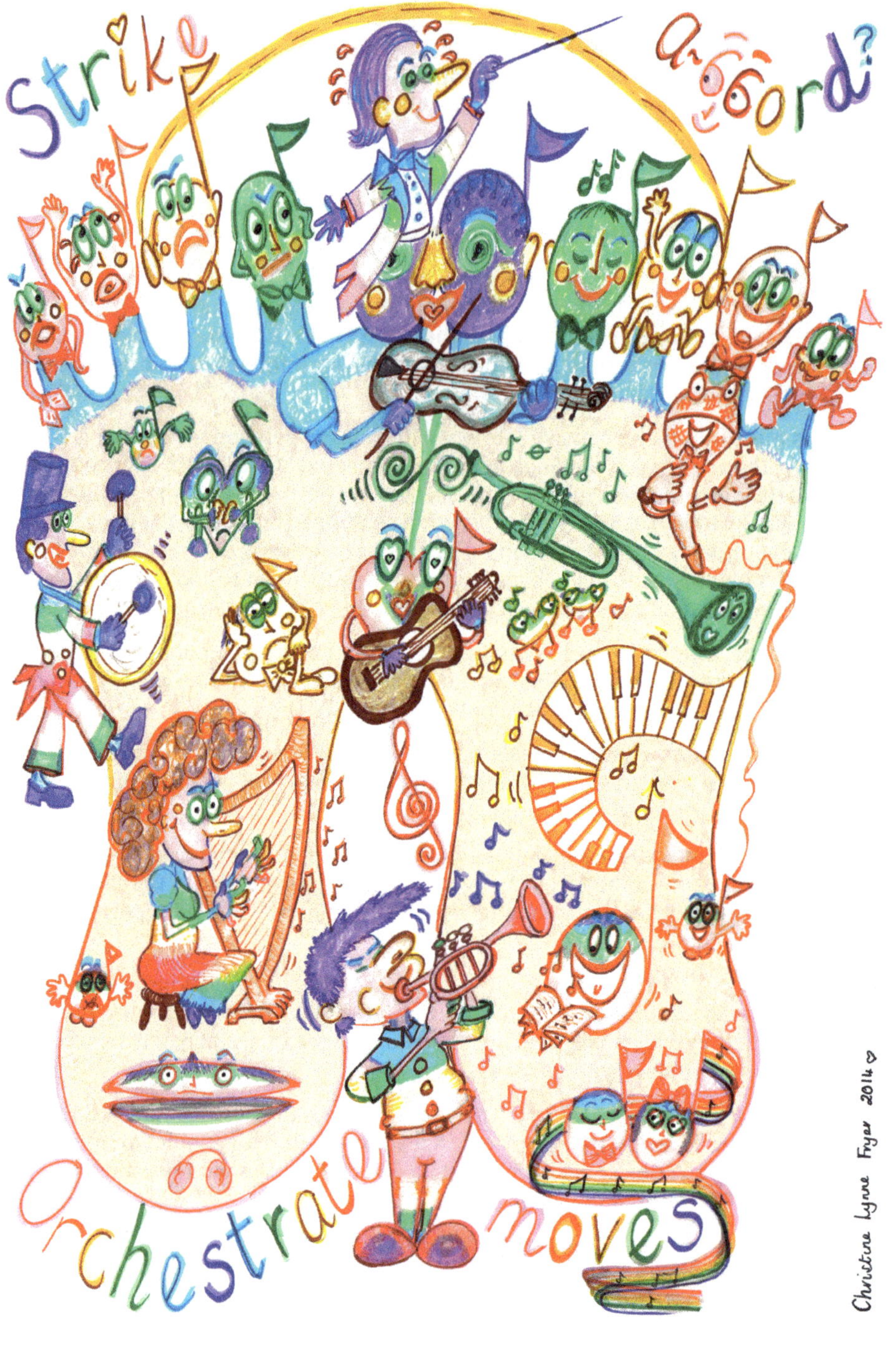
Strike
Orchestrate
moves
Christine Lynne Fryer 2014

STRIKE ACCORD – ORCHESTRATE MOVES

The endocrine system is the orchestra of the body, harmonising and balancing mind, body and Soul for inner peace and contentment.

The hypothalamus at the base of the brain is constantly alert to all ongoing undertones. As the 'composer' of the body, it masterminds the overall composition to orchestrate the best hormonal movements – once it knows the score. Choreographing interconnections and interactions requires a constant adjustment of the varying forces, tones and pitches.

The ever-fluctuating e-motions prompt these modifications, enticing hormones to either increase the tempo and speed when hypoactive, or slow it down and inhibit the body's processes when hyperactive.

Under the direction of the conductor of the body's inbuilt orchestra is the master gland, the pituitary gland. Being in control of all movements it ensures that each endocrinal gland strikes the most appropriate chord at the most suitable moment according to the role it plays.

The nearby pineal gland reputed for producing crystal-clear cyclic movements is akin to the tinkling of the triangle. As the psychic third eye, this seat of intuition and clairvoyance is a symbol of Spiritual awakening.

Shaped like a butterfly, the thyroid gland symbolises transformation between the non-physical and physical. Just like a violin, it serves as the perfect outlet for repressed feelings, or for the open expression of innermost sentiments.

The thymus gland, being the seat of the Soul, is as mystical as the breezes speaking through wind instruments and the magical flute. Beating the chest, as gorillas and warriors do before battle, stimulates this gland, preparing it for any eventuality.

Pulling at the heartstrings is the guitar, a fretted musical instrument with a hollow chamber that projects its vibrating sounds throughout. Evoked e-motions are a sentimental reminder of heartening events that either have the heartbeat subdued by sadness or exhilarated with joy.

Drumming up enthusiasm and resilience are the adrenal glands, to prevent proceeding in a humdrum sort of way. Accompanied by the black and white of the pianoforte, it is a relief to have a variety of keys and notes to lift the mood when 'facing the music' and 'all that jazz'.

Extracting joy and pleasure out of melodic sounds is the pancreas, providing the harmony and feedback as to how the overall performance is going, whether or not it is fully appreciated.

Gently celebrating the ability to create new concepts, the female ovaries use bells, chimes and whistles, while the testes take great pride in 'blowing their own trumpets'.

With new, exciting compositions constantly being composed, the ensuing vibrations are ideal for encouraging energy shifts. The arrangements that follow ensure that something new is always created from something old.

Music is the Universal language!

Foot at another's Neck!

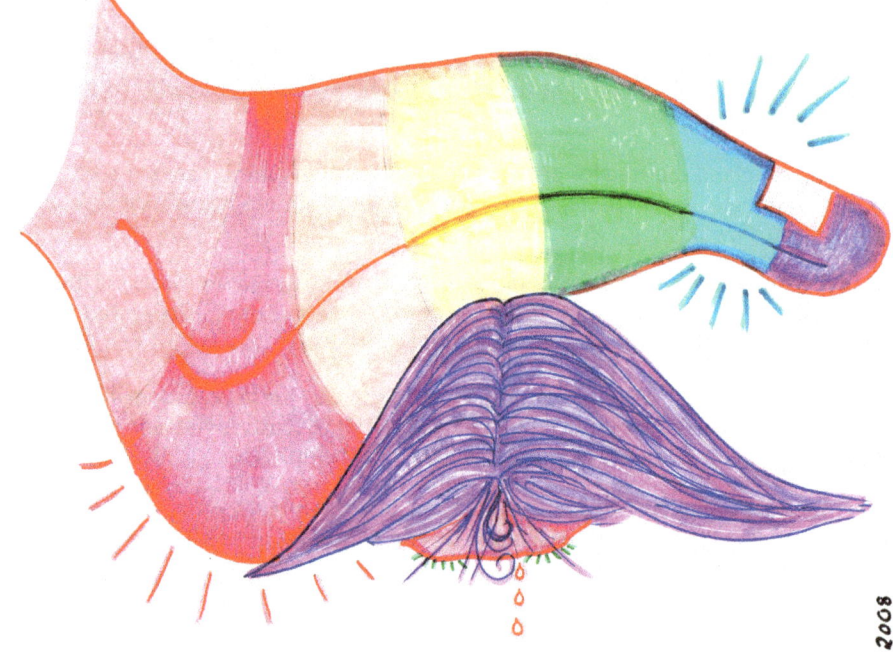

Stifling Ex-press-i-on!

Christine Lynne Stormer~Fryer 2008

A FOOT AT THE NECK

Linking the realm of thought with the realm of sensation, the neck acts as an avenue of expression. This integration of mind and body is an essential aspect of being human.

Less energy into thinking and more energy into action (and vice versa) causes conflict, depriving the whole of vital life force energy.

When energy gets stuck in the head, it intensifies and builds up like a pressure cooker. When trapped in the body, wisdom from the head is prevented from 'giving a helping hand'.

Social restrictions are like 'a foot at the neck', strangling and stifling creativity through fear, anger and guilt.

Choked with e-motion and unable 'to speak up', anxious that others might 'jump down the throat', or the possibility of 'getting it in the neck', causes words to be swallowed or stilled.

Self-expression is further inhibited through a dread of being ridiculed or being terrified of the consequences. The strain of integrating with others invariably leads to frustration, resentment and bewilderment.

With authentic expression being further restrained by social conditioning and unrealistic expectations, the mind is prevented from utilising and reaching its full potential.

Relied on to be flexible enough to see every point of view, a rigid neck becomes a 'pain in the neck', willing to see one way and one way only. Stubbornly refusing to 'see other points of view' results in mental rigidity, causing a host of unthinkable head issues.

A 'millstone around the neck' comes from having a negative attitude, along with self-admonishment, contributing to a range of neck difficulties. The neck gets it 'in the neck' when repulsed by a body that has been ab-used and neglected or disabled, making its physicality, personally and socially unacceptable.

As the mediator between head and body, the neck is responsible for holding the head up for a dignified and courageous look. Catering for the innermost needs, it facilitates the taking in of life force energies, air to boost e-motions; fire to inspire and provide fuel for cultivating unique notions, and water to maintain an equable balance within relationships.

In exchange, there is the outward flow of energy, through the breath and speech, as intimate feelings arise and as these energies are employed throughout life's experiences.

Thoughts and memories constantly running from the head through the body via the neck are translated into action. In return, the body's responses to the outcome return to the head to be externally expressed – the perfect balance between thoughts and actions.

Connecting the sky above with the waters below, the neck resonates to blue. It is where ether and air are exchanged and transformed. The connection between non-physical and physical is the essence that makes sure mind and body come alive and stay alive. Having the courage to 'stick the neck out' is frowned upon by an intimidated society, but it is essential for 'getting a head' in life.

Always wear a cheerful expression, no matter what!

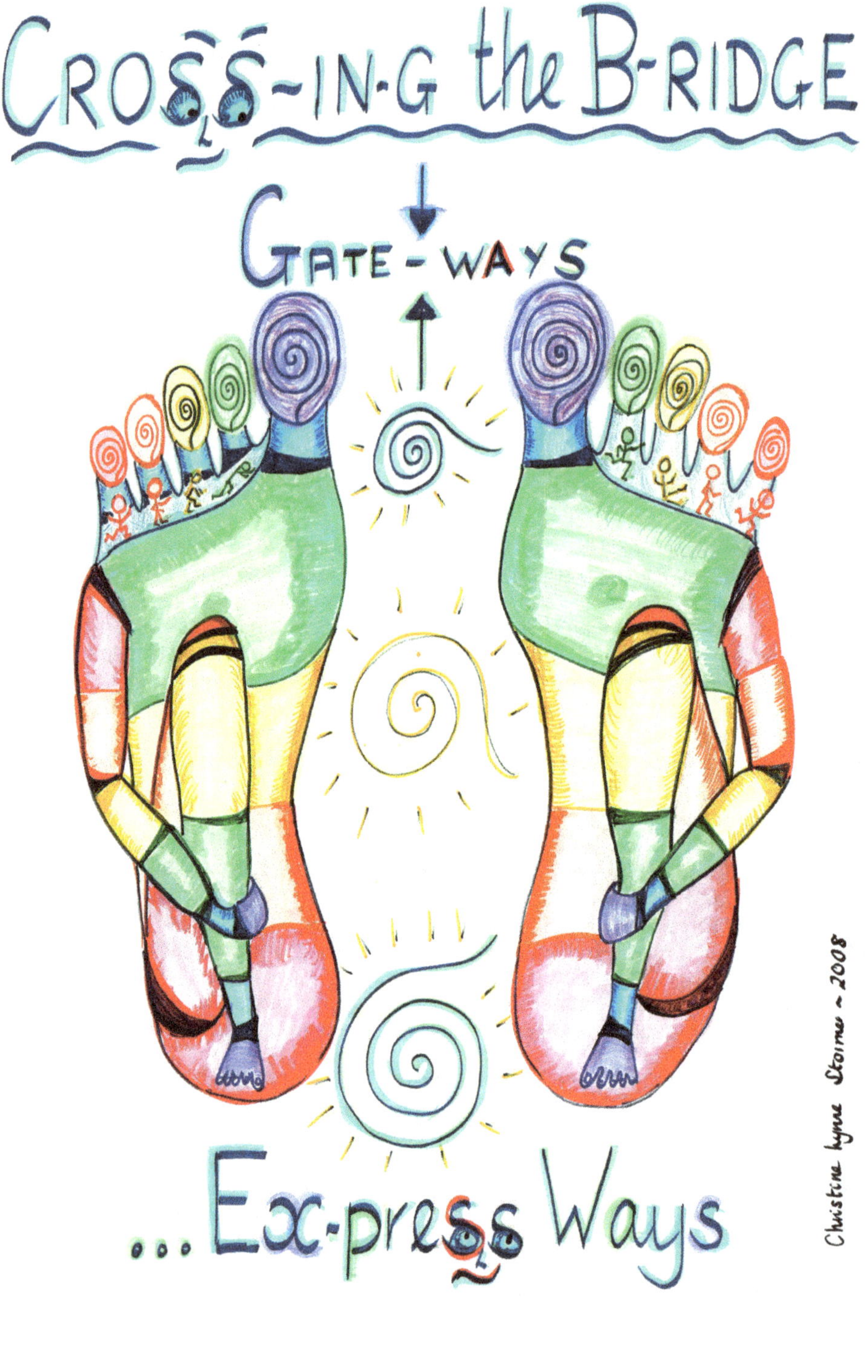
CROSS-ING the B-RIDGE
GATE-WAYS
...Ex-press Ways
Christine Lynne Stormer ~ 2008

CROSSING THE BRIDGE – EXPRESSWAYS – STIFLING EXPRESSION

The neck is the bridge between the absolute and the relative. Along with over two hundred joints, all positioned strategically around the body, it acts as an expressway. Easing movements, facilitating activities, and smoothing changes in direction, it is the bridge between the mind and the heart. Also the dwelling place of the throat chakra.

Considered the chakra of commitments, the throat chakra is linked to self-expression and authenticity. Speaking on behalf of the Spirit it connects with Higher Dimensions for reality to be meaningfully sensed with pure love. In so doing, the ideal path is provided to explore consciousness.

Having a direct link to the etheric body (where the blueprint is held), the throat is the door to another world. Holding the imprint of every vibration of all words ever spoken energetically links the throat to the solar plexus. Once personal power and Divine wisdom are one, decisions can be expedited, and appropriate actions taken. How the energy is integrated penetrates the ears, affecting clairaudience. These vibrations also influence sight, impacting the pineal gland and inner vision.

If strategic thinking is the bridge from the present into the unknown, then wisdom is the bridge that takes the mind from the unknown into the known. Meanwhile, Universal energies are the bridge from the Aquarian Age to the Golden Age.

Humanity builds too many walls and not enough bridges. Taking time to under-stand others and their cultures helps in building bridges. Once on the one side, it facilitates movement across to the other side, and vice versa.

Nestling between the eyes on the 'bridge in the nose' is the intuitive third eye, providing insight into life. Connected to the Universal truth, it is the guiding force within, contributing a sixth sense, as well as a 'gut feel', to provide direction. During problematic times, it offers a 'bridge over troubled water', along with the opportunity to steer clear of disaster. The more challenges encountered and dealt with while traversing bridges of opportunities, the greater the impact when transitioning from one state to another. Ascending the ladder of personal evolutions to a higher level of awareness and energy always entails a period of discomfort, although the rite of passage to live life more courageously and genuinely is well worth it.

'Bridging differences' reduces the space between two things, making 'crossing the bridge' and dealing with issues on the spot less complicated. It is easy to 'burn bridges', yet it takes time and effort to build them again to understand any 'water that has passed under the bridge'.

By 'bridging the gap' between bones, joint movements are perfectly orchestrated – from barely discernible to incredibly magnificent. With joints being so obliging and adaptable and constantly coping with the onslaught of daily demands, every twist and turn is taken in their stride, allowing incidents to become an invaluable learning curve. It turns the journey over many bridges into an exciting adventure.

Being fully present in the 'here and now' assists the gateways in effectively directing the energy to where it is most needed. Being forced by the Soul to progress in ways not anticipated can be fearful, not to paralyse but to liberate. The bridge between heaven and earth is an adventure in itself.

The challenge is knowing which bridge to cross and which to burn!

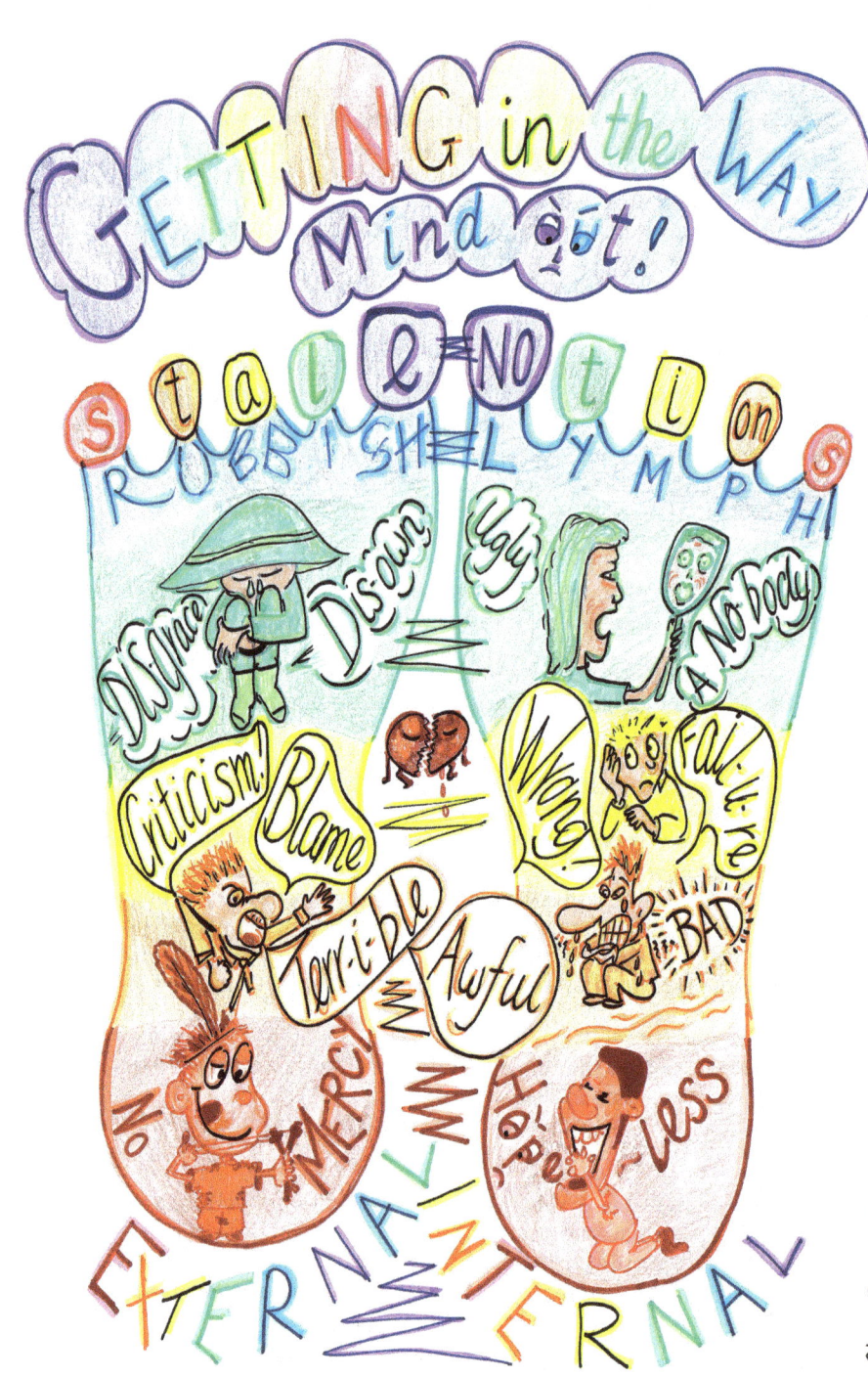

74 - CHRISTINE LYNNE STORMER-FRYER

GETTING IN THE WAY – MIND OUT

Mind out! An enormous amount of drivel gets in the way of the lymphatics. Whatever is going on externally mirrors what is going on internally, drawing attention any distressing state of affairs.

The 'stale' taste of routine purposelessness, with out-dated 'notions' being entertained for far too long, leads to a build-up of a 'load of rubbish'. As this absolute non-sense enters and leaves via the throat, the body ends up living in the psychic equivalent of a 'rubbish' dump, with the lymphatic system yearning to say 'good riddance to bad rubbish!'

Expressions of disapproval, based on perceived faults or apparent mistakes, often seem like life-sentences of condemnation. Dire criticism 'responsible for the unpleasant conflict within, generally involves some form of 'disgrace', 'disownment', or 'disagreement'.

Attempting to keep the body strong and impenetrable from these disturbing forces is the 'thymus' gland. From this 'seat of the Soul', cells migrate to the other parts of the body to form Peyer's patches, centres of lymphatic activity, safeguarding the Soul against self-flagellation.

Feeling 'ugly' when the mood turns 'ugly', 'ugly' perceptions persist. Manifesting 'ugly' is bound to have the lymph glands 'up in arms'. Belief of being 'a nobody' with no real value or worth lowers an already almost-non-existent self-esteem, eliminating any resistance when feeling under attack.

It is so easy to 'blame' for all the so-called 'wrongs', but to do so is to become powerless, blocking any hope of progress and getting in the way of the lymphatics. Resorting to 'blame' is admitting to being a 'failure'. Yet 'failure' is simply a perception, its roots deeply embedded in the 'dis-ease to please' without pleasing anyone. 'Failure', if anything, is the ideal opportunity to begin afresh!

Bringing shame or discredit through disgraceful behaviour and dishonourable actions considered to be 'terrible' or 'bad' or 'awful' brings about an embarrassing loss of reputation or respect, along with possible 'disownment' and 'rejection'.

Cast aside and abandoned, with relationships ending or being cut off without a penny, puts the lymph in a compromising position. Alert and prepared to 'fight' back, the lymphatic system attacks itself.

Important to the lymphatics is the spleen. As the warehouse and body shop, it acts as a blood filter. By synthesising antibodies in its white pulp and removing old red blood cells, it provides the essence of all that is going on.

Spreading negativity and 'feeling bad' about 'a bad apple spoiling the lot' only 'upsets the apple cart', with the situation going from bad to worse. One 'bad' thing seems to lead to another, drawing attention to what needs improving. Terrorising the living daylights out of others is a terrible state of affairs, causing alarm, dread and fear, and stopping the lymphatic flow in its tracks.

On bended knee, begging for 'mercy' is an integral concept of Divinity's compassion with humankind. Interestingly, the Divine Source never criticises, judges or condemns, yet society does.

Mercy is an event to be grateful for, providing relief from suffering and preventing something unpleasant from taking place.

Let it come! Let it go! Let it flow!

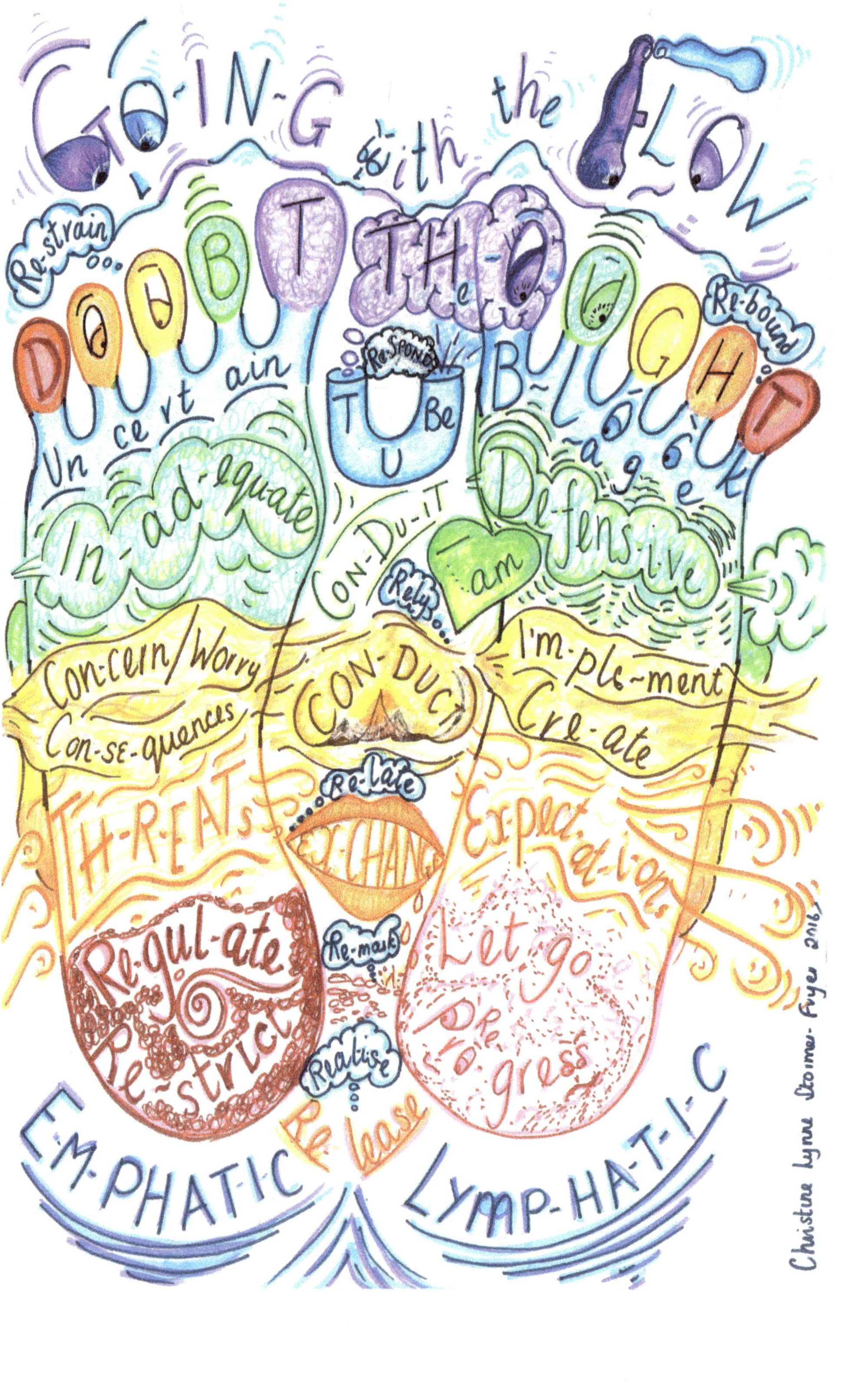
GO-IN-G with the FLOW
Re-strain
DOUBT
THOUGHT
Re-bound
Re-SPOND
TUBe
U
Un ce rt ain
In-ad-equate
Con-Du-IT
Rely
I am
Defensive
Con-cern/Worry
Con-se-quences
CON-DUCT
I'm-ple-ment
Cre-ate
Re-late
TH-R-EATs
EX-CHANGE
Ex-pect-at-i-ons
Re-mark
Re-gul-ate
Re-strict
Let go
Pro-gress
Realise
Re-lease
E-M-PHATIC
LYMP-HA-T-I-C
Christine Lynne Stormer-Fryer 2016

GOING WITH THE FLOW – EMPHATIC LYMPHATIC

'Going with the flow' is to be in tune with the lymphatic and circulatory systems. An extensive sewerage network, the lymphatic system flushes out and neutralises toxic thoughts and noxious e-motions to purify the body and make space for a fresh supply of vital life forces.

By draining tissue fluid surrounding the body's cells, this network of lymphatic vessels keeps life force energy in tip-top condition. 'Emphatically empathetic', the lymphatic system loves 'going with the flow', but things do tend to get in the way.

'Doubt' – arising from perceived obstacles, perils, risks and dangers – is 'ageing' and 'blocks' the way. Driving the mind crazy with a host of detrimental 'th-e-oughts', the inevitable indecisiveness 'restrains' the Soul, keeping it away from its intended path. So many wasted opportunities go 'down the tubes'.

With 'doubt' and action being incompatible, the more truth residing in the body, the less room there is for 'doubt'.

When it comes to 'uncertainty' in a world of 'uncertainty', the only thing that is certain is that 'nothing is certain'. There is no point in getting all 'defensive' and wishing to retaliate.

A lack of confidence and feelings of 'inadequacy' permeate from figures of authority. Altering the label to the 'I am' responsible for all that happens internally alters the perspective. It all boils down to what is in the heart. A confident 'conduit' surrounded by a pure white light inspires confidence in others.

'Worrying' over petty 'concerns' and dreaded 'consequences' that may never happen interferes with 'creating' and 'implementing' innovative concepts, which invariably has an adverse impact on the ensuing 'conduct'.

Constantly intimidated by 'threats' is Soul-destroying, yet the only 'threat' is a perceived 'threat'. The body cannot differentiate between life-threatening events and those conjured by the mind, especially when it spins endless fantasies of possible disaster, tipping the balance between health and dis-ease.

Negative 'expectations' are a dead end to thinking. There is great pain, humiliation, and a sense of inferiority when drowning in a sea of expectations. Accepting belittling expectations is so detrimental. 'Relying' on the belief that every need is met and that there is a solution to every problem boosts the morale. Developing an intimate relationship with oneself guarantees an intimate relationship with the Universe, which in turn provides the guidance to develop constructive 'exchanges' of energy and develop functional relationships with others.

'Rules' and 'regulations' are the downfall of humanity, restricting movement and 'progress' – not just outside the body but also within.

'Rebounding' back with confidence, with the courage to deviate from the norm, may be perceived as a 'threat' to society, but it's well worth it. With it comes the 'realisation' that to 'release' and 'let go' of non-significant 'remarks' 'related' to the past is such a huge 'relief'.

Breaking free from human bonds liberates the Soul, making it so much easier to 'go with the flow'.

It's not happiness that generates gratitude but gratitude that generates happiness!

78 - CHRISTINE LYNNE STORMER-FRYER

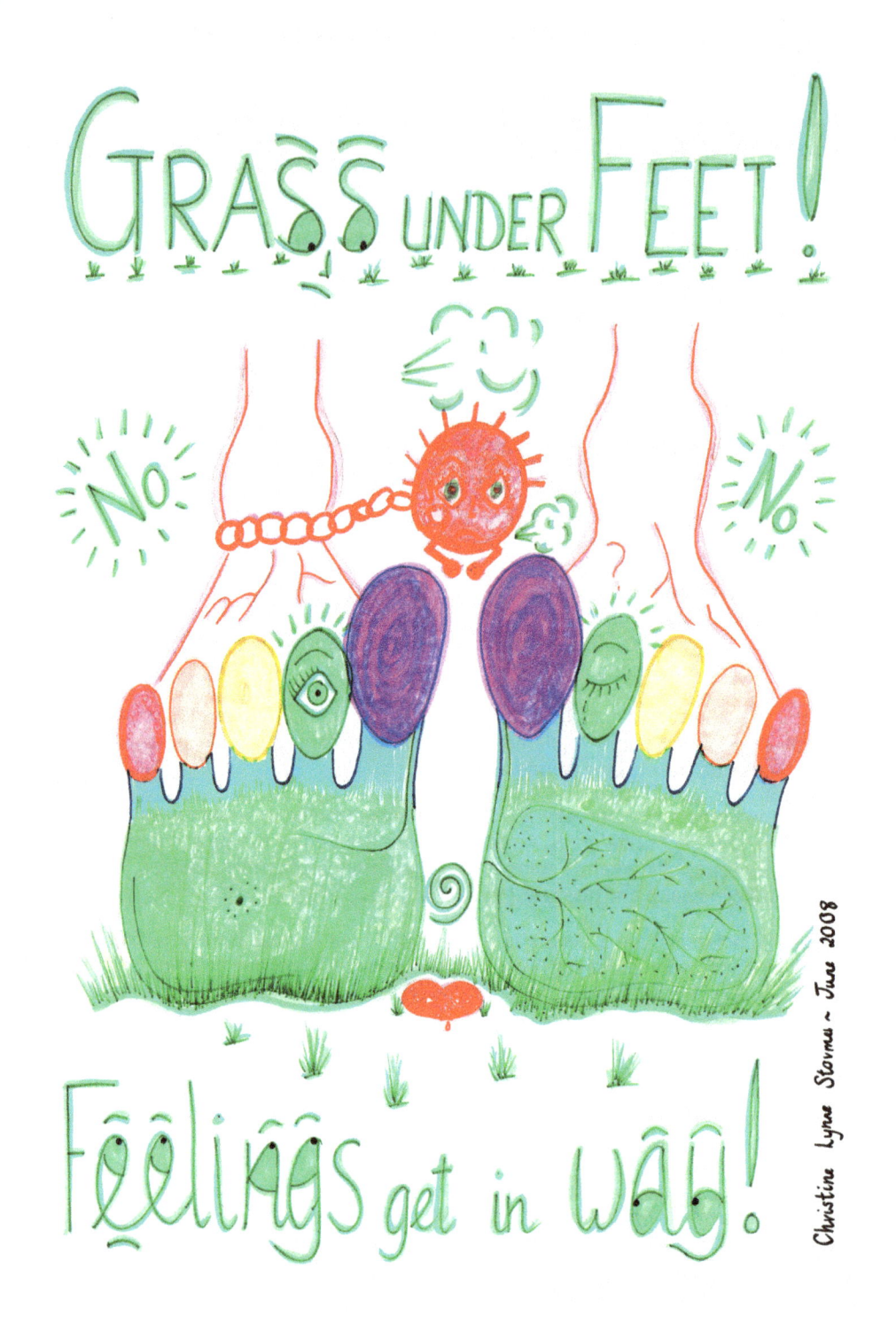

GRASS GROWING UNDER FEET – FEELINGS GET IN THE WAY!

'Growing grass under the feet' is to squander time or opportunity. Waiting to act until it is too late and slacking in getting on and doing things is what happens when 'feelings' get in the way.'

Not 'feeling good enough'. Good enough for what? Not 'feeling like it'. Like what? 'Feeling unwell'. Poorly about what? So on and so forth. All pathetic excuses not honouring the Spirit within.

Getting on and doing what needs to be done immediately and properly, without wasting time or energy grappling with much-needed challenges through productivity, is an antidote to allowing the 'grass to grow under the feet'.

Sharing many similarities are the ability to process 'th-e-oughts' and the process by which grass grows. Some ideas grow rapidly, others need more care and attention, while others grow even in the most difficult or unusual circumstances.

Grass seeds need plenty of moisture to germinate and sprout, regulated by soil temperature and depending on the type of grass. A harder outer casing can delay the process until conditions are favourable.

Likewise, a concept needs to be communicated internally and then externally, according to the Soul's temperament. Perceived obstacles invariably get in the way, with the greatest obstacle being unfavourable, hardened 'e-motions'.

Confronted with political, economic and social tension that can explode at any moment, destroying life as it was, gives all the more reason to act promptly and embrace current circumstances, making the most of every moment.

Within every body is the power (and capacity) to respond to ongoing changes when energised from 'feeling good'. It is a privilege to 'set foot on earth', especially at times of tremendous uncertainty – when it can be extremely difficult to 'find a footing'.

Despite many uncontrollable factors, circumstances can be changed for the better, starting with a changed mind and different personal view of the world. At the end of the day, it is all about 'attitude'. With so many choices to be made every day, it is attitude that determines the outcome.

Every day, three eyes must open, one to look in, and two to look out. Trusting inner guidance to show the way is to reconnect with the Higher Self and all that *is*.

'E-motions' are reactions to what happens. They are the driving force in life, ensuring that every day is lived with resolute purpose and intent.

Miracles grow out of difficulties!

80 - CHRISTINE LYNNE STORMER-FRYER

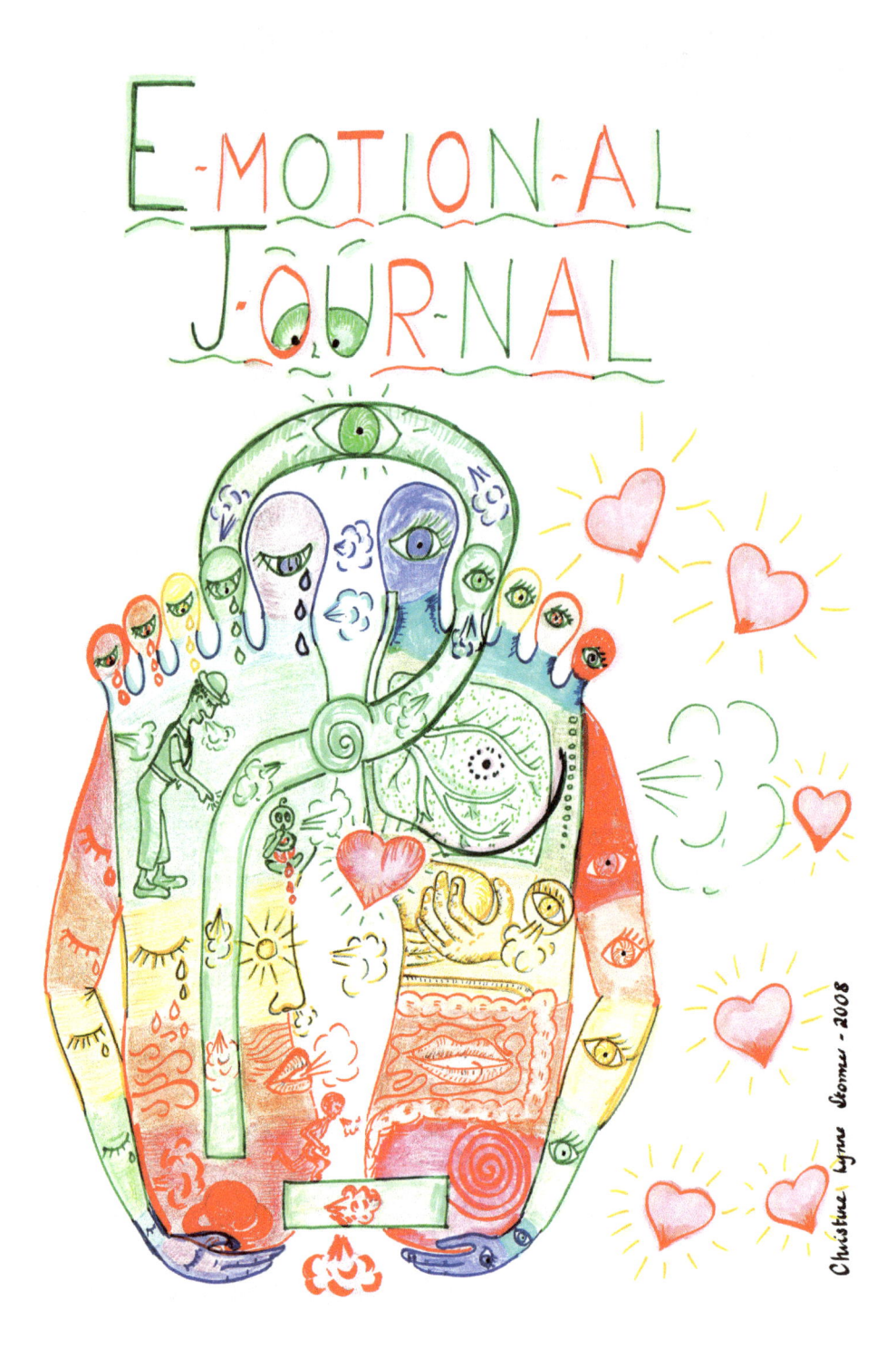

'E-MOTIONAL' JOURNEY - WILLINGNESS TO FEEL

A rollercoaster of lawless and irregular 'e-motional' reactions is responsible for some of the most breath-taking decisions.

The body itself has no feelings. It is just a lump of matter, deriving its sensitivity and consciousness from the energy of the Soul inhabiting and passing through it.

The 'e-motional' journey is never clear, constantly engendering a whole host of question marks. Linked with the highly 'e-motional' second toes and number '2' presenting through its shape one big '?'. The underlying theme is Spiritual growth through sharing and co-operating with others. Despite all the 'ups and downs', the challenge is to maintain an 'e-motional' balance.

The eyes, as 'windows to the Soul', have insight into Spirit. Able to see all aspects of life on every level, with vision provided to navigate through unknown territories.

Seeing something moving en route can arouse a variety of 'e-motional' states, bringing tears of sadness or joy to the eyes. Sights, colours and images trigger 'e-motional' responses according to previous personal experiences.

Dealing with powerful 'e-motions' is especially challenging when going through chaotic, devastating or cruel experiences. Only two options seem available. Either to let the feelings out immediately (the visceral way), or bottle them up, cramming and suppressing the 'e-motions' inside.

The truth is that there are many positive ways to deal with wayward 'e-motions'. Simply *experiencing* negative "e-motions" provides valuable insight when most needed.

Feelings arise from perceptions, and good thoughts brighten the eyes, making it clearer to see every point of view, thereby opening the mind.

As 'th-e-oughts' journey through the body, deeply ingrained memories are stirred, evoking feelings going back seven generations or more.

With feelings being self-manufactured, they can be changed simply by wishing to do so. Anybody can be as 'miser-able' or as happy as they wish to be, regardless of the circumstances encountered en route.

Honouring mind and body provides the resources to remain 'e-motionally' balanced. Evoked feelings can then be constructive, inspirational, and motivational.

Building compassion, empathy and pure love is a vital part of the 'e-motional' journey. An opportunity to be Spiritual while having a human experience.

The sole's sole purpose is to support the Soul through life by providing a firm, protective and flexible foundation from which to grow, expand, and develop, for a deeper understanding of the self and others. In so doing, the Soul feels well-supported during its journey through life on Earth.

Respect everybody as an individual entertaining their unique feelings!

82 - CHRISTINE LYNNE STORMER-FRYER

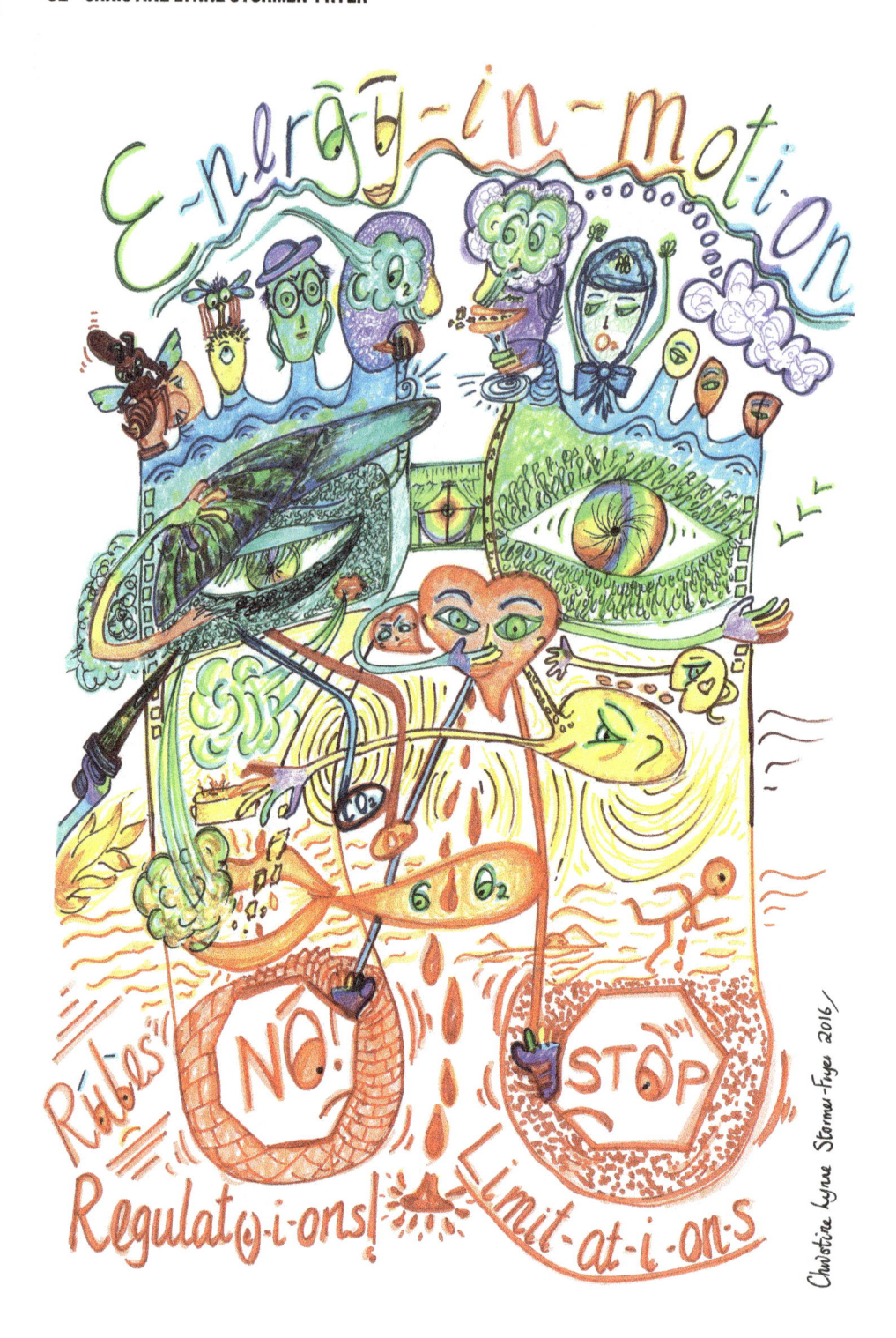

ENERGY-IN-MOTION

The 'E' representing the 'e-nergy' of 'th-e-ought' triggers a vibration when running through the body. This 'motion' shakes the molecules, loosening memories and evoking long lost feelings to generate 'e-motions'. The Soul's way of communicating and creating awareness of its essence and authentic Spirit.

Resonating to green, since it brings together two very different energies, it is the unifier of opposites, offering 'tranquillity' through 'blue', and 'excitement' through 'yellow'. Consequently, 'being in two minds' and vacillating between the logical past and creative future (as well as the unconscious and conscious) provides a much-appreciated balance. Intuition is ultimately the guiding light.

'Putting on the thinking cap' to consider all options before 'making up the mind' and then 'keeping it under the cap' could be considered a tad selfish. Far better to 'put a feather in the cap' and proudly display incredible achievements.

'To cap it all', the last straw, surpassing all that has gone before, is to submissively apologise with 'cap in hand' or even resort to collecting 'cap money' when feeling impoverished, with self-esteem 'sinking to the boots'. A 'far cry' from 'setting her cap at him', using the most becoming of bonnets to attract the attention of a favoured gentleman.

Dressed in one's 'Sunday best' or 'up to the nines' (using more material to display greater status) is to be 'made out of cloth' and entirely false or pretentious. It is all a 'load of humbug', a fraudulent deception enough to 'bug the hell' out of others and evoke heated 'e-motions'.

'Looking or speaking daggers' and openly conveying hostility, with the intention to hurt, takes the breath away, while also reducing the amount of 'oxygen' used to boost self-esteem. 'Beating the breast' in a display of guilt and public remorse, or making a show of victory or success, 'makes a clean breast' when making a full confession and concealing nothing.

Not able to 'stomach the situation' and having had a 'guts full' may result in having 'butterflies fluttering around the stomach' or the 'stomach tied up in knots'. Constantly helping itself to energy stored in the liver, the stomach relies on passion for putting ideas into action. Meanwhile, the spleen reaches out to the heart to 'get a feel' of the *dis*content, or content, being entertained in its four chambers.

Every word uttered, every expression expressed, every breath breathed, and every feeling felt is packaged into carbon dioxide. When breathed out, it fills the air, creating the atmosphere. 'Burping' and 'farting' is to 'pass wind' full of stale 'e-motions' no longer prepared to 'pay the rent'. Meanwhile, 'air embolisms' contain lethal 'e-motions' that are potentially dangerous to the body.

'E-motions' fill the air. 'Giving oneself airs' inflates self-opinion in an assuming manner (or tone of superiority), making it tempting to 'give the air' as a form of dismissal. 'Giving vent' and being 'full of hot air' is utterly absurd. While 'an air of mystery' is intriguing, an 'air of importance' prone to 'airs and graces' comes from an over-inflated ego.

STOP prevents further pretentiousness and rebelliousness. Even though 'rules' and 'regulations' can bring things to a standstill, they do not deter 'e-motions'. Lawless and irregular erratic feelings are the driving force of Spirit.

'E-motional' richness is the fuel for life!

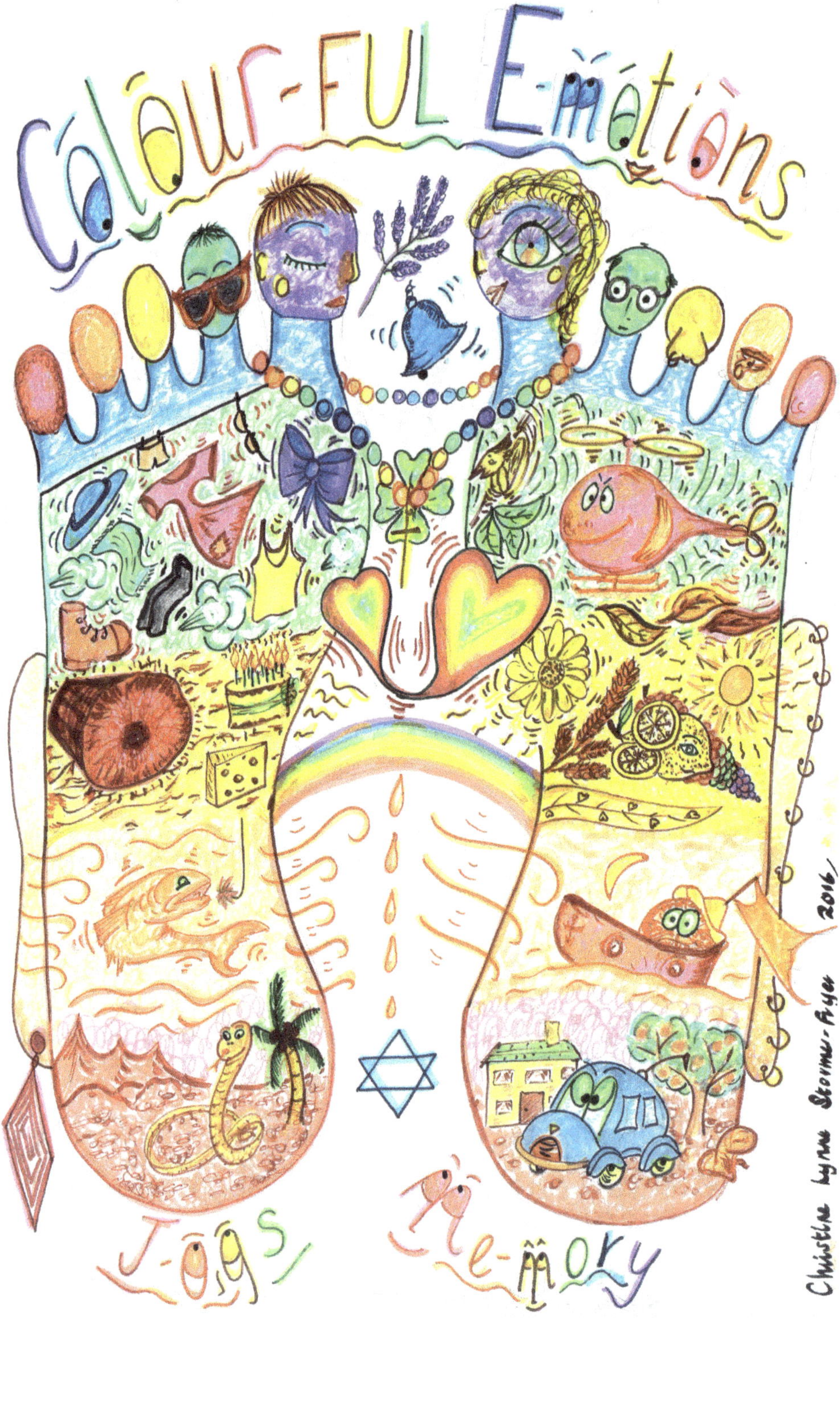
Colour-FUL E-motions
Jogs Memory
Christine Lynne Stormer-Fryer 2016

COLOURFUL EMOTIONS – JOG MEMORIES

Defining the world are wondrous displays of colour. Manifestations of light, each with its own frequency and beneficial effects.

The wide range of shades or tints has a different impact on the finely tuned body, constantly altering its chemical make-up.

The vibration of the various hues evokes memories arousing 'e-motions' in obscure ways. Swaying 'th-e-oughts' – while also affecting attitudes, disposition, and well-being – colour has a profound influence on choices made.

Darker tones bring out the serious introspective aspects of life, while lighter shades have a more calming and nurturing influence.

Sensations are awakened by eye-catching colours perceived through the eyes through a subtle language of moods, vitality and insights. The Spirit responds in many visceral ways.

Instinctive choices of colour are 'eye-opening'. Having an aversion to a particular colour highlights issues requiring attention and healing. Attraction to certain colours highlights innermost needs. These potent hues are effectively harnessed through chromotherapy (colour therapy), with individual colour frequencies used to positively motivate 'e-motions' for a renewed sense of inner harmony.

Pure white light, an amalgamation of all the colours, is cathartic on many levels, having an overall harmonising influence. When combined with pure love, it becomes even more dynamic.

Visualisation of colour during healing sessions either enhances the vitality of the body's energies – by obliterating dark, sinister memories that take the spark out of life, or calms hectic, volatile thoughts.

Shifting colourings on the skin, particularly on the soles of the feet, highlight sub-conscious 'th-e-oughts' and 'e-motional' undercurrents. With dramatic mood swings going from one extreme to another, these colours can change in the 'blink of an eye'.

Interpretation of colour provides valuable insight into the impact of 'coloured opinions'. The rule of thumb is to determine the vibrancy behind the colour, whether it is soft and gentle or harsh with darkly sinister or mysterious undertones.

There is invariably a 'change of colour' when flushed, blushing, awkward and perplexed from being found out, or 'off-colour'.

Having a 'coloured point of view' is to have a fanatical perception of a situation. 'Giving colour to the matter' makes it more plausible and 'exposes true colours' to reveal genuine characteristics, creating a likelihood of triumphing and 'coming off with flying colours'.

Colour, the sun's vital messenger, is the sensation that enriches the world!

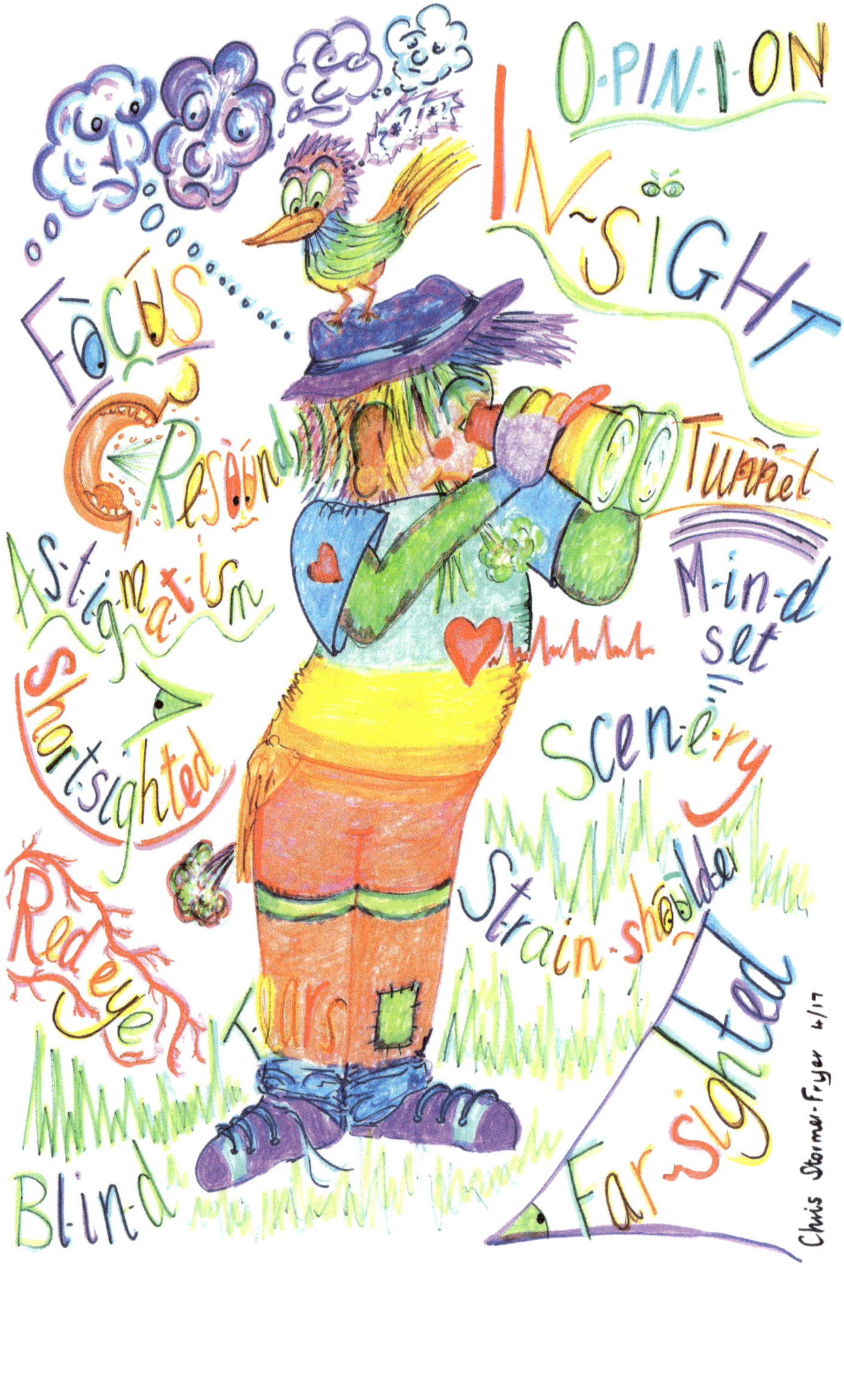
O-PIN-I-ON
IN-SIGHT
Focus
Tunnel
As-ti-g-mat-is-m
M-in-d
set
Shortsighted
Scen-e-ry
Red-eye
Blind
Far-sighted
Chris Stormer-Fryer 4/17

EYES – OPINIONS AND INSIGHTS – MAKING A SCENE!

'Making a scene' when exceptionally 'e-motional' is determined by the eyes' opinion of all that is insight. The scripts produced for each scenario are filled with heartfelt feelings of self-esteem and self-worth, with both having a significant role to play. Scenes take place in a variety of locations, with as many attempts as required to get it right. Once the issue is resolved, it is time to change and move onto the next stage of each scenario.

SCENARIO #1 Short-sightedness and retinal detachment. Constantly reviewing the outdated historical past, highlighting the need to become detached from ancient times now extinct. Setting sights in the past requires constant rewinding of 're-play', going over the same old lines and acting out the same old scenes, time and time again. Continually living in the past obliterates the present, with the future a replica of the past, usually with greater and often more-upsetting challenges, forcing the awareness to move on.

SCENARIO #2 Far- or long-sighted. Always fast-forwarding and planning ahead due to a deep concern about a time that may or may not come in the future, 'seeing life flash by' with little or 'no time to do anything'. Turning the back on the present leads to regret, frustration, resentment, anger, disillusionment and dissatisfaction, contributing to a less than adequate, even poor, quality eyesight and performance.

SCENARIO #3 Astigmatism. Not sure where to focus, with so many frenetic 'e-motional' scenes being enacted, especially at home. Irregularities, seen as defective 'e-motional' 'curve balls', dramatically change the scenes. Detrimental turns of events distort everything 'out of proportion', a means to avoid seeing what is really going on.

SCENARIO #4 Red eye (conjunctivitis). Inflamed and furious at not seeing clearly from having to contain views in a volatile environment, 'e-motions' erupt at the 'drop of a hat'. Considered highly contagious as the anger rapidly spreads, with those in the vicinity 'seeing red'.

SCENARIO #5 Blindness from constantly 'turning a blind eye' and not wishing to see. Blinded by rage (or the truth) and not wishing to witness 'e-motional' events. Many are blinded by the glare of their own personal brilliance.

SCENARIO #6 Tunnel vision. Conflict from having only one way of seeing things (one's own), while others view life through a wide-angle lens and see the bigger picture.

SCENARIO #7 Eye strain. Tired of all the 'shoulds' and 'should nots' from being expected to carry so much on the shoulders when having a completely different 'point of view'.

SCENARIO #8 Opinionated. Low opinions batter an already shattered self-esteem, with a chance of becoming even more opinionated when 'pushed around' by the opinions of others. Options are so much better.

SCENARIO #9 The present. Making the most of the here and now. Enjoying endless opportunities and cherishing each moment. Adapting and changing along the way for greater satisfaction and appreciation, with an occasional flashback to the past to admire progress made, and fast-forwarding to the future to see how to ensure that dreams still come true.

Eyes focus where the mind is focused!

88 - CHRISTINE LYNNE STORMER-FRYER

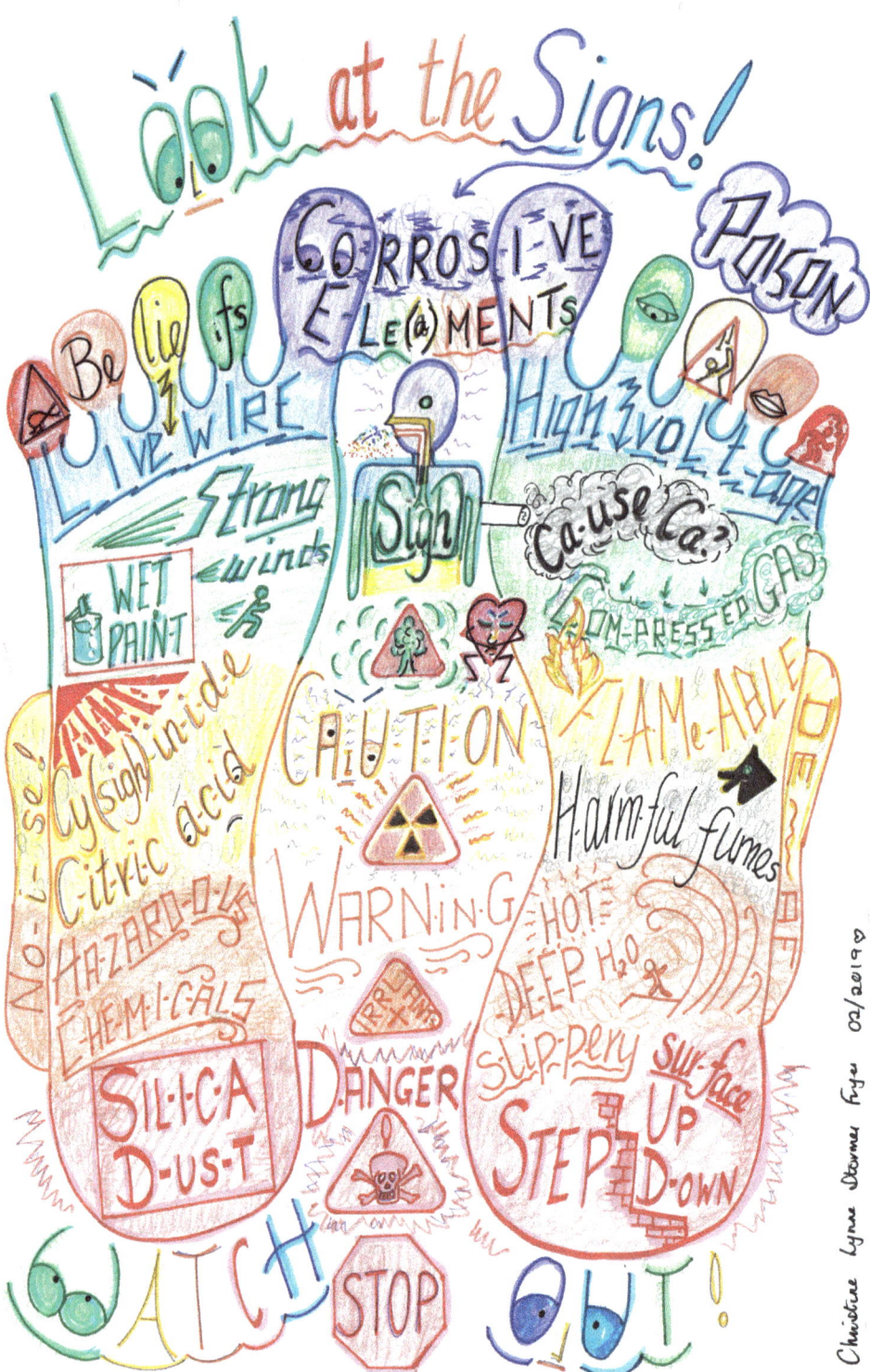

LOOK AT THE SIGNS – WATCH OUT!

Watch out! STOP before taking another step – it could be perilous. Really? Why is humanity so intent on stopping others in their tracks with such 'destructive beliefs'? Warning against some of the most 'corrosive elements' yet generating highly caustic comments through extreme criticism (in its most vicious form), usually in uncalled-for retaliation.

So, what is so 'poisonous'? Could it be toxic thoughts? Are 'th-e-oughts' 'pois'ed 'on' 'ous'? Nasty, hostile, malevolent notions entertained in the mind maliciously seeping through to contaminate the body with offensive energy.

Then there is the shock from 'live wires' with such a dangerously 'high voltage' – possibly already in shock from an explosive outburst. Tissues go into 'shock' when profoundly sad or excessively deprived of love, depriving them of vital life force energies. As a shock wave of symptoms floods the floundering body, any further shocking input causes utter confusion and a possible loss of consciousness, or even death, frequently the Soul's way of opting out of exceptionally shocking situations. At the other extreme, with nerves constantly circulating electrical currents around the body, highly motivated 'live wires' enliven the nerves with additional energy.

Just as electrical wiring is subject to safety standards, so too are the nerve connections. Acute awareness is created through volatile 'e-motions', along with dangerous temperaments, thwarting hostile comments or highly flammable chemistry between individuals. Exposure to sunlight is deemed detrimental, yet it highlights the way to enlightenment.

'Strong winds' cannot be seen, although the subsequent activity soon becomes evident. Finding out 'how the wind blows' (with developments swayed by public opinion), can 'take the wind out of the sails' when anticipated arguments, or empty, meaningless words 'take away the impetus'. The deflated chest 'heaves a sigh', with ensuing respiratory issues making the body 'cough up'.

'Wet paint' is a timorous cover-up that can be passed on if touched. Suppressed inflammable 'e-motions' in the form of 'compressed gas' become a cy(sigh) inside and, like 'cyanide', increasingly noxious. 'Throwing caution to the wind', 'harmful fumes' can become highly 'flame-able', with engendered bitterness turning into 'citric (see-I-tric-k) acid'.

'Turning a deaf ear' in hazardous relationships is a 'warning' of being in 'hot or deep water' and 'out of depth', with venomous chemical reactions between individuals. Progress is hazardous at a time when 'slippery when wet'.

Anything related to 'dust' points immediately to 'dust swept under the carpet', either within the family or society, symbolised by 'silica (still- I -see- a) dust'. Any thought of 'danger' triggers a 'Stop' sign in the mind. Yet so much hearsay is based on other's experiences. Everybody creates their own situations through ongoing beliefs. Something considered 'dangerous' to one person may be hugely exciting to another.

STOP and think. Too often, the 'blind lead the blind'. Instead of 'stepping down' in fear, take a confident 'step up'. The heights of each accomplishment will make every next step that much easier.

Trust your intuition to show you the way!

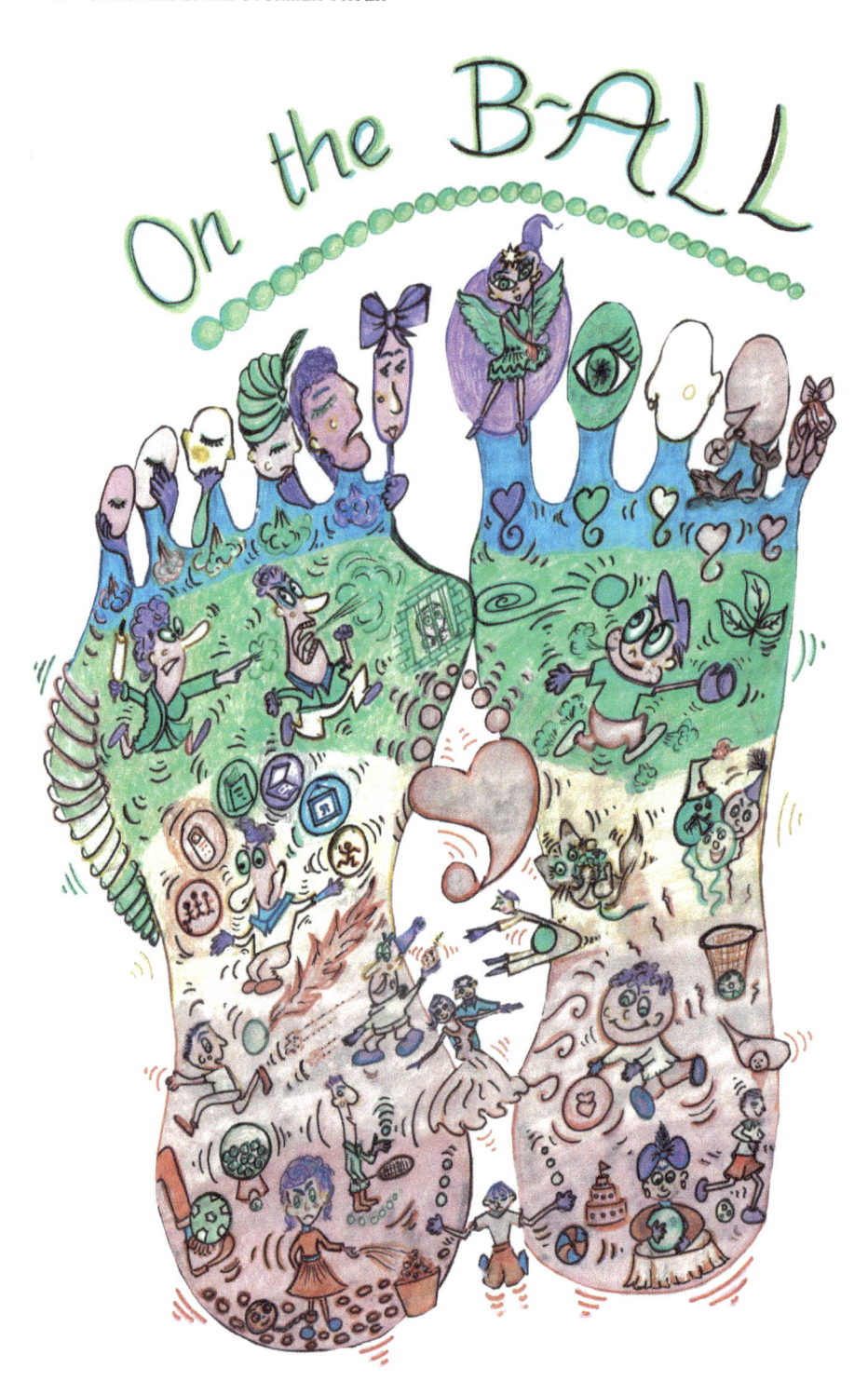

ON THE BALL

When the unexpected happens and life 'throws a curveball', staying on the 'balls of the feet' keeps the body alert and in control. Used to bearing the body's weight, the balls of the feet rely on self-sustenance from inner core strength.

Setting goals provides a sense of purpose and direction. Then, in a 'blink of an eye,' there is a 'turn of events', throwing everything into a quandary. The unexpected happens (like a worldwide lockdown), with all original expectations 'flying out the window'. 'Keeping an eye on the ball', adjusting, postponing, and setting up a whole new 'ball game' are winning ways for regaining and maintaining the balance.

Life is unpredictable at the best of times, so being 'stuck in the head' and 'digging the heels in' really are the worst possible scenarios. Adamantly defending notions 'set in cement' can lead to 'heads rolling' with non-compliance. A win-win situation is achieved by 'bouncing ideas' and filling the body with optimism and vigour.

'Th-e-oughts', once set in motion, trigger 'e-motions' to inflate and excite the Spirit. With the 'ball on a roll', it is easier to 'go full steam ahead' on the Soul's journey through life. Relying heavily on the treasure chest of 'e-motions', reflected onto the balls of the feet, the body is alert to heavy sentiments weighing everything down into the doldrums, knowing that happy, buoyant feelings soon bounce back to lighten the load.

Many vital and important body structures are reflected onto the balls of the feet. Major blood vessels convey an ample supply of sentiments to and from the heart to be adjusted and played with, inflatable lungs that tussle with disconcerting feelings 'kept close to the chest', and rounded breasts to provide comfort when 'pride is injured' or 'losing sight of the game'.

On the corresponding tops of the feet, the upper back reflexes reveal the amount of 'e-motional' backing and support available. When others 'don't play ball', unshed tears are concealed in noticeable mounds of puffiness. Meanwhile, the stress of 'being a sport' and reluctantly holding things together puts a strain on the upper back, with strained dorsal ligaments trying to provide additional backing.

An important endocrine reflex residing in the balls of the feet is the thymus gland. As the 'seat of the Soul,' it reveals the Spiritual essence that enlivens the body, making it feel good. Nearby, the solar plexus reflexes in the central hollows under both 'balls of the feet' reflects the abdominal brain. Sunburn on the corresponding tops of the feet draws attention to 'burning issues'.

With so many 'balls in the air' and a lot going on, there is a greater chance of a 'balls-up' bungling and messing things up. 'Not having the balls' and being too terrified or 'rolling up into a ball', even with all the 'balls at the feet', 'takes balls' to confidently and courageously 'start the ball rolling' again.

The knack is to 'stay on the ball' and maintain momentum while still 'playing ball' and cooperating, 'passing the ball' and sharing responsibilities when 'the ball is in one's court'. Everything rebounds back to self-esteem and self-worth, boosted by the breath, and shared with all the cells via the blood. Curveballs are inevitable, essential for keeping the body 'on its toes' and 'having a ball'.

It takes balls to participate in the human race!

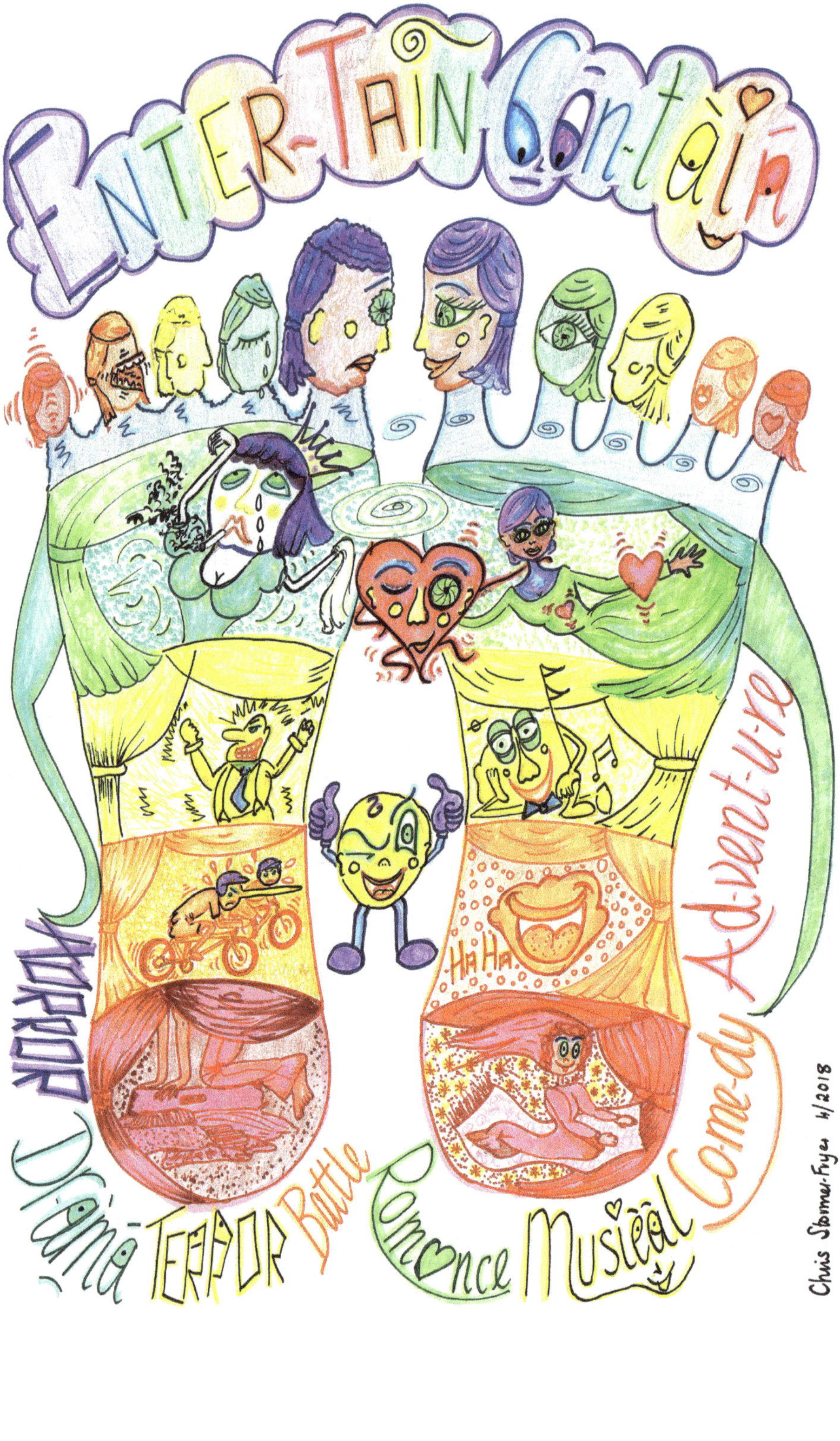
Enter-Tain Con-tain
Horror
Drama
Terror
Battle
Romance
Musical
Come-dy
Ad-vent-u-re
Ha Ha
Chris Stormer-Fryer 4/2018

ENTERTAIN – CONTAIN

'Entertain the thought'! Whatever thoughts the mind entertains captivates its audience, the bodily cells. Holding their attention and interest always engenders a reaction, be it pleasurable or deeply concerning. Every act performed externally is then enacted internally, and vice versa.

Taking a peek at the personal selection of favourite books, videos, CDs, movies and choices of television programs provides insight into what regularly regales the mind via the senses. Whether through choice, attitude or patterns of thought, drama is unconsciously attracted. No matter how disastrous, it can also be exciting and stimulating. However, once the thrill of the pandemonium has worn off, the Soul often becomes frustrated.

Everybody is continually playing out their own personal drama. Indulging in external 'horror' is one way to 'act out' the fear, dismay, revulsion, shock, disgust and dread that has been accommodated within for too long. Belief in being a victim of fate and decrying the Universe as responsible for malevolent chaotic circumstances is frequently viewed to be some form of punishment.

The conviction that a serene joyful life is boring often contributes to the addiction to drama. The subconscious mind's need to cause commotion generally stems from the mayhem and confusion caused by hurt feelings, the so-called 'baddies'. These troublemakers take great pleasure in terrorising the 'living daylights' out of the Soul. Scallywags constantly on the lookout for ways to 'put the fear of God' into gullible Souls.

The satisfaction derived from witnessing battles and war scenes compensates for not having to face internal struggles. The 'bloody outcome' helps lance deep sadness and extreme unhappiness from unresolved conflict, rivalry and feuding in the past. The rush of adrenaline can be thrilling and even exhilarating. The most difficult drama to make a dramatic exit from, however, is the family drama. The fear of being disinherited for not playing a key role in the family dynamic is terrifying.

A whole different scenario 'tickling the fancy' is romance. To love oneself is the beginning of a lifelong romance. It is often enticing to fall prey to the *idea* of romance rather than the actual experience of it. The conceptualising of true love is a multimillion-dollar industry, little of which leads to an authentic experience of love. Foot tapping, heart beating musicals also have a big role to play in setting the body's tone, with the brain's interpretation influenced by memories that range from soothing to irritating.

The entertainment industry has escalated enormously over the years, reaching a far wider audience, serving as an outlet for contained feelings that have been 'bottled up'. This is not a coincidence; it is a sub-conscious choice.

Bursting out laughing is the medicine of life. It is easy enough to laugh when feeling good, but it is when the world appears dim that laughter is needed the most. A good old belly laugh, coming from the core of every cell, permeates the whole before radiating outwards, making the adventure of life that much more epic. An adventure of the mind makes anything possible. The energy, enthusiasm, and interest generated through escapades engenders further interest and anticipation, and a yearning for more.

If all desires were fulfilled, there would be nothing to look forward to!

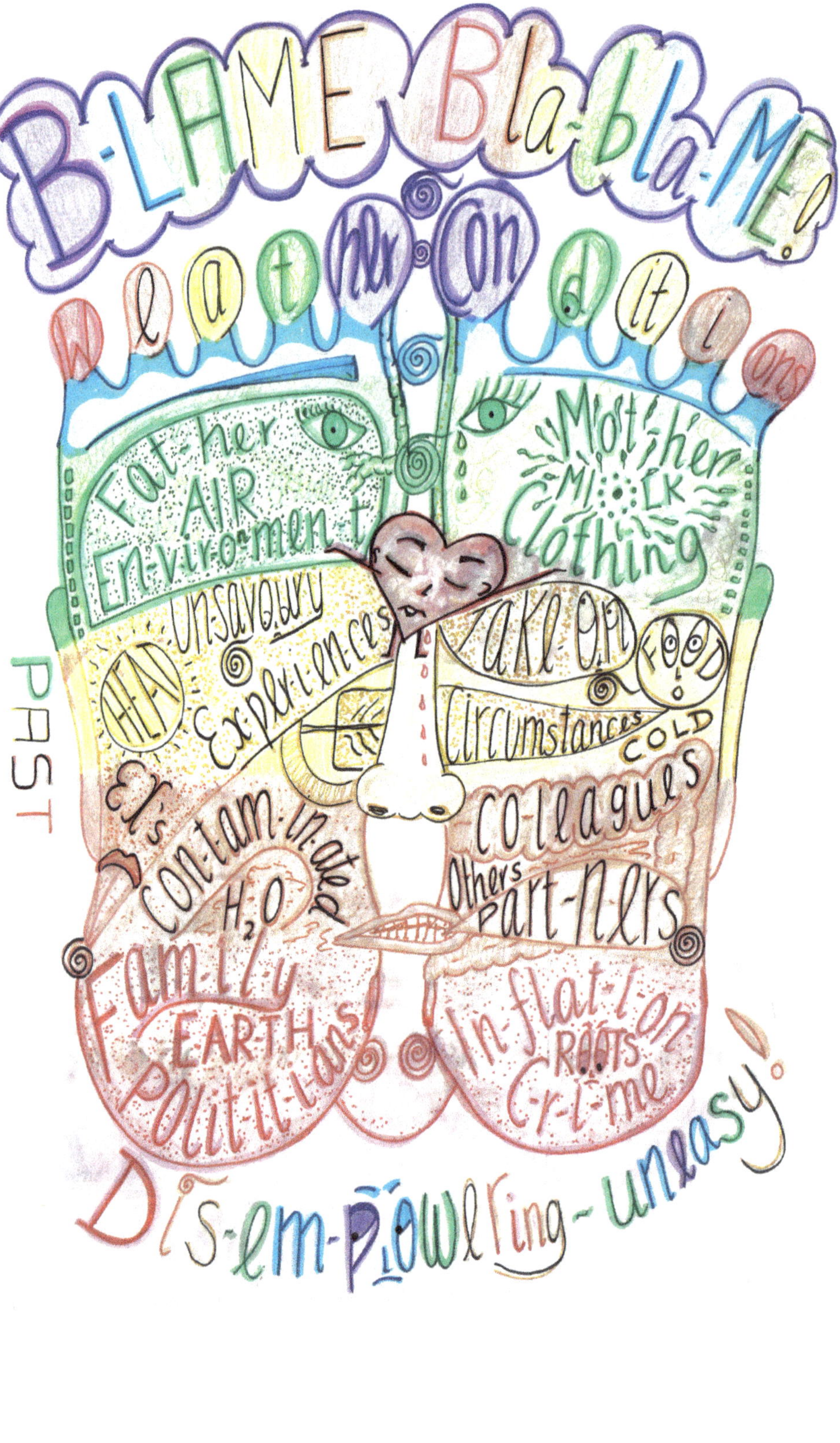
B-LAME Bla-bla-ME!
Fat-her
AIR
En-viro-n-men-t
Mot-her
MI LK
Clothing
Un-savoury
HEAT
Experi-en-ces
FOOD
Circumstances
COLD
PAST
Ex's
Con-tam-in-ated
H_2O
Co-lea-gues
Others
Part-ners
Family
EARTH
Polit-it-ians!
In-flat-i-on
ROOTS
Cr-i-me
Dis-em-power-ing-uneasy!

BLAME – SO DISEMPOWERING

Not taking responsibility becomes a nasty habit when it is easier and less traumatic to blame circumstances, rather than face the consequences. But to 'blame' is to 'be lame'. Popular targets 'taking the heat' are weather, food, drink, clothing, neighbours, colleagues and the government. Also held responsible for personal deficiencies are parents, partners, and loved ones.

Quick to blame others, the accuser is placed in a vulnerable position. With the solution beyond reach and in other's hands is to completely lose control. It is extremely disempowering, creating a lot of uneasiness within.

Not only does blaming complicate matters, but it makes it difficult to move ahead under such a burdensome feeling of guilt and shame. Fear and anxiety from being so vulnerable, and in such a disadvantageous situation, compromises the immune system's ability to defend the body. When it ends up attacking itself for being a failure, auto-immune uneasiness is a possible outcome.

Other people, circumstances and conditions are not to blame for personal situations. The physical world simply highlights deep personal issues already manifesting in the tissues. 'T-issues' reveal 'the issues' of too much or too little sensitivity, or too much or too little tolerance. What is being blamed, and why it is blamed, provides incredible insight.

When 'heavy weather' is seen to be the culprit, it soon becomes obvious who is making life 'heavy going'. Bitter winds 'go straight to the chest', bringing to the fore problems from holding embittered feelings 'close to the chest'. Any resentment, especially when engendered by sentiments regarding the father-figure, 'fills the air' and pollutes the atmosphere.

Complaints about the heat or the cold depend on one's temperament when dealing with unreliable situations that constantly change. Clothing is also a highly evocative subject. Decisions of what to wear are based on feelings, the energy of which becomes increasingly fabricated throughout the day.

Issues produced by milk immediately point to maternal matters. Realising these issues go back several generations is not to blame, but to understand the source of distress. Mammoth maternal memories are constantly diarised in the 'mammary glands'.

As for food causing digestive disorders, it all boils down to unsavoury circumstances around what is being 'stomached' and 'processed'. An intake perceived to be far from pleasant leaves the body 'cold'. Begrudgingly complaining about jobs or tasks around the house taking up too much time and energy is to admit that inherent problems are taking too long and require too much effort to 'work out'.

Blame attached to any form of fluid instantly draws attention to communications and relationship issues – such as prejudiced interactions within contaminated affiliations. 'Exes' invariably 'bear the brunt' with so much 'water under the bridge'. The repetitive cycle of self-destructive behaviour keeps the Soul imprisoned in the ego.

It is a crime to keep blaming others unjustly before sorting out one's own political situation of inflated dissatisfaction within. Family, being so familiar, provide lots of clues as to where the blame stems from. Trusting the Universe is to know that there are more than enough inner resources to find a solution for any situation as it arises. It is best just to deal with it.

Looking within means never having to go without!

96 - CHRISTINE LYNNE STORMER-FRYER

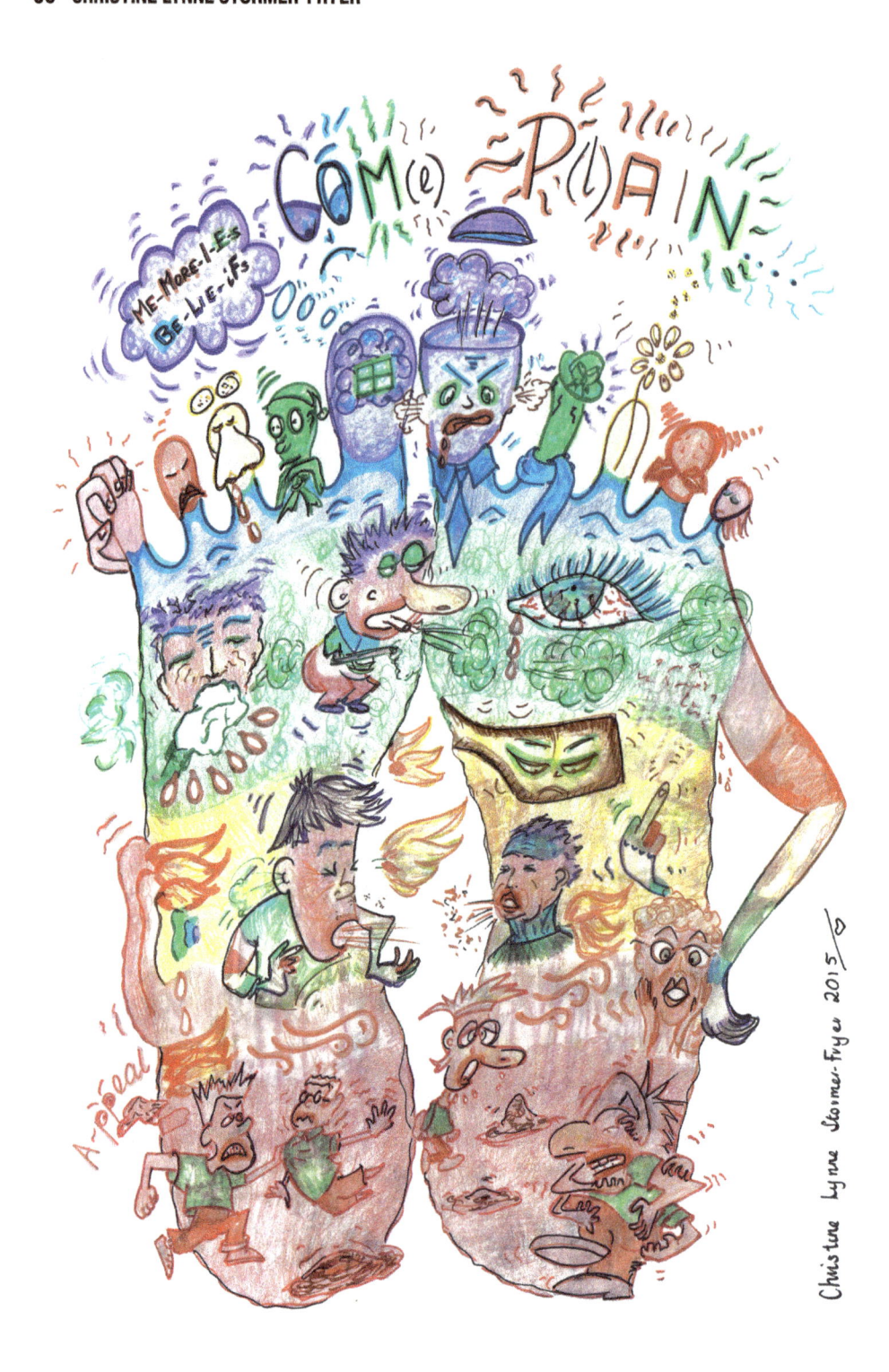

COMPLAIN – COME PAIN

Complain, complain, complain, 'come pain', 'come pain', 'come pain'! Complaining is an absolute pain not just for those in the vicinity but also for the body. There is no way it improves a situation. In fact, it makes it worse. 'Feeling sorry for oneself' does not help either. It just wastes a huge amount of energy.

Whatever is given out always returns. Magnetically drawn back to create reality. Lashing out with negativity only attracts more negativity. It is pointless and disempowering. The helplessness of believing that there is no choice and that nothing can be done only makes matters worse.

Finding problems every which way and complaining is indicative of life 'not working out' as expected. Extreme unhappiness creates so much inner turmoil, constantly 'rocking the boat'. Complaining does not offer a solution.

It constantly 'tears down' undesirable structures to make space for something new, but without creating 'something new', thus the process remains incomplete. The danger is that the remnants become a stagnant destructive force within, with one destroyed structure piling on top of another, placing unnecessary burdens on mind and body.

Focusing on others' perceived faults is not the solution either. Criticising others rarely changes them or their behaviour. This is only a possibility when shown by example.

Transforming complaining into something useful is a twofold process. Firstly, to use the critical eye to see what can be fixed. Then to fix it. Shifting the perspective and taking positive action channels a negative habit into a creative process. An energy that changes the world in a positive way.

> "Today before saying an unkind word - think of someone who can't speak.
> Before complaining about the taste of food - think of someone who has nothing to eat.
> Before complaining about your spouse - think of someone desperate for a companion.
> Today before complaining about life - think of someone taken too early to heaven.
> Before complaining about your children - think of someone who is barren.
> Before complaining about your dirty house - think of those living on the street.
> Before whinging how far you drive - think of someone who walks the same with their feet."

Anon

Yesterday was the deadline for all complaints!

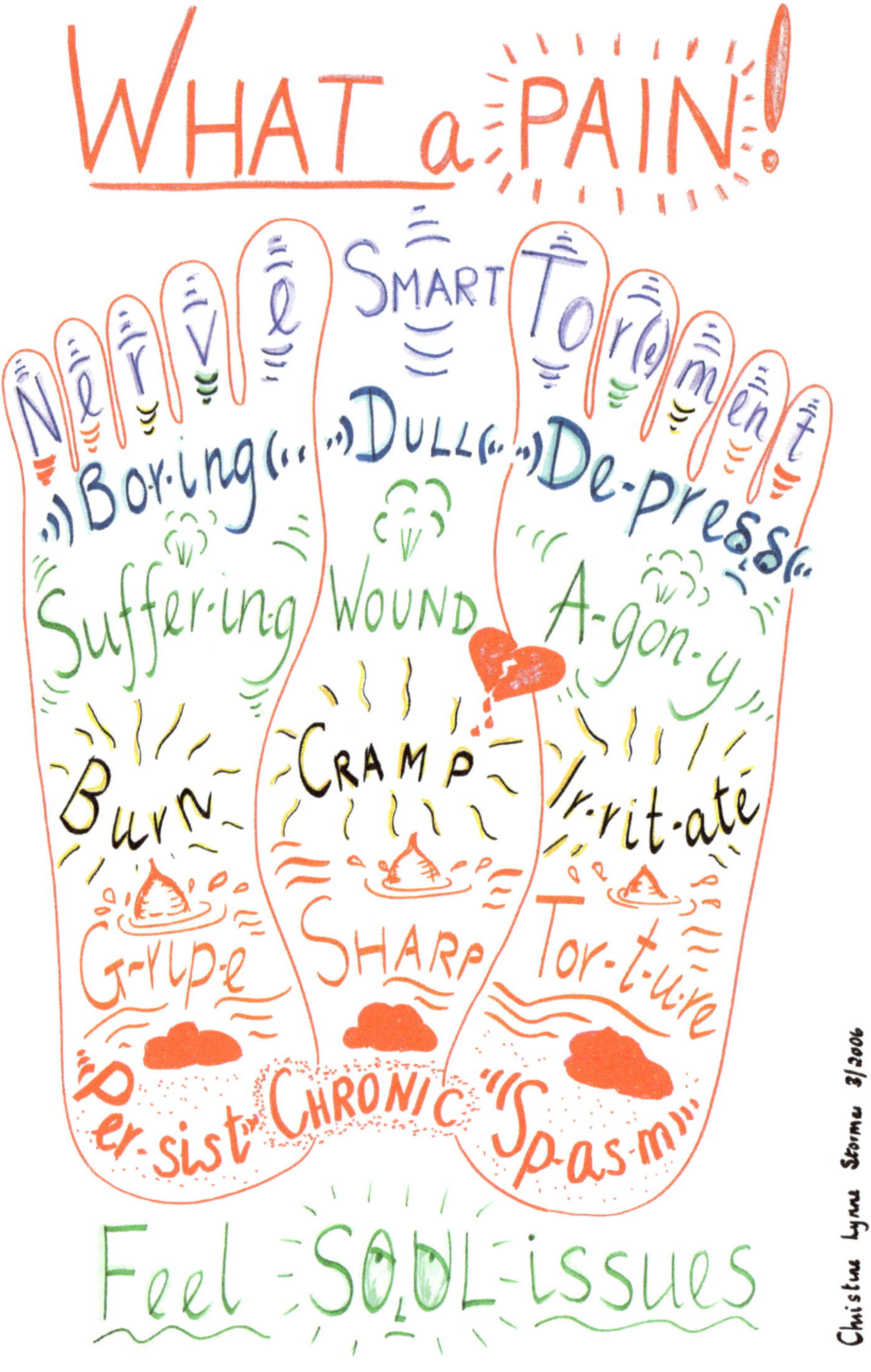
WHAT a PAIN!
Nerve
Smart
Torment
Bor·ing
Dull
De-press
Suffer·ing
Wound
A-gon-y
Burn
Cramp
Ir·rit-ate
G-rip-e
Sharp
Tor-t-u-re
Per-sist
Chronic
Sp-as-m
Feel SOUL issues
Christine Lynne Stormer 3/2006

WHAT A PAIN – FEEL SOUL ISSUES

Nothing outside the body causes pain. Judging and perceiving painful memories and beliefs as 'bad' evokes incredible discomfort. A disturbing feeling that unsettles mind and body pain stems from an underlying issue, with its roots residing in the base chakra.

'Pa-in' stems mainly from 'Pa's' circumstances and upbringing. Society's condemnation and stern disapproval of wimpish behaviour in males engendered the belief that 'big boys don't cry'. With no feasible outlet, all hurt sentiments are passed on for future generations to 'work out'. It takes a sensitive member of the family, usually 'fe-males', to pick up on the suffering and process 'Pa's energy', working it through the system until 'the issue' no longer affects the 't-issue'.

It is not dis-ease that brings pain but the uneasiness of the Soul. A dampened Spirit mercilessly disrupts life force energies in an effort to get attention. 'Smarting' pain 'gets on the nerves and 'comes to a head' when 'tormented', 'torn mentally' apart by impertinence, and disrespect for personal notions entertained in the traumatised mind. Feeling 'bored stiff' or 'depressed' and 'down in the dumps' brings on a 'dull' throbbing pain of dissatisfaction.

Physical pain is not the only kind of pain. 'E-motional pain' provides valuable insight into the psyche. Denial and fear – the pain of hating oneself – affects everything, consciously and unconsciously. Pain from an 'e-motional' 'wound' comes from preoccupation with the 'agony' and 'suffering' of past hurts, making it difficult to heal. The reality is that nobody and nothing can hurt unless given the power to do so'. It may be hurtful to know, but ultimately it is 'hurt feelings' that 'rub salt in the wound'.

'Cramping one's style' and being restricted or hampered has muscles contorted in torturous contractions. 'Burning' resentment may erupt and become inflamed with fury over what happened or did not happen. 'Irritated' beyond words at rash behaviour aggravates the annoyance of being inconvenienced. As issues surface, pressure is put onto the highly sensitive sensory nerve endings. The nerves, in turn, get infuriated by the intrusion of chemical mediators (other people inflaming the issue).

Having a 'gripe' and complaining about the 'sharpness' of the tongue can be torturous, inflicting deep anguish on the protesting intestines already 'tied up in knots' of anxiety. Constant 'persistence', harping on and on about the 'same old, same old', becomes a chronic problem to the bowels of the body. 'Spasms' from feeling 'spastic' and helpless make muscles 'contract' as energy is withdrawn in fear.

Yet pain is a 'blessing in disguise'. It creates an awareness that something is drastically wrong and that radical steps are required. A warning signal to the mind. Should it become an all-consuming matter with pain feeding the pain, the situation 'gets worse' instead of 'getting better'.

It is natural to want to resist pain. It takes courage to face the terror of stoking the fires of pain, but it is in times of crippling pain that true strength is born through greater understanding. In healing the pain and using it constructively, there is newfound faith, positivity, hope and opportunity.

When painful circumstances become intolerable, then change is the best remedy!

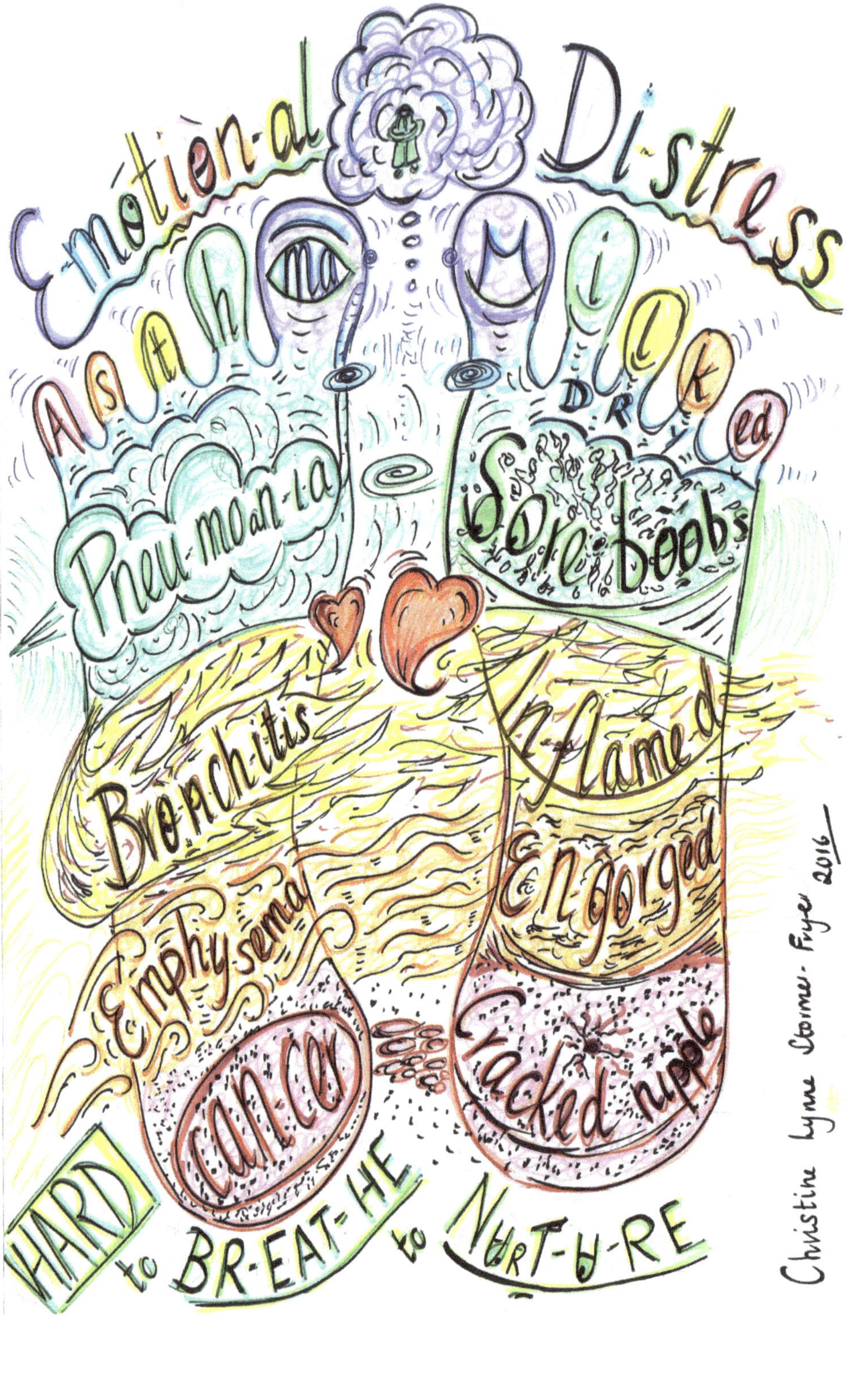
Emotion-al Distress
Asthma
Milked
DRY
Pneu-moan-ia
Sore boobs
Bronchitis
Inflamed
Engorged
Emphysema
cancer
Cracked nipple
HARD
to BR-EAT-HE
to NURT-U-RE
Christine Lynne Stormer-Fryer 2016

EMOTIONAL DISTRESS – HARD TO BREATHE

Feelings, pervasive in everyday life, can be extremely challenging, constantly affecting perceptions, reasoning and behaviour.

Happening everywhere and at any time, it is when 'e-motions' become overwhelming, extreme and harmful, that mind and body take umbrage. For instance, every body experiences anger as a release valve for pent-up feelings, but when uncontrolled, it can become a destructive and unpleasant force.

Undergoing intense 'e-motions' and overpowering 'e-motional' responses, without knowing why, makes it difficult to know how to soothe the distressed mind and anguished heart. With overly inflated egos building up impure 'e-motions' inside, each exhaled breath gradually pollutes and contaminates the atmosphere, making it increasingly difficult to breathe.

Holding back 'e-motions' is of no help. An overwhelming flood of feelings takes over, coursing through the body and becoming all-consuming and incapacitating. Whatever is resisted persists. Whatever is released is the catalyst for a much larger, much-needed catharsis.

Lungs are affected by distressed 'e-motions' involving men. If the right lung, it is more likely interference from the older generation. If the left lung, it points to an issue with the younger generation. 'As-th-ma' draws attention to being 'e-motionally' smothered 'as the ma', compounded by breath-taking resentment at being 'antagonised'. The distress caused makes it hard to take in air.

'Pneu-mon-ia' inflicts the body when having 'nothing new to moan about'. The chest has become used to being deflated. Having happened many times before, this time 'that is it'. Not 'able to take any more', self-flagellating lungs lose the desire to carry on and often 'call it quits'.

Otherwise, if the fury and rage of what went on without personal permission or approval are too much to contain, it can set light to the fires of discontent in the form of 'bronchitis'. 'Passing the buck' has proven, once again, not to be the solution.

'Emphasising' the distress and trying to fill the 'emptiness' within is 'emphysema'. 'Drowning in sorrow', the 'emphasis' is once again on 'ma'. The mounting discontent can grow out of proportion and become malignant and spiteful, or benign and benevolent, forming unhappy growths known as 'cancer'.

On the other side are female-related issues, frequently involving breast complications. 'Sore boobs' carry the hurt of all the 'boo-boos' after being downtrodden and belittled. Often swelling with indignation, the pain of not being noticed and 'taken for granted' can be overwhelming.

Feeling 'milked', exploited and taken advantage of, breasts get infuriation and inflamed. The tendency is then to 'take on too much' and become 'engorged' when trying to overcompensate. Nipples 'crack' when pulled apart and divided, not knowing which baby to nurture, the 'big baby' feeling neglected or the 'newborn' hogging all the attention.

It is essential to acknowledge, understand and release pent-up 'e-motions' for a smoother, less complicated ride.

Give a voice to feelings to rediscover 'e-motional' equilibrium!

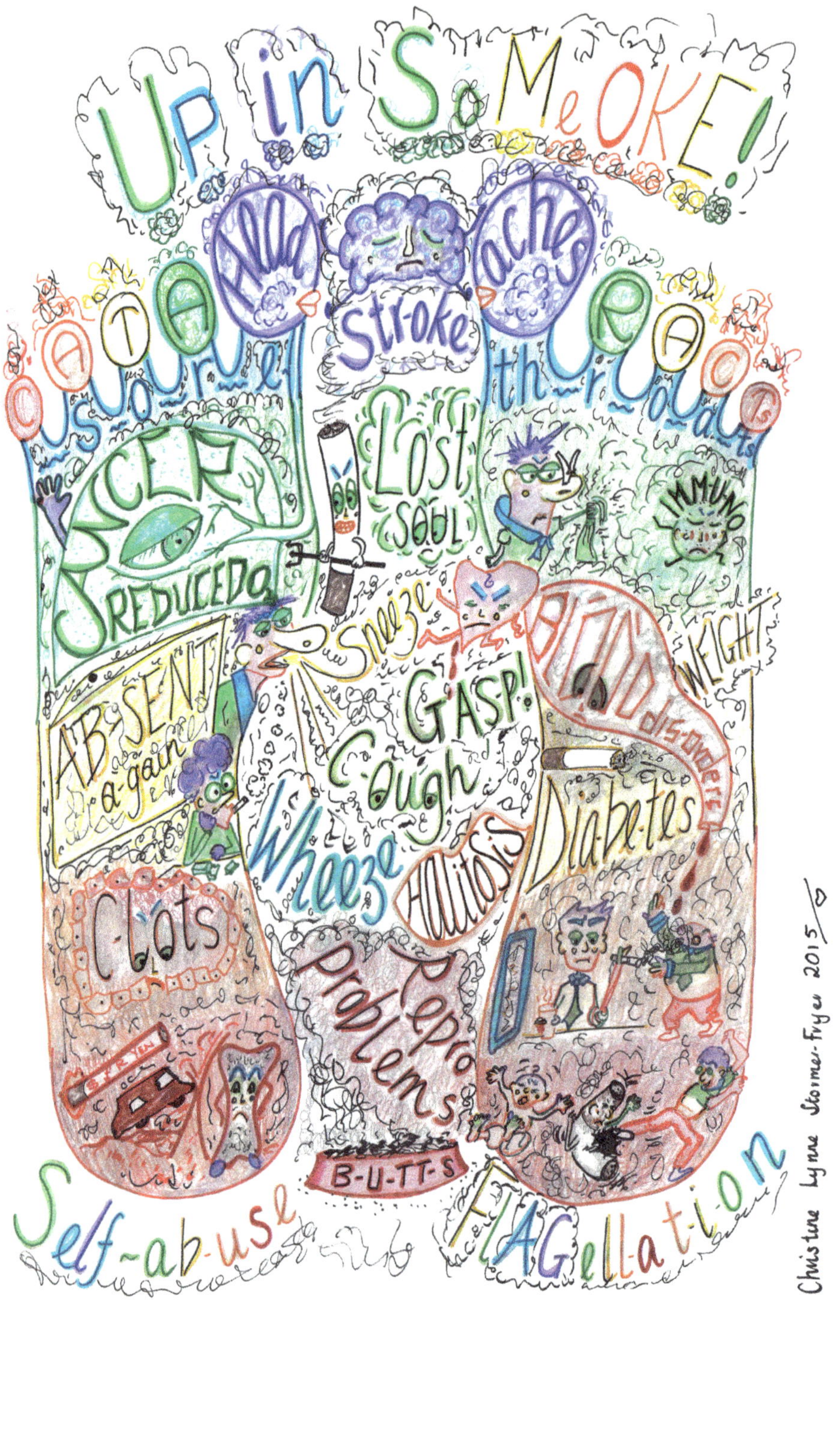
Up in SMOKE!
Head aches
Str-oke
Lost soul
REDUCED
AB-SENT a-gain
Sneeze
GASP!
C-ough
Wheeze
Halitosis
Dia-be-tes
dis-orders
WEIGHT
IMMUNO
C-Lots
Repro problems
B-U-TT-S
Self-ab-use
FLAGell-at-i-on
Christine Lynne Stormer-Fryer 2015

UP IN SMOKE – SELF ABUSE

A practice that dates back to 5000BC, smoking is part of tribal rituals in several cultures. Altering the state of consciousness, shamans often use it for Spiritual enlightenment. By going into a deep trance, it is possible 'to go out of the mind' and be transported to other realms of awareness.

Perceptions of smoking range from 'holy and sophisticated' to 'sinful and vulgar'. Although now generally viewed in a negative light, 'smoking' in itself is not harmful. It is the motive behind all the puffing that is ultimately the lethal weapon, either to appear cool, unruffled and sexy when lacking self-confidence, or to prevent the inner grappling of hectic 'e-motions' 'gaining the upper hand'.

Ideal for ultra-sensitive Souls, cigarettes and cigars form the perfect smokescreen. Clouds of smoke successfully conceal deep-set feelings and intimate 'e-motions', while de-sensitising related thoughts.

Creating an illusional air of mysticism is invariably bewildering to others intentionally kept at a distance. The pseudo front of confidence is perfect for concealing unaccepted personal inadequacies.

Smoke signals are sent out to deliberately mislead others, sending them way off track so that the truth never has to come out into the open. Terrified of losing a crutch and being exposed when giving up smoking, weight is piled on instead as a cover-up.

Cigars, synonymous with success, were, and still *are*, used as prizes and awards. The expression 'close, but no cigar' implies getting near but falling short of the goal towards the end. Enough to play on the psyche and consider taking up smoking.

In the 19th century, oblique complaints about items being overpriced resulted in the saying 'a good five-cent cigar' implying a 'sensibly priced item.'

Blaming cigars and cigarettes for chest disorders and lung cancer throws the scent 'way off track', distracting from seeing the real issue of why smoking was taken up in the first place.

Used to draw attention towards or away from the self, there is an 'air of pretence' with the authentic Soul concealed in copious amounts of smoke. Nicotine, a 'feel-good' chemical with the ability to mimic one of the brain's neurotransmitters, helps in fooling mind and body along with the outside world.

Exhaled 'e-motions' left unresolved and 'hanging in the air', cloaked in 'smoke and daggers', contaminate the atmosphere.

Moving beyond the 'smoke and mirrors' helps to clear the air with a glimpse of what is really going on, allowing the true essence of the Spirit within to be fully appreciated.

Truth and openness are valuable assets!

104 - CHRISTINE LYNNE STORMER-FRYER

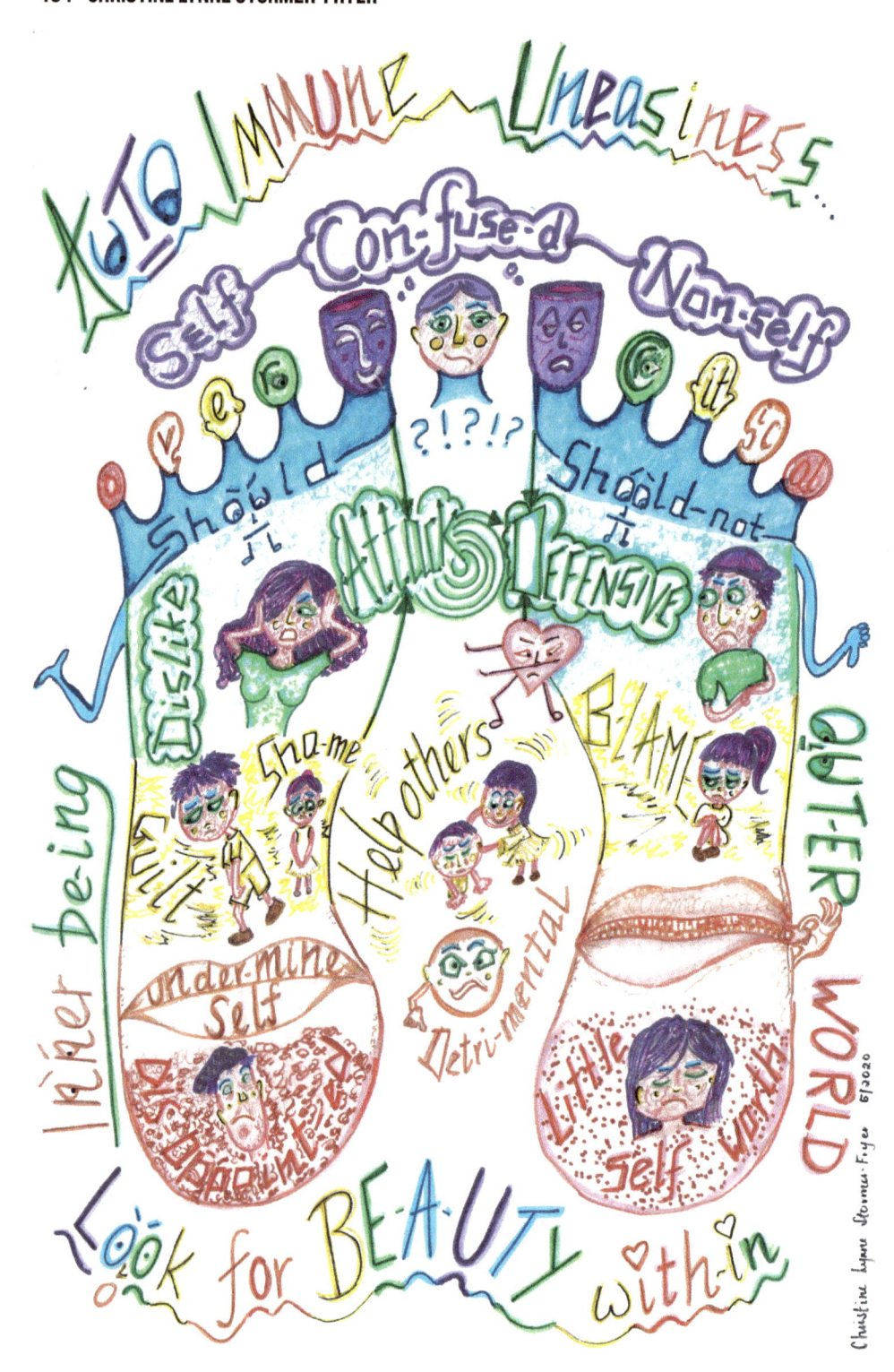

AUTOIMMUNE DIS-EASE – LOOK FOR BEAUTY WITHIN

There are no inherited 'dis-eases' only inherited *belief systems* handed from generation to generation that continually make mind and body uneasy. Triggered by intense noxious feelings 'filling the air', an unhealthy atmosphere at home is inevitable, with things gradually going from 'bad to worse'.

All eighty or so autoimmune 'dis-eases' have common ground, confusion between the 'self' and the 'non-self' causing 'e-motional' conflict between the 'inner being' and the 'outer world'.

Then come all the 'shoulds' and 'should nots', weighing heavily on the 'should-ers' and interfering with the lymphatic flow, often making it impossible to 'let go' of worn-out beliefs. Constant 'criticism', unspoken and spoken, fills mind and body with a sense of self-loathing and self-hatred, along with the belief that something is inherently wrong.

'Disliking' the self and longing to be somebody else, but not sure who, adds to the feeling of being valueless and worthless. With little or no regard for personal well-being, self-worth sinks further and further 'into the boots', even choosing to stay in a toxic relationship to prove a point.

At times of utter despair, the temptation is to resort to self-destructive behaviour. The mind, no longer impervious to being belittled, takes it all on board. Not knowing what else to do when feelings of not being 'good enough' take control, 'defensive' feelings 'attack' and destroy parts of the body.

Despite symptoms of unworthiness coming and going, the continual agitation and fanatical behaviour, compounded by impatience, frequently contribute to a low-grade fever. 'Tired' of the 'same old, same old', yet too dissatisfied, uneasy and melancholy to 'feel well' enough to do anything about it and to feel better about life, is constantly used as an excuse.

Aching muscles long to get along with each other without any unnecessary pressure or expectations. Joints take on the pain of inflexibility, preventing progress. Then there is the perceived imprudent and thoughtless behaviour among 'kin' 'getting under the s-kin' and flaring up in rashes.

All the 'guilt', 'shame' and 'blame' cannot be eliminated, even when compelled to 'reach out and help others'. It is impossible for the red blood cells to distribute joy and happiness in such a miserable, self-flagellating environment.

Adding to the 'doom and gloom,' the thyroid gland bemoans its fate at having no space for self-expression. Despite knowing how 'detrimental' resentment and constantly 'undermining the self' are, the thymus gland has no option but to keep attacking itself. Feeling so useless just increases overall vulnerability, with a life filled with ongoing disappointments.

So, what can be done? A change of mind with small steps taken to building a healthier and more appreciative relationship with oneself has the molecules 'jumping for joy', eager to assist in making things better.

Positive self-talk, along with small gestures such as giving oneself and others compliments. Smiling is the best tonic of all, along with heartfelt gratitude also to boost well-being throughout. Focusing on and acknowledging accomplishments make mind and body buoyant with pride. In time the brain translates this to 'I am beautiful'.

Be BEAUTIFUL ! BE-yoU- To the -FULL!

106 - CHRISTINE LYNNE STORMER-FRYER

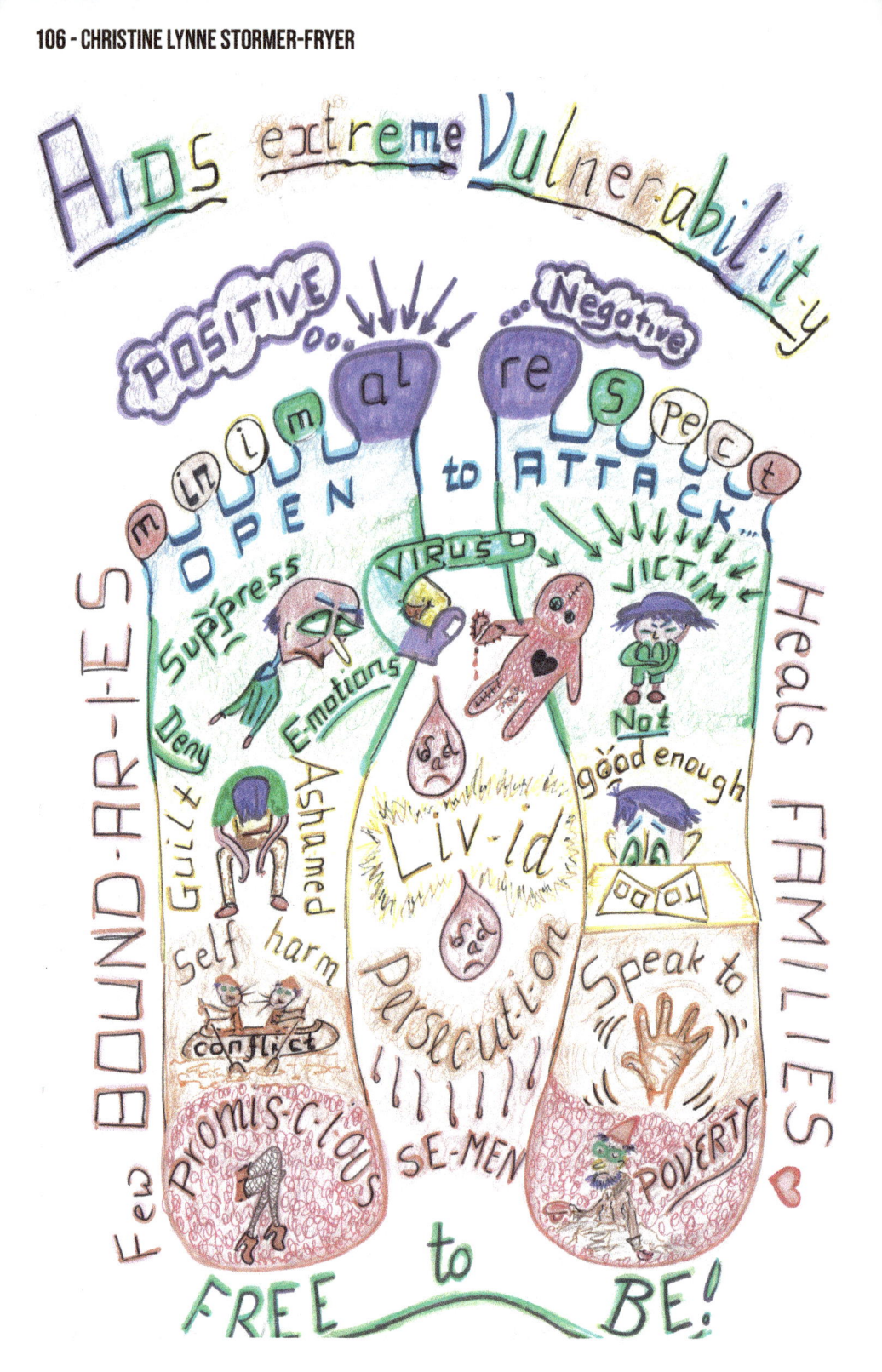

AIDS – EXTREME VULNERABILITY

'A void' that is 'avoided' is subconsciously filled with substitutes to comfort the Soul, but should the Soul remain dissatisfied with being fobbed off, it will still feel the lack. Aware of the Soul's uneasiness, the body uses symptoms to draw attention to what requires healing. As perceived deficiencies weaken the Soul, the body succumbs to becoming increasingly vulnerable. It needs all the 'aid' it can get to fully express itself creatively and free itself from the shackles of prejudice and suppression.

'Minimal respect' for oneself is an open invitation to the outer world to do the same. Showing compassion for the inner child and respecting the reasons for past incidents generates the respect the Soul deserves.

An overwhelming, all-consuming craving to be loved and accepted is at the root of so much uneasiness. Ironically, AIDS spreads through two love channels, blood (responsible for distributing love and joy throughout), and sexual juices. Issues arise when these roles become distorted or misconstrued.

'Suppressing' or 'denying' heartfelt feelings is to 'point a finger' at oneself for feeling 'hard-done-by' and an unworthy 'victim'. Overpowered by crushed 'e-motions' makes the Soul uneasy, opening it up to a viral attack from a perceived dreaded source to mirror what is happening internally.

'Guilty' and 'ashamed' at performing socially unacceptable acts makes the liver livid, often leading to 'self-harm'. Not feeling 'good enough' 'to do' something to change critical and judgemental minds only makes matters worse, giving the wrong impression.

Inner 'conflict' and 'paddling' in the opposite direction to others gets frustrating. Mad at being persecuted, with nobody taking the time to *really* listen, is enough to engender 'talk to the hand' gestures.

The more 'poverty' conscious the Soul, the more 'promiscuous' the body becomes in a vain attempt to prove self-worth. Liberal 'sex' is futile and meaningless, being devoid of true love and genuine acceptance. 'Sex' is a backdrop for acting out feelings of entrapment when personal creativity has stagnated. 'Sex' is possible with anybody, but 'love-making' is a sacred bonding with a 'loved one'.

In most same-sex orientated Souls, there is a missing piece, usually a biological parent. Either because of being physically absent, or mentally just not 'getting it'. On different wavelengths, estrangement confirms the belief of not being worthy enough to be loved.

The male/female imbalance, with an overpowering dominance of men, is stressed through AIDS. Resentment at being repressed takes on many forms, to the detriment of the offspring, particularly little boys forced to 'be a man' with comments such as "boys don't play with dolls". Being estranged from feminine qualities of intuition, nurturing, peace-making and pure love is confusing. The best way to equalise these energies is to honour these innate qualities.

Choosing same-sex intimate relationships is a way of balancing out the yin/yang elements, healing the female within every man, and the male in every woman. As the base chakra heals, the need for physical stimulation falls away to make space for more evolved Spiritual partnerships.

Love above all is a gift to oneself!

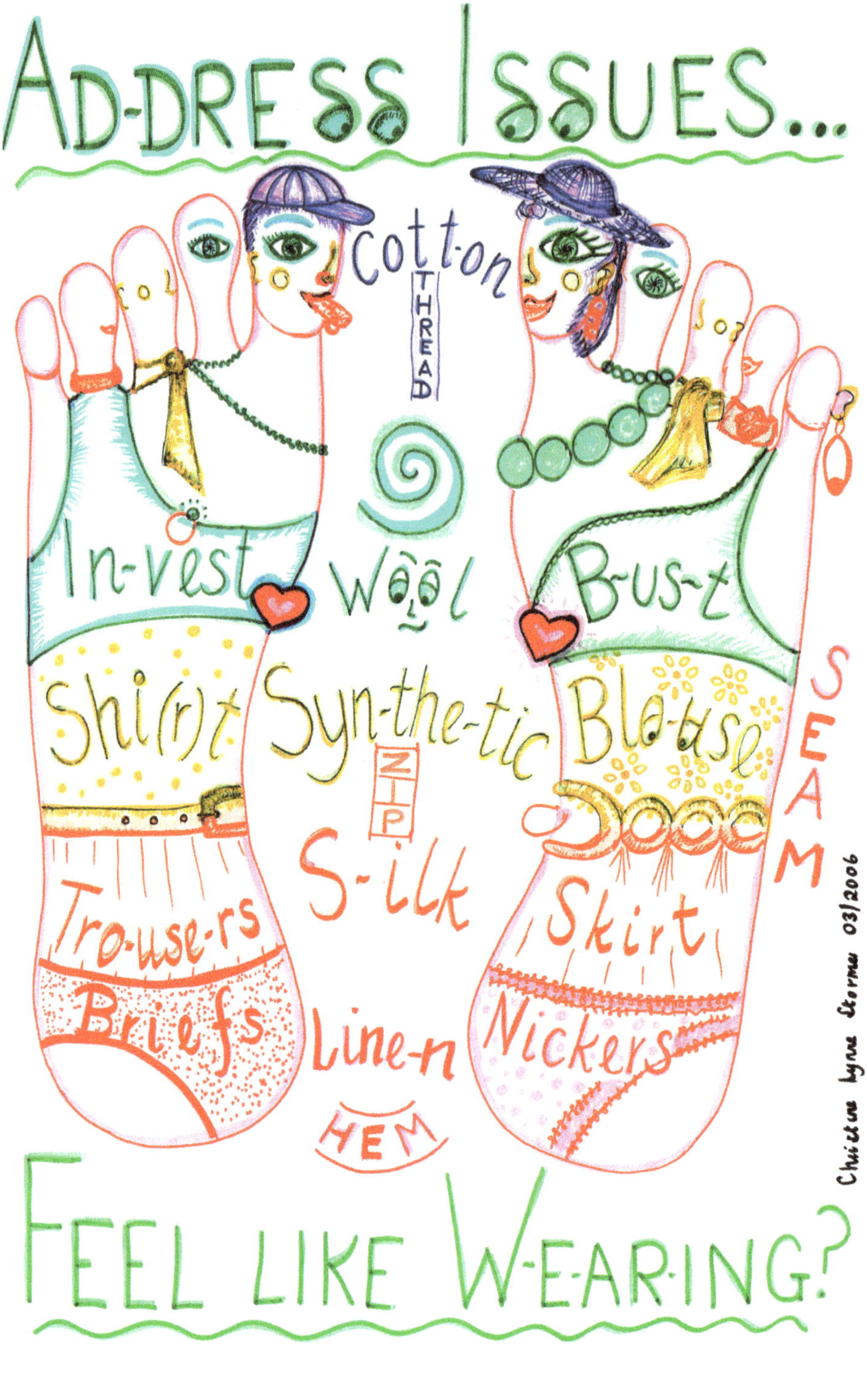
AD-DRESS ISSUES...
Cot-t-on
THREAD
In-vest
Wool
B-us-t
Shi(r)t
Syn-the-tic
Blo-use
ZIP
SEAM
S-ilk
Tro-use-rs
Skirt
Briefs
Line-n
Nickers
HEM
Christine Lynne Stormer 03/2006
FEEL LIKE W-E-AR-ING?

ADDRESS ISSUE – FEEL LIKE WEARING?

Prepared for all the 'cloaks and daggers' in life, the Soul has a clothed body, dressed ready for many an occasion. Frequently misled by 'ideas cloaked in words' or taken aback with 'clothes taken from the back', the 'backcloths' conceal what is really going on to engender a false sense of security. In contrast, 'a face clothed in smiles' is a welcome relief.

'Keeping it under the hat' (or a variety of 'headgear' these days) conceals what is 'on the mind'. 'Think it, but don't say it' being the motto prevents many innovative ideas from being addressed. 'Hanging onto clothing' in case it comes back into fashion is symbolic of old worn-out ideas hanging in the closet, taking up useful space. A cluttered mind 'clothed' with useless notions has great difficulty in 'cottoning on', especially when only a 'thread of truth' is accessible. Further strangling any semblance of authenticity is tying a noose around the neck with a tie, representing commitment.

'Pulling the wool over the eyes', 'wrapped in cotton wool', or 'wrapped in self-importance', all make for an insignificant 'e-motional' package. A 'chest of drawers' jam-packed full of feelings kept 'out of sight' reveals the type of 'in-vest-ments' in self-worth. 'Going for bust' and being 'busted' before the 'cup runneth over' exposes unresolved maternal 'boo-boos' bursting to get attention and sympathy. The more flesh shown, the more the Soul reaches out for love and affection.

Closets stuffed with an unprecedented amount of clothing hold a mound of lofty secrets and 'e-motions' around inadequacy stored in the lungs, along with some long-forgotten 'skeletons in the closet'. 'Skirting the issue', many women now 'wear the trousers', taking over a bulk of male responsibilities to sort out the mess. Materialism puts artificial demands on life. Wearing 'synthetic' materials can rub some 'up the wrong way' when a lack of sincerity is detected. Having to 'conform' to a 'dress code' engenders a range of feelings, from 'pride' to 'frustration', especially when 'made out of whole cloth' and being entirely false or imaginary. 'Dressed to kill', 'dressed up to the nines', or 'dressed flamboyantly' to put on 'airs and graces', to stand out and be noticed, is so different from wearing set uniforms to be identified as belonging to a group.

Being 'shirty' and obnoxious makes it difficult 'to keep the shirt on' and stay calm, a far cry from 'taking the shirt off' to show respect, or at having something 'under the belt' to be proud of. Anything 'below the belt', be it an action or a comment submitted in an unscrupulous or cowardly way, is generally extremely hurtful and a good time to 'belt up' and be quiet. Instead of 'tightening the belt' to reduce expenditure and 'cutting the coat according to the cloth', it is so much better to 'hold the belt' and be a champion.

In short, wearing trousers, slacks, jeans or denims keeps the legs warm, while also 'going to great lengths' to conceal the ability to move 'a-head'. 'All mouth and no trousers', full of boastful, arrogant talk that cannot be delivered, is like 'trailing the coat' to deliberately pick a quarrel. Situations that need handling with 'silk gloves'.

'Falling apart at the seams' and 'torn apart' when 'all is not what it seems' externally, exposes areas that are 'in shreds' and require fixing. Darning holes in socks signifies gaps from being 'worn out' but not having the means to replace with something new. 'Linen' is the pits when it came to ironing out 'creases of concern'. Feeling 'hemmed-in', skirt lengths have been drastically reduced to expose the next 'leg of the journey'. Keeping it 'brief' 'knickers in a twist' tie the mind up in knots, underwear being the department that knows what is going on 'behind closed doors'.

The body is only fully dressed when it wears a smile.

110 - CHRISTINE LYNNE STORMER-FRYER

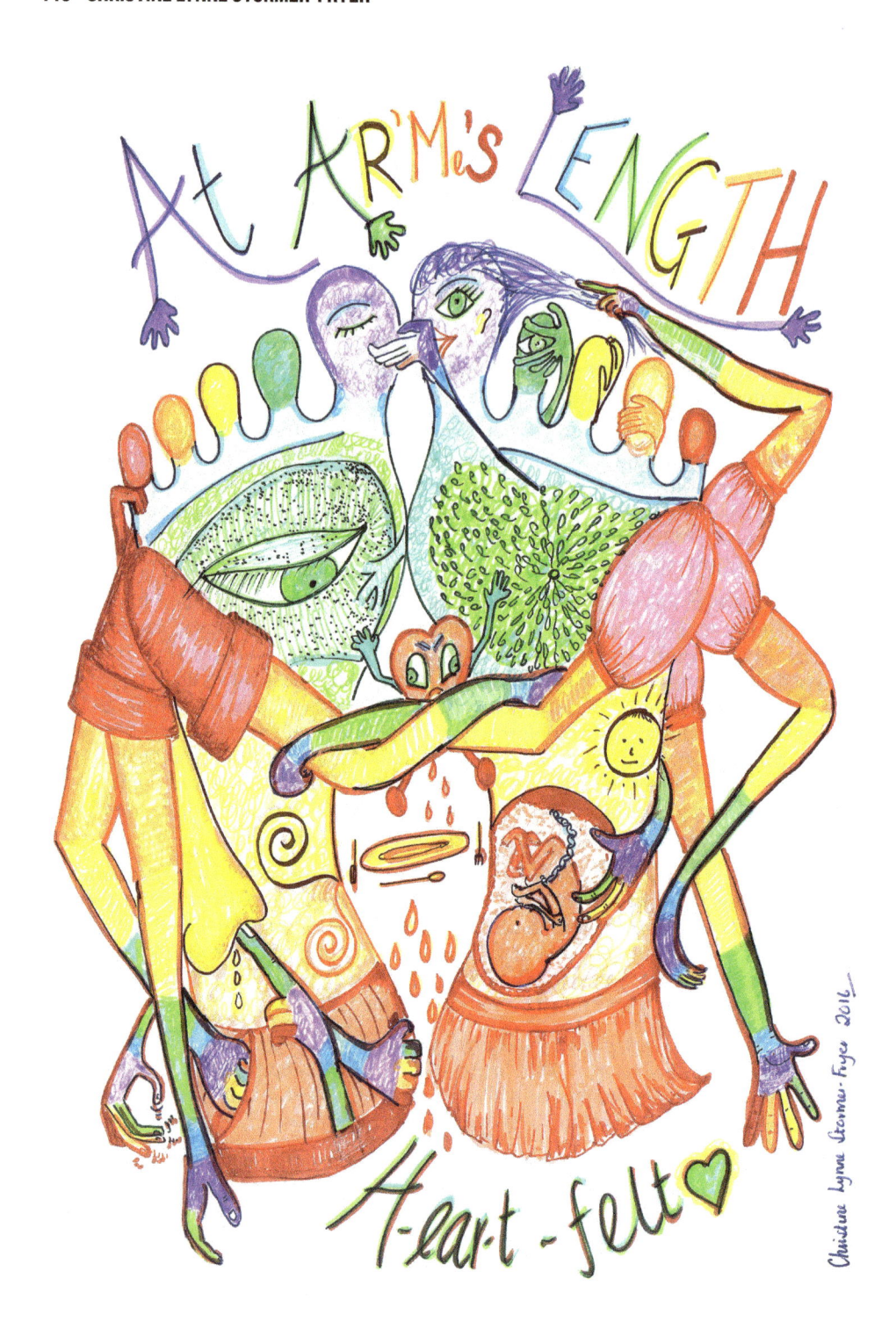

AT ARM'S LENGTH

Always on duty, arms convey and express the heart's energy, extending out into the world through hugging, touching, articulating and caressing. 'E-motionally' involved in all that happens, arms embrace life experiences, gathering and pulling love towards the heart, holding on to keep cherished ones 'close to the heart'.

Able to freely give and receive, arms remain extremely flexible, allowing creative energy to flow to the hands through a whole range of arm movements. Keeping arms in place are the upper arms. These tend to become 'flabby' when no longer able to embrace or hang onto loved ones who have moved out of reach.

Hands, as 'tools of creativity', have the wherewithal to manifest inner desires, longings and yearnings. Issues arise when there is conflict in the way situations are being handled, when 'the hands are tied', or when wishing to reach out and touch but too fearful of the consequences from feeling too insecure.

Handling 'e-motional' rejection is challenging. Constantly pushing away, keeping others at 'arm's length' to avoid familiarity, has a profound impact on both arms and the heart. The arms stiffen and become heavy, 'aching' to reach out but holding back instead.

Arms control everything within the personal space. 'Armed to the hilt', prepared to retaliate when 'up in arms', and feeling highly indignant or rebellious it is 'up to the arms' to defend the body, knowing how to lash out in self-defence ' attacking, denying, rejecting or repelling when required.

The 'long arm of the law' extends far and wide, even 'making a long arm' to prolong things unnecessarily. 'Pinned to the side or the ground' renders the body completely helpless. 'A shot in the arm' generally 'does the trick' to get things moving again.

'Chancing an arm' and taking a huge risk is better than 'giving the right arm' to satisfy selfish whims. Anything 'costing an arm and a leg', a saying stemming from the high price paid by servicemen suffering the amputation of an arm and a leg in battle, is ridiculously exorbitant.

Folded or crossed arms keep 'e-motions' close to the chest in an endeavour to protect the heart. Forming a barrier warning others to 'stay clear', 'keep a distance', or to state 'intimacy not wanted', effectively shuts others out 'e-motionally'.

'Twisting the arm' to persuade otherwise is easier when having 'a rubber arm' and effortlessly manipulated. Far better is to 'lay down arms', ceasing hostilities and surrendering. Meanwhile, many families are proud to have a 'coat of arms' to serve as a personal emblem.

Arms serve mind and body, day and night. The more open they are, the more life's wonders can be embraced, accepted and welcomed. Trusting in the many invisible arms that are there to support, no matter what, is to know that nobody walks alone. Everybody is all one.

Reaching out to dreams, arms manifest deep desires and passions!

112 - CHRISTINE LYNNE STORMER-FRYER

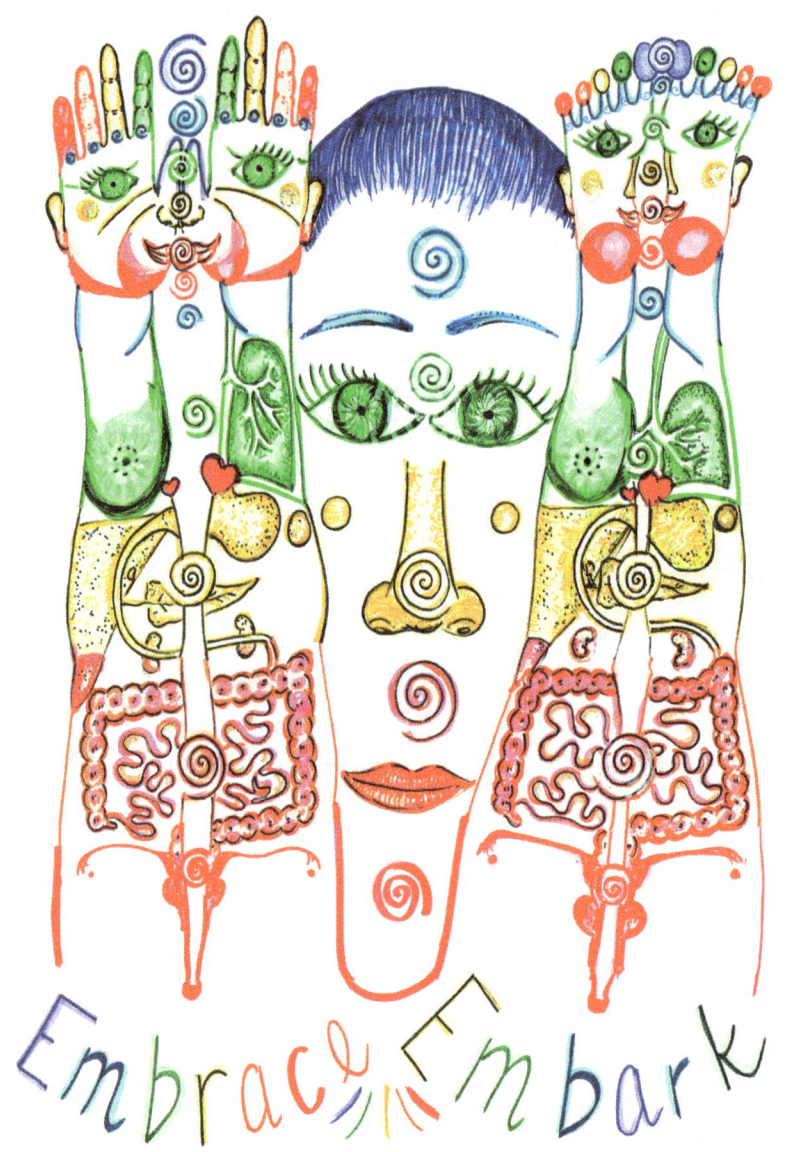

OUT ON A LIMB – EMBRACE / EMBARK

Human dexterity is relatively unique. Arms actively reach out to embrace the fullness of life, using a wide range of distances and angles for specialised hand movements to get a grip and finely manipulate 'th-e-oughts'. Assisted by the resourceful and powerful two-legged locomotion provided by the legs, the body has the strength to fend and stand up for itself.

As the body's vehicles, and with a remarkable agility to move through space, limbs are the ideal means to relate to the outer world. Supported by the shoulders, the forelimbs can lovingly embrace the true meaning of life. Meanwhile, the hind legs offer the pelvic girdle plenty of mobility to move ahead and attain personal goals.

Venturing forward is often complicated by a jumble of 'e-motions' left hanging carelessly in the air. Every step taken also means leaving something behind.

As the limbs extend outwards, they take it upon themselves to reflect the impact of every thought and 'e-motion'. The upper surfaces of the arms and the anterior parts of the legs reflect the back of the body, while the front of the body is mirrored onto the more tender interiors of both arms and behind the legs.

> Hands and feet, as extensions to the brain openly exhibit ideas before getting them out there. Wrists and ankles have an incredible amount of flexibility, just like the neck. The lower halves of both lower arms and either calf reveal the state of the ribcage and all its contents. The upper halves of both lower arms and either calf show what is going on in the upper part of the abdomen, occupied mainly by the upper digestive organs.

> The lower halves of both upper arms and thighs mirror the lower region of the abdomen filled, to a large extent, by intestines and the colon. The upper halves of both upper arms and thighs replicate the pelvis, with a mixture of some of the excretory and part of the reproductive systems.

The capacity to orchestrate these movements takes wisdom, knowledge and experiences to venture onto the next stage of the journey.

Yet, when deciding to take the next step, pride often gets in the way bringing to the fore concern about 'looking stupid', 'things not working out' or 'not the right thing to do.'

With life in constant, energetic motion, ongoing change is inevitable. Any transitional phase involves movement. An opportunity to move beyond dimensions of illusion into dimensions of awareness.

From each electron spinning around the nucleus of an atom, to planets spinning around suns in galaxies, life is in a perpetual state of movement and an ongoing process of creation. It is the work of individuals that is the spark moving every body forward. Each movement is significant, so it helps to make it worthwhile.

'Limb-er' up and be free!

The Gift of Love through the Feet

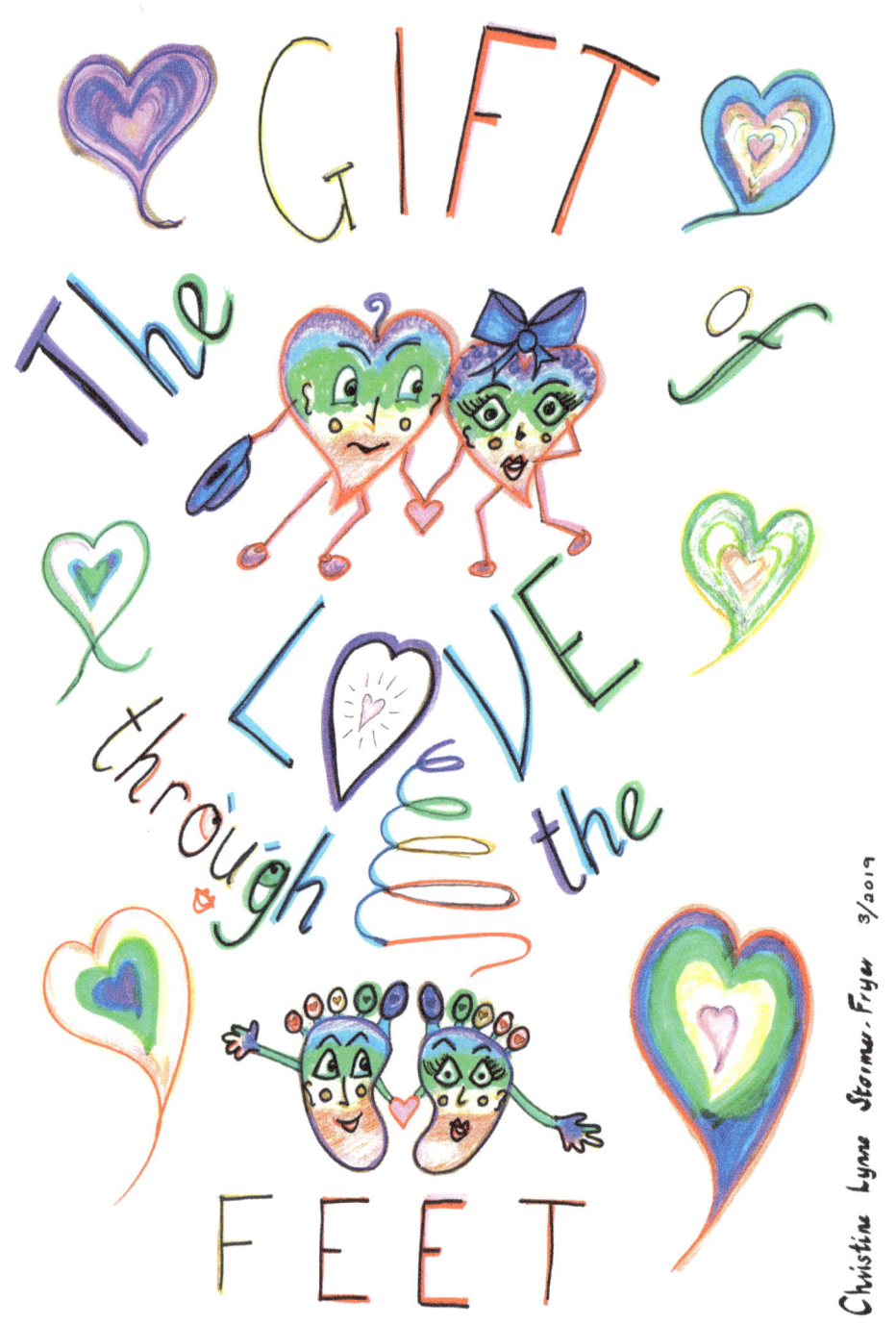

Christine Lynne Stormer-Fryer 3/2019

GIFT OF LOVE

No force is more potent than love. It is one of the greatest mysteries of life shared with every body through a web that brings everything together. A fabulous gift given to oneself and others.

Not just an 'e-motion', true love is a tool, a foundation of strength, a source of faith and trust, and a well of solutions when in doubt about the meaning of life. Love is a means of connecting the known with the unknown. Love is a Soul mate. A faithful and keen companion, smoothing the way in desperate times.

Without love, life is drab, meaningless and unfulfilling. Echoing with emptiness, being unloving and feeling unloved reinforces negative perceptions of self-worth. 'Dis-ease' from uneasiness within arises from a lack of self-love.

Love cannot hurt, it does not know how. It is the *lack* of love that breaks and aches the heart. Removing all negative, unloving thoughts, and banning destructive, critical inner voices allows the love of the Spirit within to shine through, even during times of hardship. Love hoarded dwindles, but when given away, it grows.

Vibrating with warmth and encouragement, love cures all ills. The most memorable and wonderful times, when life is lived to the full, stand out when infiltrated with pure love.

Learning to love is learning to live, the most important ingredient for success. Beginning with the self, only by experiencing self-love is it possible to know what love truly is.

The lessons of love are many. Yet every body deserves love, whether perceivably deserving of it or not. It symbolises the Soul's true nature, a creative energy that encourages the Soul and the world to evolve. It is an irresistible desire to be desired.

Pure love manifests as compassion, understanding, and utilisation of energy in a practical and responsible manner. A loving atmosphere at home is the foundation for life.

Love is far greater than can be imagined. It expects no rewards, knows no fear, makes no demands, and thinks no evil. It just *is*.

Love knows no fear. There is no motive. Divine love is always giving and never demanding. To love is to share and serve purely and unconditionally. Pure Divine love is attained when tapping into the Universal Source of Love.

Waves of love are currently transforming the planet, creating Fields of Possibility. Love makes the world go round. Acting as a glue, love keeps the world together.

The more it is given away, the more it multiplies, with so much more then becoming available.

All the love, happiness, security and stability ever wished for is within, and can never be taken away. A heart in love with beauty never grows old.

Believe in love at first sight!

Those who love are wise and believe in the impossible when knowing I am possible!

116 - CHRISTINE LYNNE STORMER-FRYER

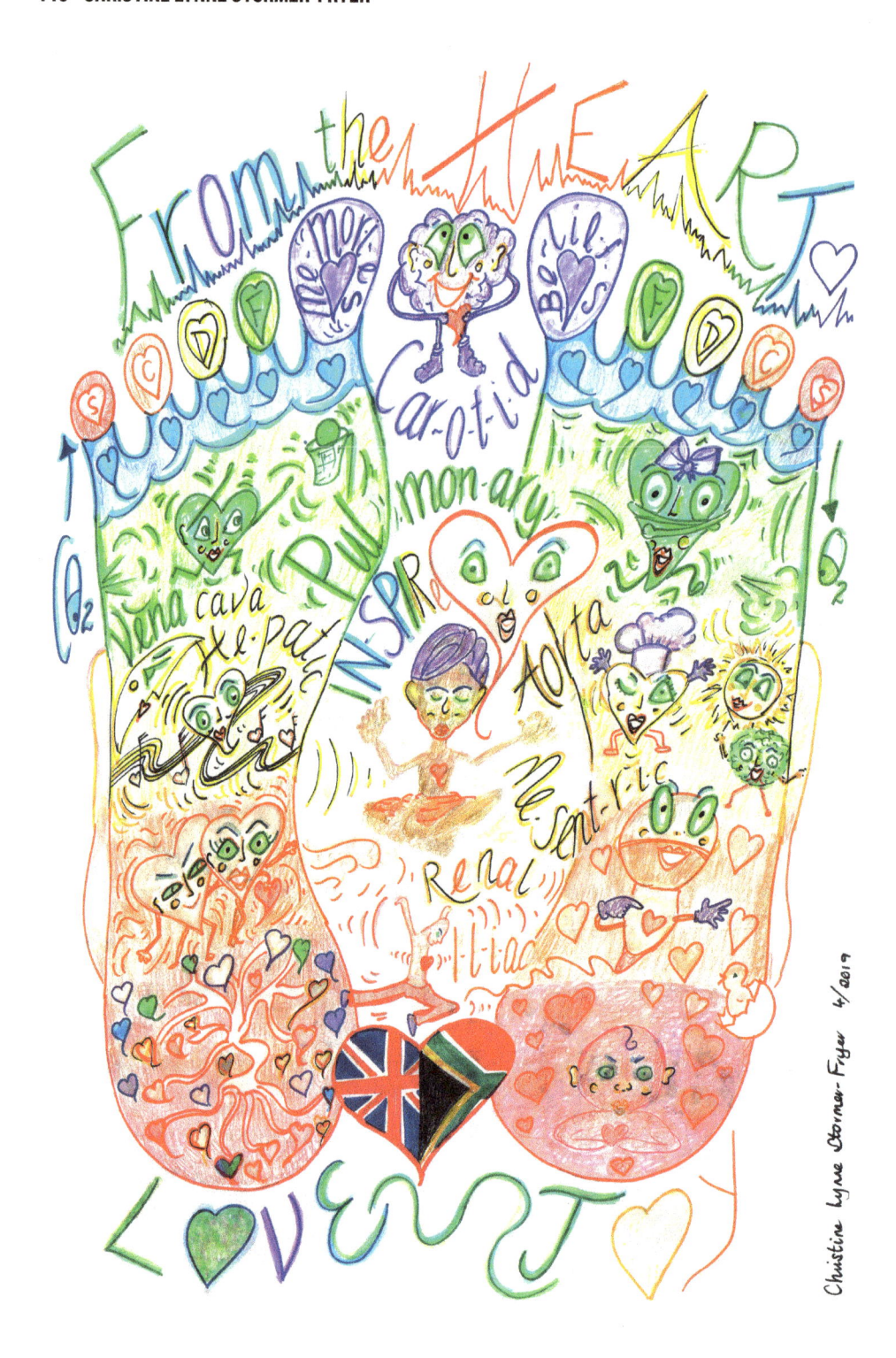

FROM THE HEART

Emanating from the heart, love tenderly fosters every miniscule atom throughout the body via the blood. To 'have a heart' every body 'needs a heart'. The heart is the 'guru', 'Gee-yoU-aRe-yoU' of the body, while the head processes information. It is a choice to either be 'the heart of the matter' or the 'head of the matter'.

Third world cultures tend to place more value in the head, listening and responding from the neck upwards. The remainder of the body has little or no say in the matter. This over-ruling masculine energy makes it difficult for the 'carotid' artery (the 'car' being man's pride and joy) to 'get through to the nut' and 'rid' itself of 'rotted' notions to replace them with a fresh supply of 'nu-trients' – 'new trends'.

It is up to the 'vena cava' to drain the brain of worked-through 'e-motions', but with so much obstinacy this becomes a mission. 'Caving' in under the strain is the *precaval* anterior 'vena cava', while at the other end of the spectrum, and 'getting a bum deal', is the *posterior* vena cava. It is a struggle to get things moving with little or no input from the 'powers that be' above.

The 'pulmonary' artery, 'pulled' by 'monetary' issues of self-worth, gets overwhelmed by all the moans and groans of not having enough. Sapped of energy and already feeling exhausted, it becomes an effort, and takes 'overtime', to expel the mass of noxious 'e-motions'. This puts huge stress on the heart, making it difficult for it to distribute the free flow of life force energy throughout. Any problem of the heart becomes a problem of the matter (and vice versa), with profound issues governed by a lust, victim, poverty or hate consciousness.

One of the most vulnerable organs in the body, the heart holds the most fear, along with a lot of old pain and repressed energy. Consequently, it carries plenty of wounds constantly conveyed to the liver via the hepatic artery, 'he pathetic' when 'he' lacks the courage and is too 'pathetic' to 'stand up' and 'be a man'. No judgement, just an observation. Within 'hepatitis' are many strains of suppressed anger flaring up and 'spreading like wildfire' when 'battling' and 'fighting' past injustices and demons.

With the brain masterfully imposing structure and order, the heart's wisdom is essential for survival. It is the only viable way to soften the logical grids of the brain and to perceive the interconnectedness underlying everything. The heart 'oughta' be proud of itself for using the 'aorta' to convey 'love' and 'joy' around the body, provided all the 'oughts', 'musts' and 'have tos' do not get in the way and slow down the process.

Conflict is inevitable when beliefs and modes of being contrast powerfully. It is a 'fat lot of good' to keep arguing 'adding fat to a fire'. 'Fatty substances', overstuffed constituents, keep scattering 'plaques' of commemoration all over certain walls. This first narrows, then 'blocks', the mesenteric intestinal artery, leaving little room to celebrate the true meaning of life. The renal artery and the common iliac artery then have to work exceptionally hard to make a worthwhile contribution.

Casting aside judgments and blame to embrace adversity with an open heart laden with compassion engenders mutual respect. As the heart becomes less covered with hurt, the more the Soul is able to dwell comfortably in its chambers and enjoy the sweetness of the present. The highest kind of living comes from the bottom of the heart. Loving thoughts filling the mind are then conveyed to the heart for the influence of love to be felt everywhere.

There is no exercise better for the heart than reaching down and lifting others up!

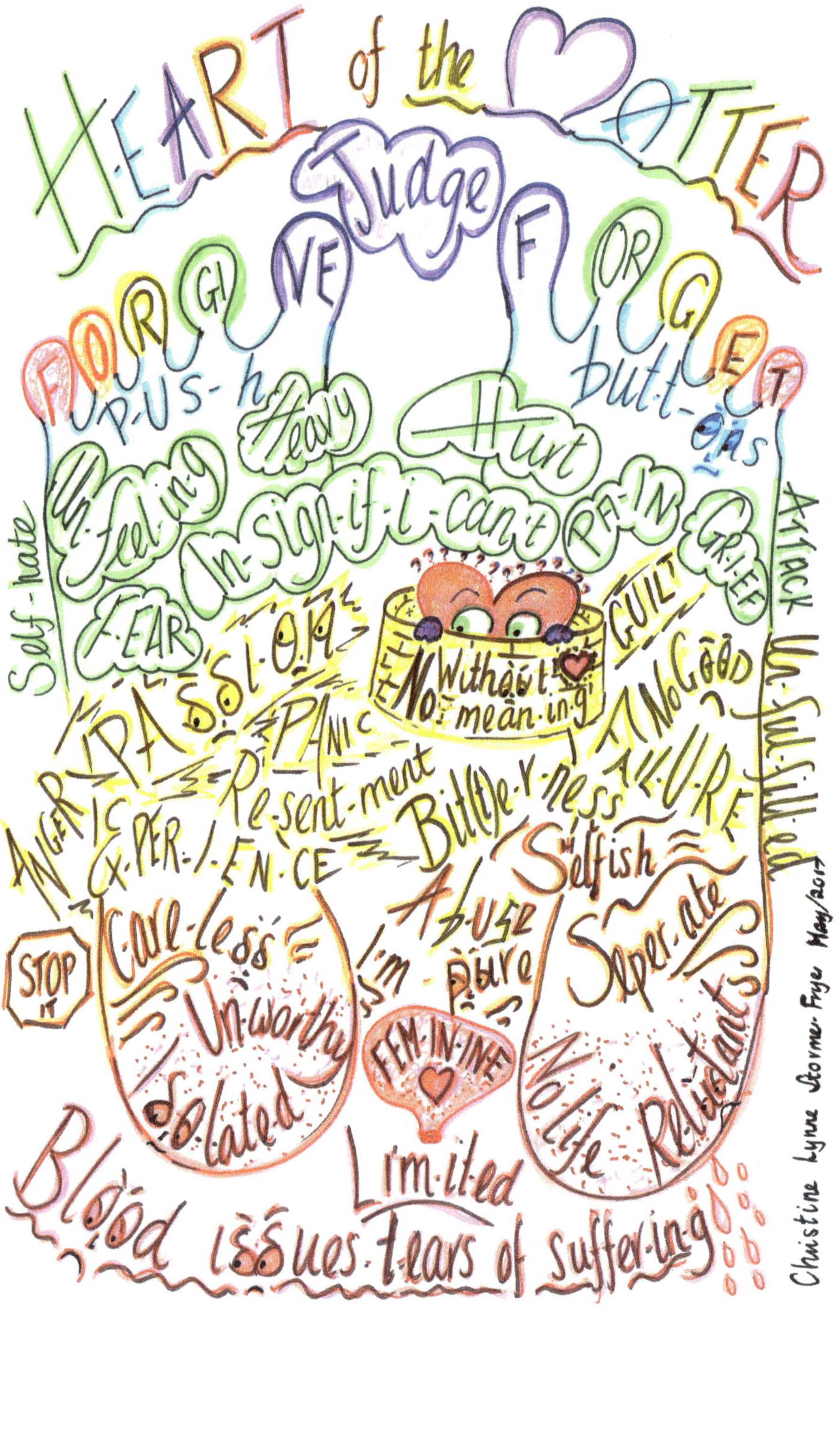
HEART of the MATTER
Judge
FORGIVE
FORGET
P-U-S-h
butt-ons
Heavy
Hurt
Un-feel-ing
In-sign-if-i-can't
PA-IN
GR-I-EF
Self-hate
ATTACK
F-EAR
PASSI-ON
GUILT
No
Without meaning
NoGood
Un-ful-fill-ed
PANIC
ANGER
Re-sent-ment
Bit(t)er-ness
EX-PER-I-EN-CE
Selfish
Abuse
Care-less
I'm pure
Seper-ate
STOP IT
Un-worthy
Isolated
FEM-IN-INE
No Life
Reluctant
Lim-it-ed
Blood issues
Tears of suffer-ing
Christine Lynne Stormer-Fryer May/2017

HEART OF THE MATTER

At the 'heart of the matter' is the very centre of life, with the 'heart of the matter' always being a 'matter of the heart'. Anything that 'matters' affects the 'matter' of the body. If 'it does not matter', there is no impact on the 'matter'. Choosing to live with an open heart is to live a life filled with love, happiness and healing, enhanced by wisdom every step of the way.

Telling a hard-hearted, 'judgmental' person to 'forgive and forget' is like 'bashing the head against a brick wall'. Instead, it may 'push buttons' of 'self-hatred' tender spots around 'insignificance', having been pushed once too many times already.

Having the 'heart in the right place' is be kind, considerate and well-meaning, but when life has 'little or no meaning', the heart has precious little or nothing to get excited about. 'Hurt', 'pain', 'grief' and 'fear' all contribute to a 'heavy' heart, agonising it with 'angina'. The more 'anger' directed towards the past and carried in the heart, the more difficult it is to be loving in the present.

A backlog of detrimental 'e-motions', with a build-up of 'resentment' and 'bitterness' at feeling a 'failure', 'panics' and 'attacks' the heart. Having to over-compensate through greed, together with an overwhelming desire for material possessions, places great pressure on the heart until it ends up striking out at itself for 'not being good enough'. Any outpourings of blood are tears of sadness from the heart.

Rather than 'eat the heart out', or brood or pine with grief or jealousy, or 'cry the heart out' with the 'heart in the mouth' ' or even allow the heart to slump into the 'boots', 'giving heart and Soul' to everything and doing the very best possible is massively heart-warming.

'Bridging the gap' between many worlds, Spiritual and physical, super-conscious and conscious, upper and lower worlds, the heart, as the 'e-motional brain', is the 'transformer' of the body. As the Spirit's mind, it loves refining feelings to make everything better.

A significant centre of intelligence, the heart is an extremely important endocrine gland, producing hormonal secretions that profoundly influence every operation in the limbic structure, as well as the hippocampal area where memory and learning take place.

Thinking with the heart is a delightful prospect, with its neurological tissue being an extremely powerful electromagnetic generator. Surrounding the body with an electromagnetic holographic field makes it possible to have ongoing 'e-motional' experiences of the world.

When heart and mind merge science and Spirit. This is where the truth of all that is becomes evident in the perfect alignment of all Souls. Similar resonances will, in time, ultimately merge to form a mass of heart consciousness.

'At heart' in the 'heart of hearts', it 'does the heart good' to have the 'heart in the right place' through kindness, thoughtfulness and good intentions, while keeping cherished ones 'close to the heart'. Doing everything with the utmost sincerity 'from the bottom of the heart', fulfilling the 'heart's desire', thrills every single molecule to their 'heart's delight'. Sentimental events have a knack of 'pulling at the heartstrings', while 'wearing the heart on the sleeve' is to openly display these loving feelings.

Walk into every day with a heart full of love!

120 - CHRISTINE LYNNE STORMER-FRYER

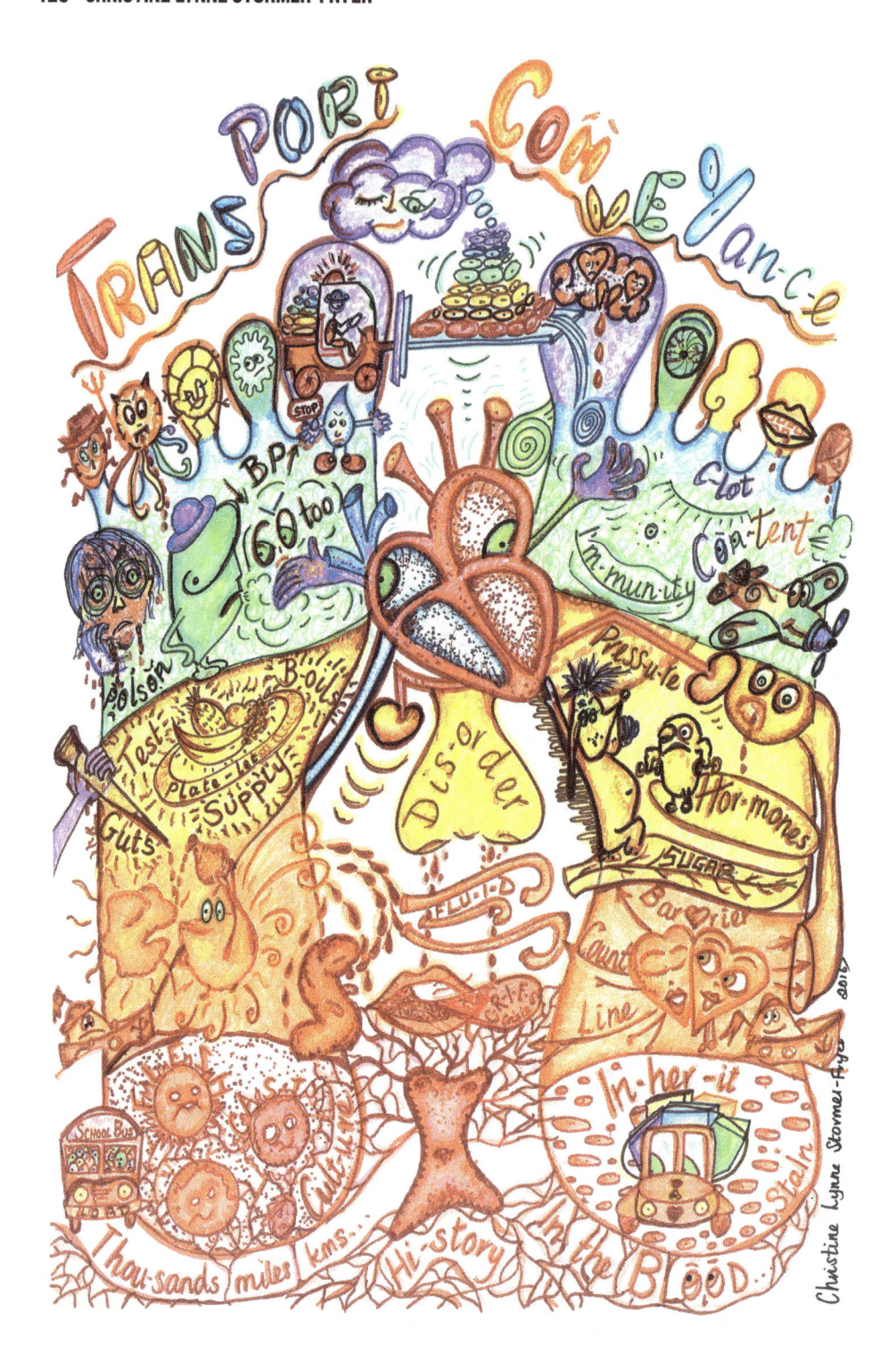

TRANSPORT – CONVEYANCE

Every body is an 'offshoot' of the 'go-to' One Universal Mind. As the seat of perception, the mind knows how to 'transport' the body into blissful Spiritual realms through meditation, a space where there is no past, present or future, no anger, sorrow or anxiety, just peace. A silent shuttle of thoughts, constantly weaving in and out of cells, shares a myriad of moods throughout, via the nerves.

Substances are consistently 'transported' into and out of the body, as well as between cells, to sustain life, either passively or actively, using 'hormones' or the electrochemical gradient. An attempt to be in complete control with no 'give' hardens and narrows the arteries. The strain raises the blood 'pressure' and slows the flow, increasing the chances of thrombosis when feeling a stupid 'clot'.

With the body making its own blood, its 'content' or discontent is greatly influenced by past, present and future Spiritual, both beneficial and detrimental. The energy of deep 'in-her-it'ed discontent is passed via the blood 'line' from generation to generation until the issue is resolved.

White blood cells (leukocytes) are extremely intolerant of any 'poisonous' 'e-motions' that are a threat to personal well-being, making sure that necessary additional reinforcements are rallied to get rid of the perpetrator.

Blood steadily transports life-giving components around the body to inflate self-esteem and provide 'immunity'. 'Making the blood boil' is aggression getting the 'upper hand', the indignation of constantly being 'put to the test' to see if there is any 'disorderly' behaviour raises the temperature.

'Slogging one's guts out' for little or no recognition is 'like getting thumped on the nose' and ending up with a 'blood nose'. Incessantly 'supplying' and circulating joy and happiness in a sceptical body insistent on entertaining worst-case scenarios puts a huge amount of 'pressure' on blood vessels. As their lumens narrow to force the reluctant blood through, the body becomes fraught with 'hypertension'.

Extreme sadness during childhood 'with little or no oomph left' has the opposite effect of 'hypotension', an unnaturally low blood 'pressure'. Attention is instantly drawn to any damage of 't-he issue' through haemorrhaging. Platelets (thrombocytes) rush to the rescue to stem the outpouring of unhappiness, before feeling a 'clot'.

Blood 'counts' on passion being injected into the body when getting on with the process of living life to the full. With no mental 'barriers' to prevent this process from taking place, the pleasure derived is extricated by the pancreas. Used to boost 'blood sugar' and spread ecstasy around the body, this delightful organ invariably 'lifts the Spirit'.

Originating in the 'b-one' blood loves to 'Be-ONE' of a kind. When the spleen insists on going all out to please everybody to the detriment of itself, the body, drained of enthusiasm, is left feeling flat and anaemic.

After 120 days of constantly serving day in day out and circuiting thousands of kilometres of blood vessels around the body, the red blood cells gracefully retire. The energy attained through a multitude of experiences is broken down and stored in the liver, later used to determine the characteristics of new blood. It also provides the passion to move onto the next stage.

A powerful vibration and healing force, love instigates and conveys magnificence!

122 - CHRISTINE LYNNE STORMER-FRYER

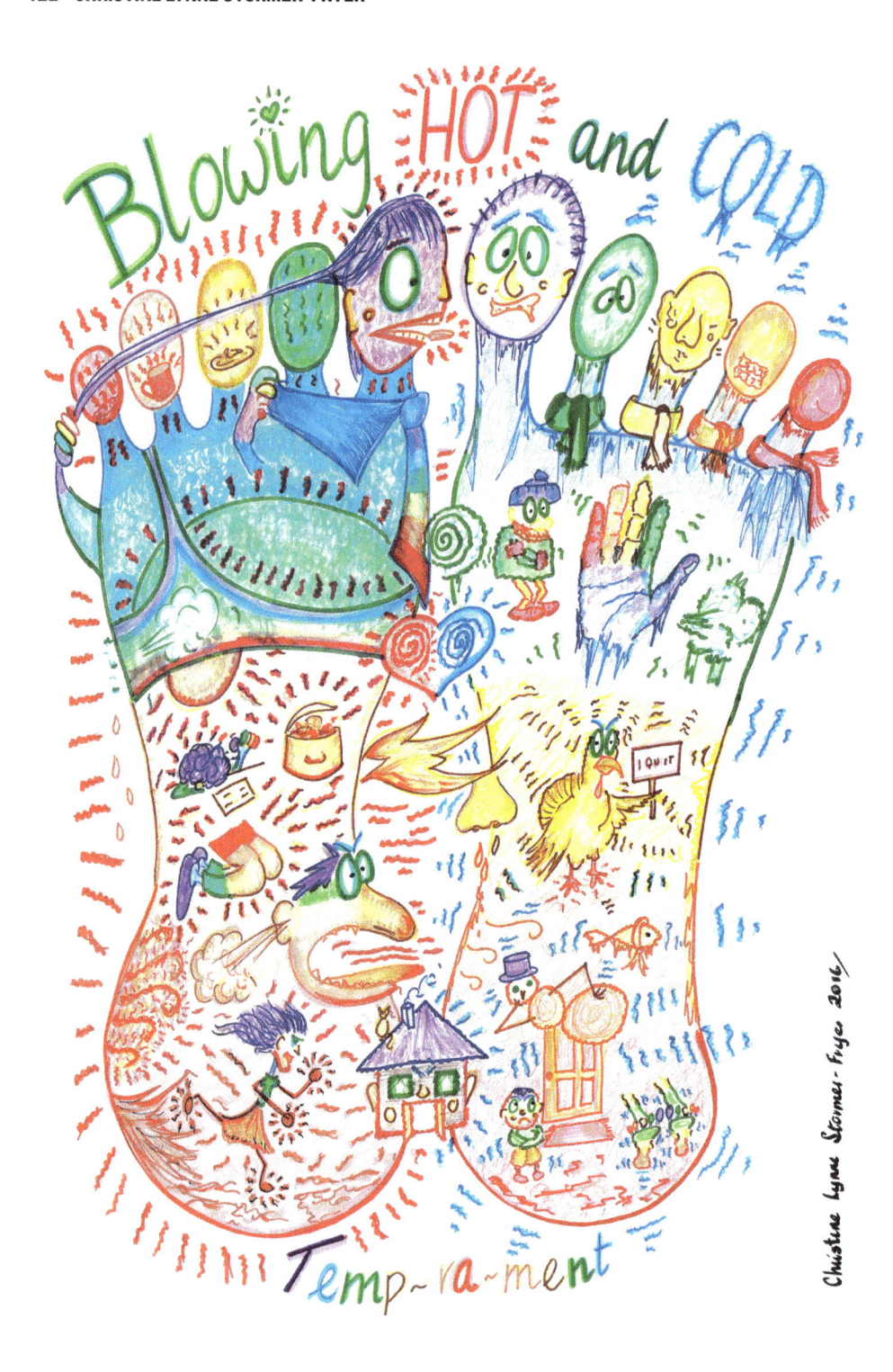

BLOWING HOT AND COLD

'Blowing hot and cold' is to be highly unpredictable, frustratingly inconsistent, and maddeningly irresolute.

Unable to 'make up the mind' is enough to make the body 'blow its top', lose its temper, and even 'blow up' and explode as the body breaks out into a 'cold sweat' of terror and fear.

As the mind 'toys with all options' and debates each matter, it is 'neither here nor there'. The environment gets uncomfortable with the blood rushing to the cheeks in utter embarrassment.

'Blowing off steam' and getting rid of superfluous annoyance, especially when 'full of hot air' one moment, then getting 'cold feet' the next, makes the body 'blow hot and cold' in frustration.

Hoping that flammable matters 'will soon blow over' after having been 'blown sky-high' with 'a good scolding' requires 'seeing which way the wind blows'.

'Give it to them hot', firmly chastising and reprimanding then going 'cold liver' and uncaring, makes 'going cold turkey' and 'quitting while ahead' a tempting option.

Previously hurt 'e-motionally', 'blowing hot and cold' becomes a defence mechanism. Excited one minute then too terrified to step out the next for fear of being miffed again or wishing to do something to make a situation better, but too terrified to do so.

Even when 'hot-blooded', passionate and ardent, it can be difficult to enthuse a 'cold-blooded' Soul, often making the 'blood curdle' instead.

Being 'hot stuff' and a 'hot favourite' is so exhilarating initially, even surreal, as if 'floating on a cloud' after a flurry of achievements. But when the excitement dies down, and the accolades diminish, a nagging doubt about the ability to achieve outstanding success again results in 'withdrawing into the cold'.

Too scared to do anything worthwhile while 'shivering in the boots', or simply too anxious and timid to get a move on, the heated embarrassment becomes awkward. Scenarios constantly played through the mind, going through the smallest, most insignificant details, and eventually opting out, has the head shaking in dismay.

'Blowing hot and cold', fluctuating between two extremes is confusing and downright exhausting. A 'cold front' moving in, bringing a 'cold snap' after warm weather, often brings on 'colds' and 'flu'. Temperatures rage and 'teeth-chatter' uncontrollably as the body rids itself of 'non-sense' for a personal transition and promotion to the next stage.

Difficult to second guess what happens next as burning issues could come to the fore, feet burn in frustration and discomfort. The 'burning question' under hot discussion is whether to 'burn the fingers' and suffer loss and misfortune, or get exhausted when begrudgingly 'burning the midnight oil'.

Or to 'burn with enthusiasm' and get on and do what the heart desires, and just 'go for it'.

Be a fundamentalist - ensure that the fun always comes before the mental on the list!

124 - CHRISTINE LYNNE STORMER-FRYER

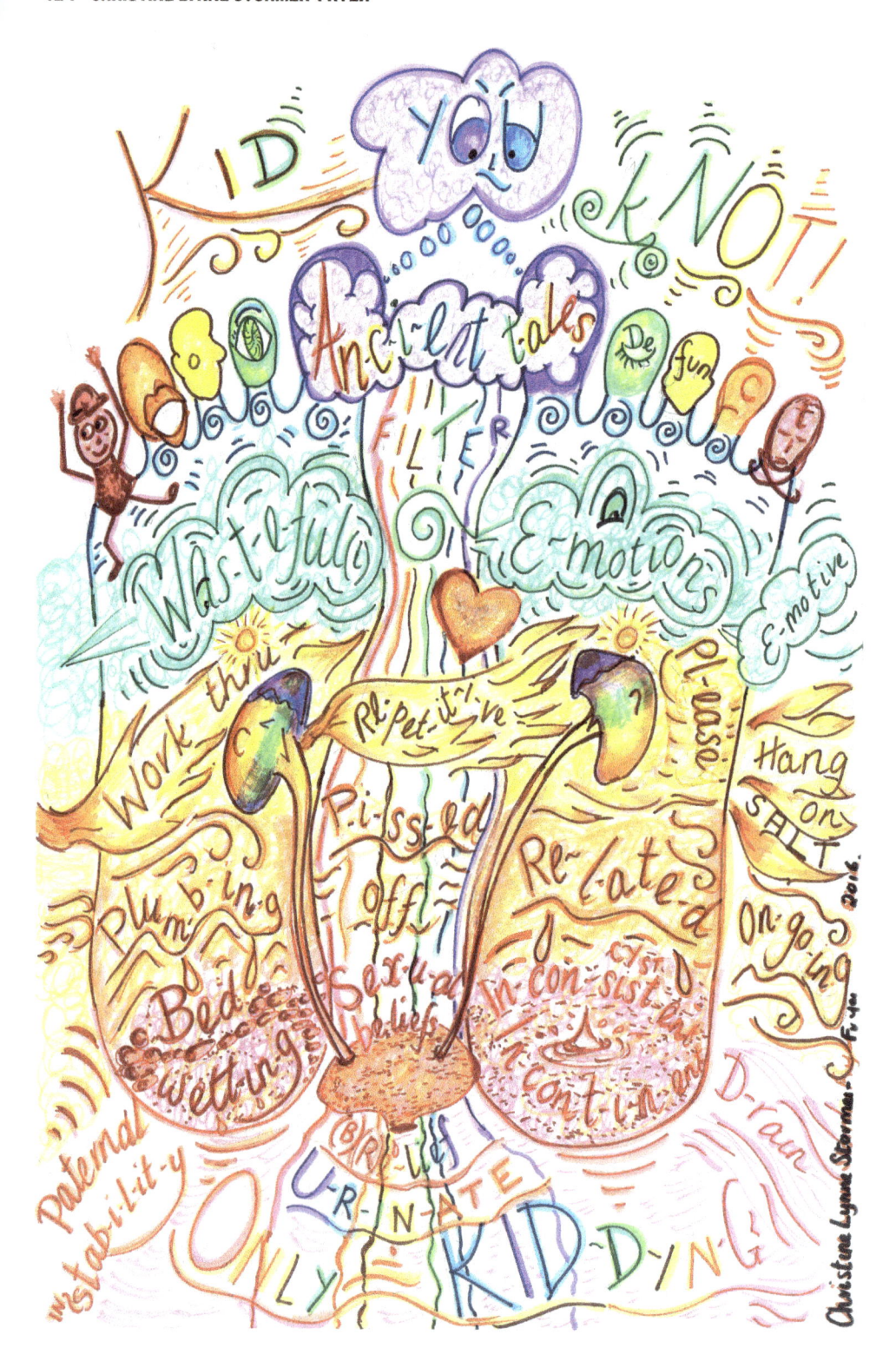

KID YOU KNOT

'Kid you not', the kidney's equilibrium is quickly unsettled when adults behave like 'kids'. 'Throwing tantrums' and 'stamping feet' when 'disappointed' or 'disillusioned' would have deserved a 'good hiding' in times gone by.

There is not much 'good' achieved from a 'good hiding' though. Relentlessly ribbed, cruelly teased, mercilessly mocked, remorselessly ridiculed, and persistently joked about, even when nonchalantly dismissed with an 'I was only kidding', is all too much for highly sensitive Souls. Exasperated by spiteful vindictiveness, the agitated kidneys 'twist and turn' writhing in agony. Tired of running the same wasteful 'e-motions' and dissatisfied notions through their systems, the convoluted tubes get increasingly irate and 'pee-ed' off.

Disheartened and disenchanted about being 'let down' time and time again 'gets the knickers in a twist'. It becomes increasingly difficult for the distraught kidneys to rummage through all the thwarted energy continually sent their way. Resorting to 'trying to please' to counteract meanness, only makes matters worse.

'Rubbing salt' into the 'e-motional' 'wound' is hanging onto excess water, bloating the cells when overwhelmed with a sense of drowning in work or relationships. If persistent, the body's 'plumbing system' gets 'pissed off' until it reaches bursting point.

The strain of repeatedly dealing with stacks of unresolved 'ancient tales' eventually clogs the system. Slowed down to almost a standstill, residue sediments gradually stick together, forming kidney stones. The pain of being blocked and prevented from moving onto the next stage is excruciating.

As embarrassing as 'bedwetting' may seem, the reasons are waterproof. Stemming from excessive anxiety about 'father's' unstable circumstances makes 'hanging on' with little or no 'purse strings' problematic. 'Incontinence' among the elderly comes with inconsistency or when no longer feeling 'in control'. 'Losing their grip' when others take over can be draining.

'A far cry' from the usual ease of sifting through nullified thoughts and processed 'e-motions', anything still worth hanging onto is 'run through the system' again, while the remainder is eliminated in the form of urine.

The right kidney is anatomically lower down and slightly more central than the left due to the bulky presence of the liver. It deals more with past feelings, about what was done or not done, while the left kidney is more connected with notions of what is happening now and how best to sift through current circumstances.

Kidney transplants are possible when issues to be processed are the same, hence having to find matching 't-issues' to avoid rejection. It is possible to be born with an extra kidney when additional assistance is required to wade through a watershed of unresolved family issues.

Storing the 'jing', a vital essence involved in reproduction, kidneys are the shock absorbers, bottle washers and waterworks of the body. Particularly sensitive to the balance of power and sense of empowerment, these master chemists of the internal environment constantly filter relationships, hanging onto some and letting go of others.

To keep the body running harmoniously, a tune-up is often needed!

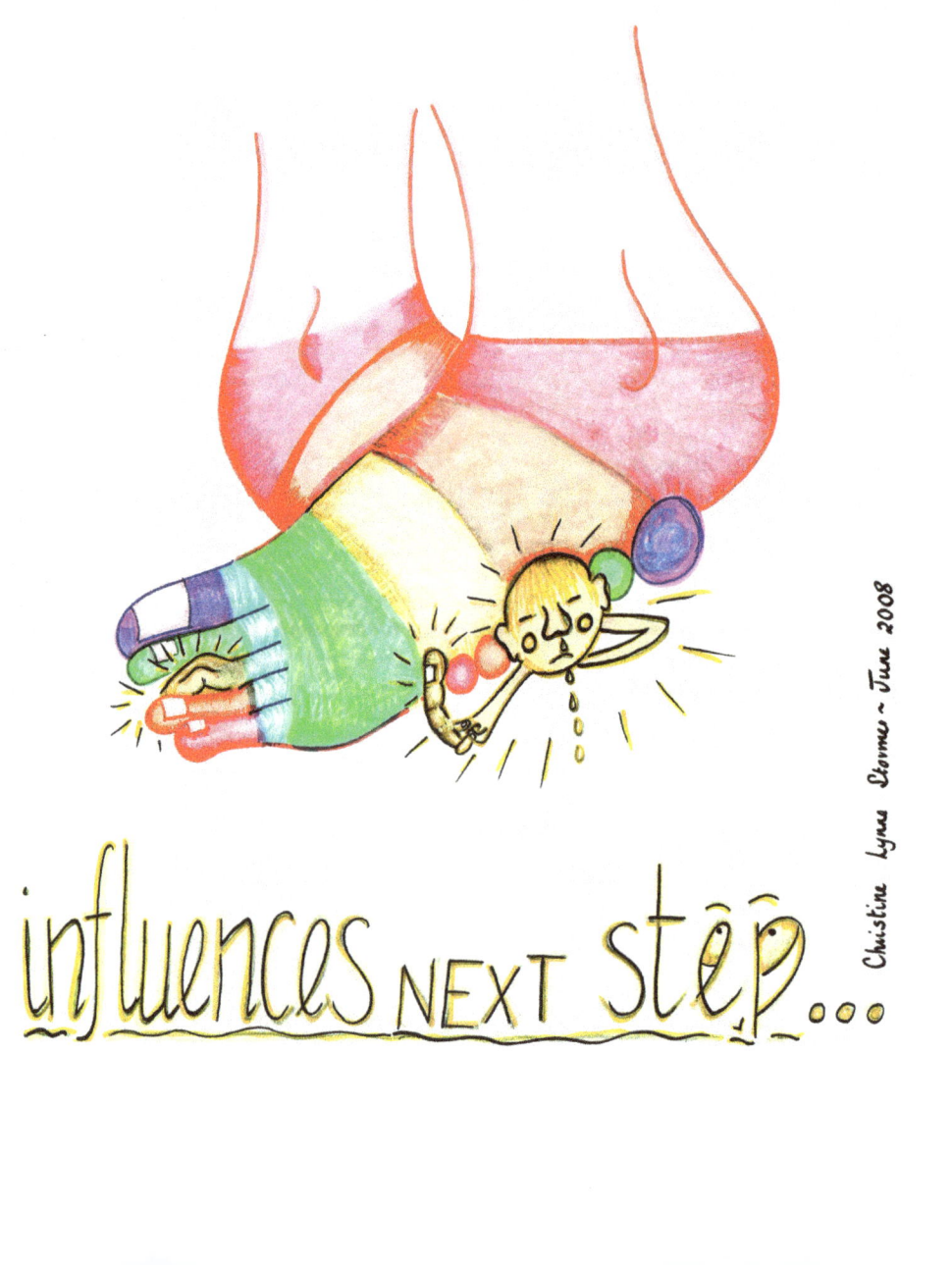

Get off on Wrong Foot!

influences next step...

Christine Lynne Stormer ~ June 2008

GETTING OFF ON THE WRONG FOOT – INFLUENCES THE NEXT STEP

'Getting off on the wrong foot' originated from an ancient Roman superstition that it was bad luck to enter a house with the left foot, to the point that footmen were placed at the front door. Also, a metaphor from the military drill where the rule is to step off on the left foot. If a soldier starts with the right foot, he is out of step with the rest. Furthermore, bogeymen are depicted with their feet turned the wrong way round.

Many 'lost and bewildered Souls' continue to wander around 'in the dark', 'unsure of their footing'. Others, 'rushed off the feet', get 'hopping mad' when anybody 'puts the foot in it!' Not sure of 'where they stand' and having no idea of 'what on earth is going on' is 'knocking many off their feet'

The incredible confusion and chaos worldwide is due to accelerated Universal energies propelling every body through the tunnel of transformation for the next evolutionary phase of humankind. With life moving at such a pace and putting every body under a tremendous amount of strain, it is difficult for the feet to know whether they are 'coming or going'.

Never before has it been so important to 'find the feet' and get 'back on track' to keep pace with escalating changes. Instead of 'running around in circles' and 'getting nowhere fast' feet point mind and body 'in the best direction' for significant progress to be made.

'Putting the foot down' and 'the best foot forward' makes it possible to 'get a foot in the door', with all solutions being only two feet away. Being so attached to the torso means feet 'know every move' – not to mention the motivation behind it.

When disillusioned, life is heavy-going. It is a real drag with the feet 'bearing the brunt'. Yet feet 'under-stand' and know everything 'going on at 'grassroots level', including what is happening 'beneath the surface'. Despite relying on having 'feet on the ground', they are often 'downtrodden' and 'sniffed at'.

Feelings towards feet reveal subconscious thoughts about the current position in life. Not being able 'to stand' feet – and 'turning the nose up' at the thought of looking at or touching them – indicates 'running oneself down' or 'tripping over one's own two feet'. Not liking specific parts of feet pin-points areas of deep dissatisfaction desperately seeking attention.

Liking certain aspects of the feet highlights strong points and talents that can be built upon and developed. With a 'change of mind' and a change of attitude, the characteristics of the feet also change. A positive, more understanding approach to life 'takes a weight off the mind' as well as the feet. When happy, there is 'a spring in the step', the body is 'light on the feet' and positively dances with joy.

Despite being relatively small, feet are incredibly versatile and dependable. 'Covering a tremendous amount of ground' and 'paving the way' by 'blazing a trail of their own', they love to 'step out of line' and 'create new pathways' for ongoing human advancement. 'The going may get tough', but that is 'when the tough gets going'. Feet love resourceful, innovative ways to keep them 'on their toes', despite the odds.

The journey of a thousand miles begins with but a single footstep!

In·ci·dents and Ad·vent·u·res

INCIDENTS AND ADVENTURE

The number 3 indicates an awareness of the Divine aspects of mind, body and Spirit. A spinning vortex of magic as 'th-e-oughts' are set in motion, offering fields of endless opportunities. Uniting past, present, and future, the three are enclosed in a ring of eternity. Just as night and day have twilight and dawn, so the in-betweens often go unseen and, just like this distinct unison, they blend so delightfully into each another.

'Incidents' 'I -c(see) – 'I- dent' 'myself' in an instance' 'invariably disturb the usual course of events, but not by accident. Every 'incident' is an experience. Although a hard teacher, testing first and teaching later – the true essence comes to the fore. The 'incident' is a jewel acquired at great cost, yet it offers priceless insights.

The continuation of unpleasant circumstances is fuelled by hatred, judgement and resentment. These three 'e-motions' intensify and mirror everything detested in life. After a perceivably regrettable occurrence, the constant replay in the mind eventually becomes a stumbling block. Stoical blinkers, seeing the 'incident' as 'bad', prevent it from being perceived as an opportunity with numerous invisible possibilities.

The greater the resistance to new beginnings, the more turbulent and chaotic life becomes. All occurrences highlight the impact of innermost thoughts swayed by memories and beliefs featured through personal behaviour. It is highly unlikely that anybody has exactly the same perceptions as another, even of a shared encounter.

The middle finger, taller than its counterparts and centred poignantly amid the others, represents the 'self'. In ancient times, extending this finger was used to avert the evil eye since it was assumed to have apotropaic potency. Later, it gained sexual connotations, with neighbouring digits representing the testicles. Used in a manner to degrade, intimidate or threaten, a gesture still used today to communicate moderate to extreme contempt, it can also be used humorously or playfully.

The reaction can take on many forms, from a 'punch on the nose', a 'box on the ears', an exclamation of horror at the 'cheek of it,' or a condescending smile, often arising from utter disbelief. Constructive, innovative and adventurous thoughts are ideal for keeping these parts otherwise occupied, improving their overall performance and ensuring that they stay 'in good working order' for guaranteed personal satisfaction and ultimate fulfilment. The nose points the digestive track in the most appetising direction to make sure innovative thoughts stay on track. Cheeks love bold concepts that explore novel ways of implementing ideas. Meanwhile, ears keep the mind alert to new input and lively ways to manifest concepts. The external ears absorb and listen out for sounds outside the body, mingling them with internal sounds detected by the inner ears to obtain a bigger picture.

Every event raises consciousness, bringing with it inner expansion and greater wisdom. Near-death experiences are life-transforming, catapulting the mind to new levels of enlightenment beyond anything dreamed possible.

Every incident and adventure ensures Spiritual growth and evolution. All life experiences are an ongoing breeding ground for transformation, contributing to larger planetary developments and group consciousness. Perfect stepping-stones arranged in Divine order, all occurrences powerfully determine the quality of life

No incident or experience is wasted – use them wisely!

130 - CHRISTINE LYNNE STORMER-FRYER

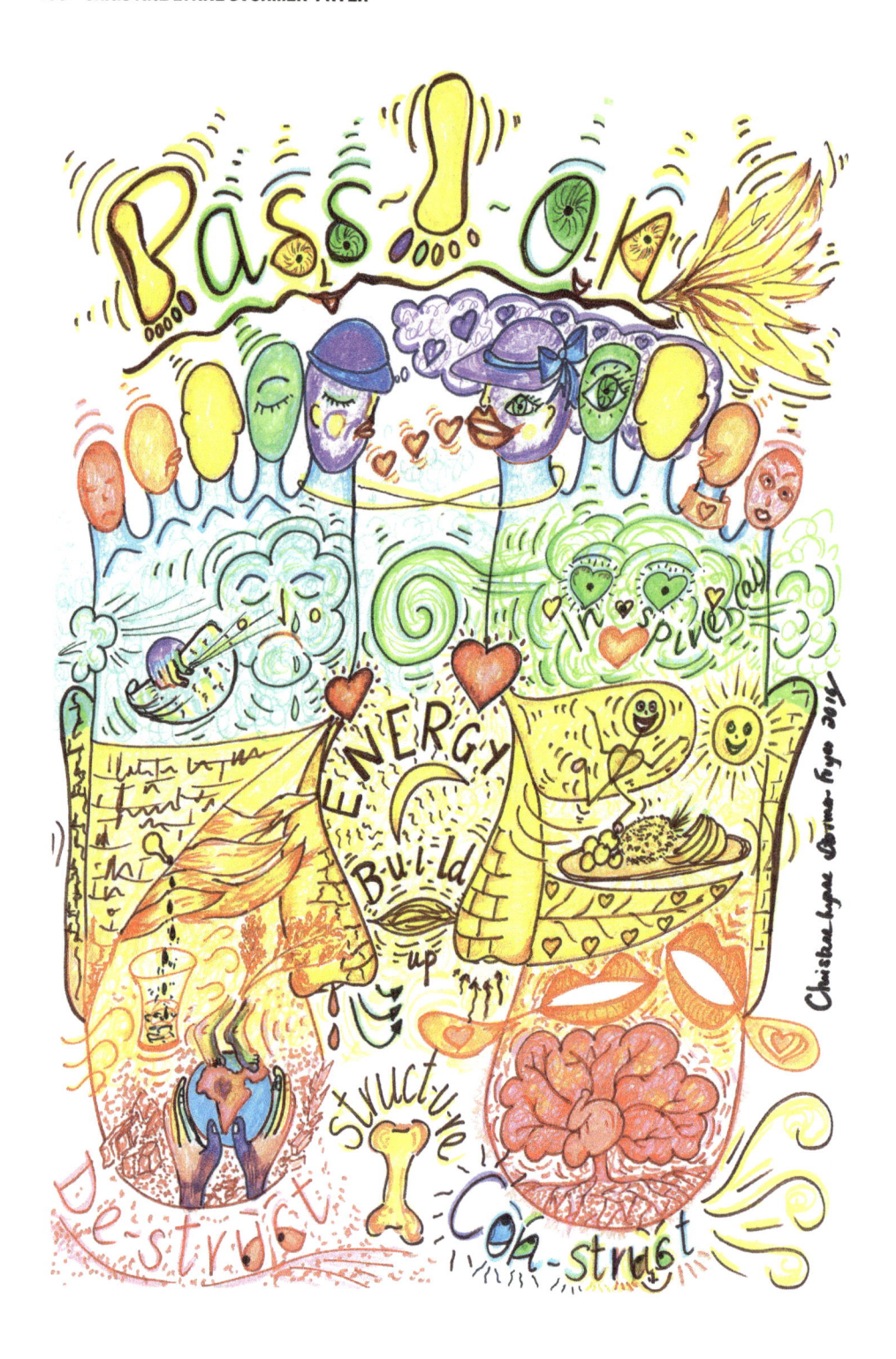

PASSION – DESTRUCT – CONSTRUCT

Passion is the key to living a fulfilled and satisfactory existence, 'pass- I -on' what I 'ate' (experienced). A vast range of different passions stems from a wide variety of motives, some destructive, others creative.

Working hard without passion creates stress while working hard with passion is exhilarating. Being passionate inspires others to pass the 'passion' on. True compassion recognises all limitations to be an illusion. It sees the deep connectedness between everybody and everything. It understands passionate displays of frustration and inconsideration. It sees how fear, stress and irritability create absolute havoc, including acts of violence. Within everybody's heart and mind are dark places that still need healing.

There is no room for judgement, just under-standing and love. Focusing on the light dissipates the dark. Every molecule in the body knows that performing without ardour is a form of self-sabotage. Without passion, there is no energy; without energy, there is nothing and no quality to life.

Every great dream begins with the dreamer. Within are the strength, patience and passion to 'reach for the stars' and passionately change everything for the better.

All great leaders have looked inwards to tell a good story about authenticity and passion. Our beloved Nelson Mandela said, "There is no passion to be found playing small, in settling for a life less than the one you are capable of living". What else is there to do other than follow the passions of the heart? Many things will catch the eye, but only a few will capture the heart, these are the ones to pursue with passion.

Finding creative passion is about finding the authentic spark to ignite the flames, with an intense zest and enthusiasm that is exceptionally compelling and inspiring. Everything done becomes effortless. Hours whizz by, with tiredness and fatigue taking a backseat.

Passion is energy. The power that comes from focusing on the Soul's innermost needs. Passion has to be acted out first before its drive is felt. It is impossible to explain this to somebody who has never experienced passion; it is up to them to find ways to attain this incredible force of life.

True passion can never be extinguished. Ranging from eager interest to intense desire, passion is far deeper and more encompassing than lust. It is an exhilarating feeling that excites the heart and Soul. Passion knows no bounds or boundaries.

Motivated by the Soul, passion and desire go hand in hand. The power behind great achievements, it is the key to inner strength and personal excellence. Passion cannot be faked. It is either there, or it isn't. Passion makes life happen, with heart and Soul united as one.

Developing a passion for learning means the Soul never ceases to grow. Believing in passion turns dreams into reality. It is the very essence of being. With passion, anything is possible. Passion in all walks of life is the key to living a fulfilled and satisfactory existence.

Passion opens the door to joy and abundance!

132 - CHRISTINE LYNNE STORMER-FRYER

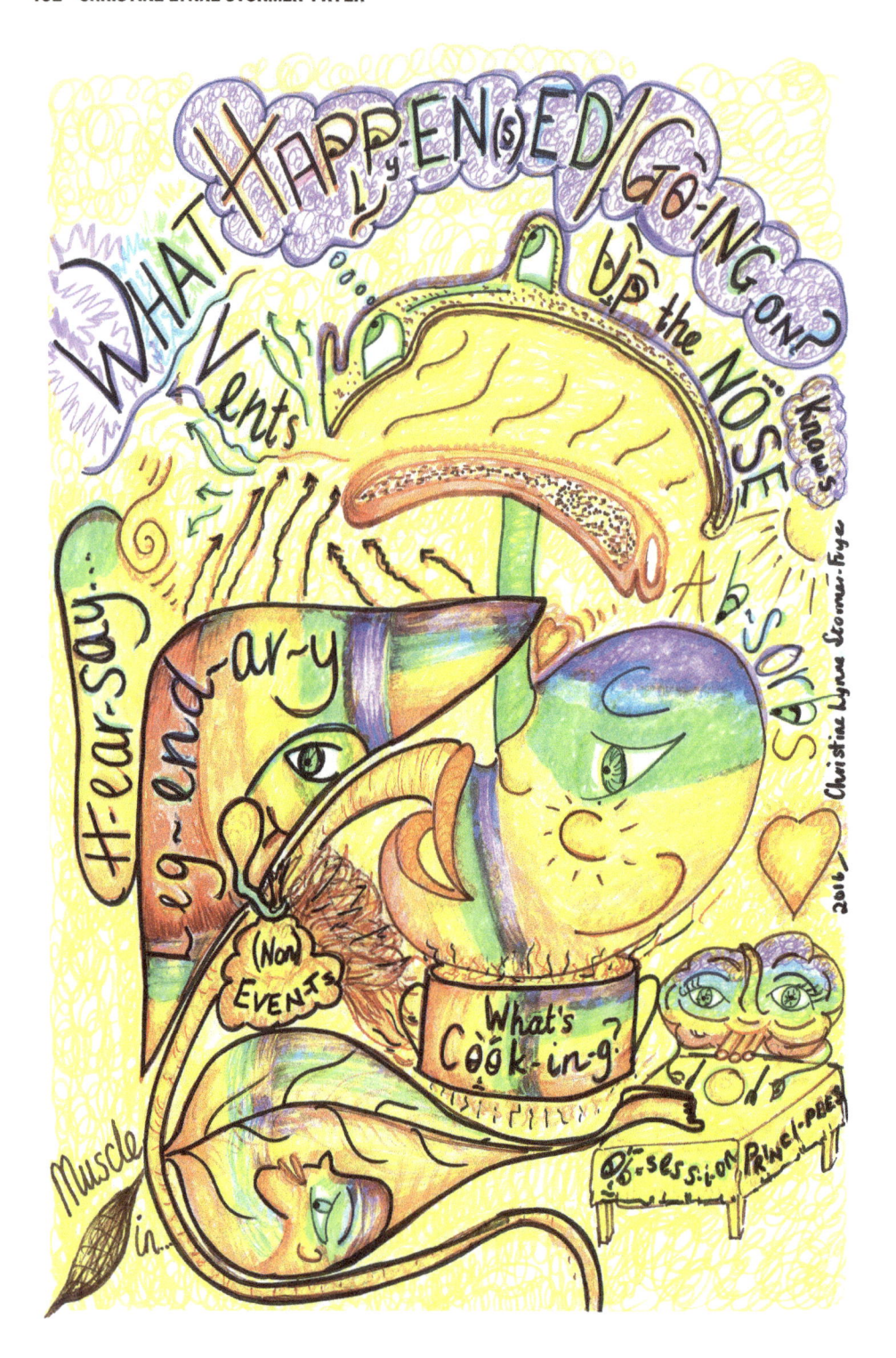

WHAT HAPPENS OR HAPPENED - CONSIDER THE BULK OF EACH PRODUCTION

Everybody is an energy waiting to happen. Each physical experience is ideal for actively and energetically processing thoughts, ideas and concepts before putting them into action. To stay balanced requires a caring head and a wholesome heart.

Whatever happens or does not happen attracts and emits a vibration that is important and sacred. Responsible for the bulk of each production is the body's torso, created with the express purpose of becoming reacquainted with the authenticity of the Spirit. It is a great feeling to be comfortable in the body, making the production so much better.

The 'nose' 'knows' how to 'vent' its case, making required adjustments before permitting any air into the body. Meanwhile, the 'ears' process variances within the wavelengths to offer 'sound', and not so 'sound', advice to the mind, for it to decide what to do or not do next.

Energy derived from legendary events and non-events is stored in the liver to provide the incentive to keep going, no matter what. Knowing 'what's cooking' helps in 'stomaching' the new intake of life's opportunities. Absorption of the 'content' or 'discontent' of 'new trends' offered by 'nu-trients' determines the amount of progress made when it comes to digesting what is going on.

The spleen is more prone to being a tad obsessive. Being so highly principled can 'pose a problem' when adamant about the 'dis-ease to please'. Meanwhile, the pancreas does its best to extract as much joy and happiness as possible to make the journey more pleasurable.

Happiness does not just happen. It is getting on and making things 'happen' that creates 'happiness'. It is the small daily happenings that make life spectacular. Whatever happens, happens for a reason. Yet the quality of life is determined not by what happens but how it is handled. Every body has the power to choose how to react to the perception of 'whatever happened'.

Enormous modifications are currently required as genetic intelligence and encoded memory patterns are being re-awakened to be healed. For this to happen past restrictions, limitations and imperfections must first be released.

Every one has been given a body in which to live and learn. With beliefs creating its biology, all actions and reactions are in the hands of its owner and at the mercy of the mind. The human body is its own best apothecary with the most successful prescriptions being those filled by the body itself.

True happiness comes from making things happen!

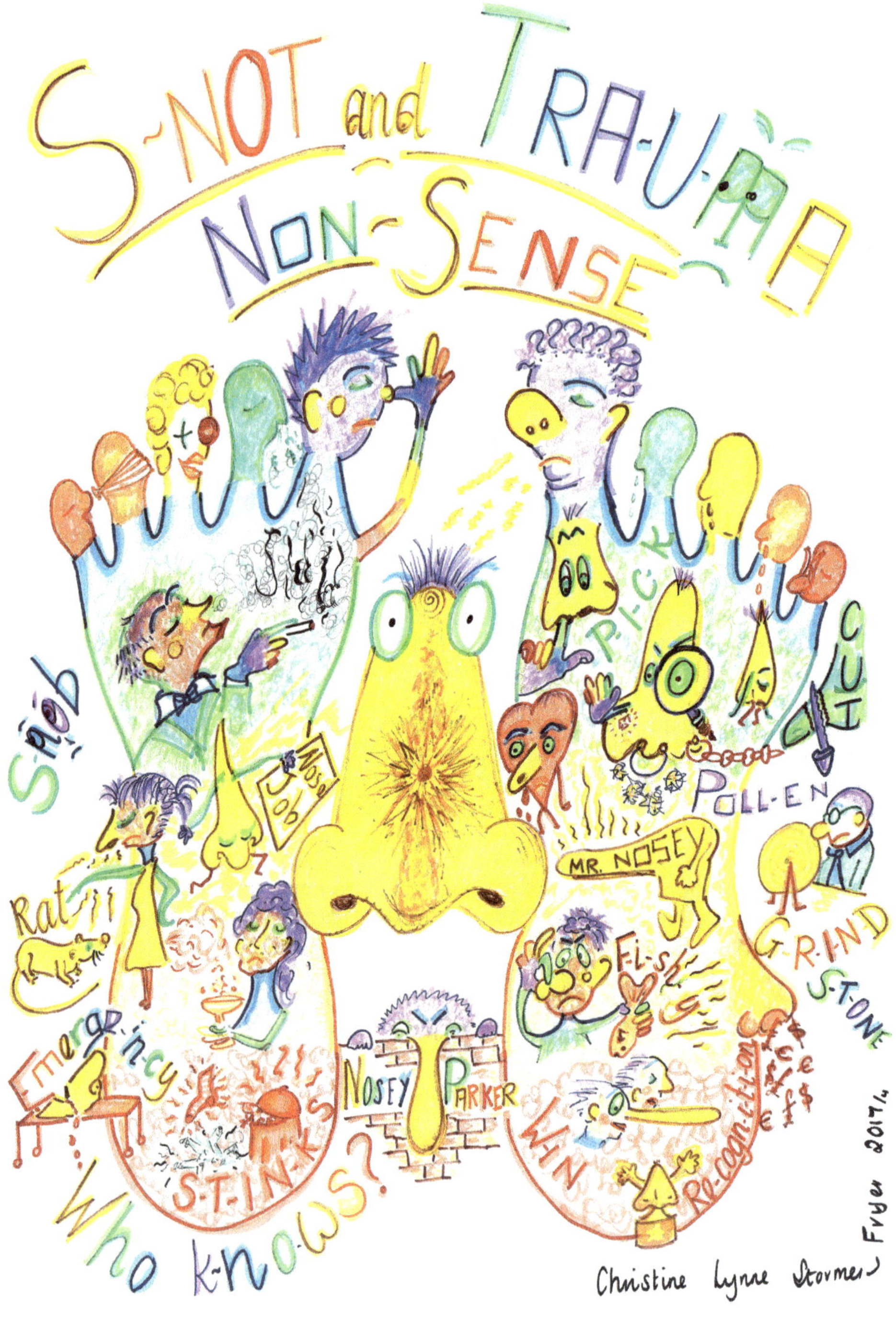
S-NOT and TRA-U-MA
NON-SENSE
Nose Job
Rat
P-I-C-K
POLL-EN
MR. NOSEY
G-R-I-N-D S-T-ONE
F-I-S-H-Y
Emergency
S-T-I-N-K-S
NOSEY PARKER
WIN
Re-cogn-i-t-i-on
Who k-n-o-w-s?
Christine Lynne Stormer-Fryer 2017

S-NOT AND TRA-U-MA NON-SENSE

Hysterical shows of 'snot and trauma' really do 'get up the nose'. All that 'tra ra ra ra' nonsense of blaming 'u' and 'ma' for all the 'tr-ials and tr-ibulations', dragged through dribbling tr-ails of 'poor me'. The nose willingly rids itself of meaningless absurdity left needlessly 'hanging in the air'. It is also highly intolerant of ridiculous beliefs considered to be untrue, silly or lacking coherence. 'S-not' nobly comes to the rescue.

Constantly analysing whether the content or discontent of incoming breath is perceivably friendly or not, the nose decides what to take on board. Its work is really cut out when faced with actual trauma. Desperately flushing away upsetting energies, it is a great relief to have its flaring nostrils alleviated by the continual blowing of the nose.

'Dust swept under the carpet', concealing a pile of derelict grime from previous generations, is so irritating. 'Sneezing' prevents past filth and previous irrational behaviour from 'getting up the nose'.

With a 'good sense of smell', 'a rat can be smelt a mile away'. Suspicions are aroused when non-physical smells are detected, 'sending shivers down the spine'. With smell being the most evocative of all senses, conjured-up memories and remnant feelings from the past flood the mind.

'Lead by the nose' following dominant characters without question is to have a 'wax nose' and be easily influenced, often ending up 'paying through the nose', with nostrils flaring in frustration. 'Looking down the nose' in superior contempt or disdain is to soon 'lose the sense of smell' and end up way off track with the Soul's purpose. Any 'e-merge-n-cy', like a 'nose-bleed', is indicative of outpourings of sadness clearing the way for new 'e-nergy' to 'emerge'.

'Not seeing further than the end of the nose', lacking insight and foresight makes it impossible to notice what is so obviously 'in front of the nose'. 'Keeping the nose to the grindstone' 'working diligently and continually is excellent for 'keeping the nose clean' and staying out of trouble, or getting involved in dubious activities. Perfectionists are invariably agitated by pollen 'getting up the nose', irritated that others are not picking up on their pedantic way of doing things.

Prominently positioned on the face, the nose takes the lead, sniffing out the best opportunities for the Soul's journey. Being 'on the nose' and intuitively knowing how to acknowledge the inner essence, it has a much-appreciated connection with the Divine source.

The nose and its 'snot' are essential for survival. Intellectually recognising the true self through personal achievements sharpens its sense of smell, as consciousness and self-awareness evolve.

When discouraged, just keep the schnozzle up!

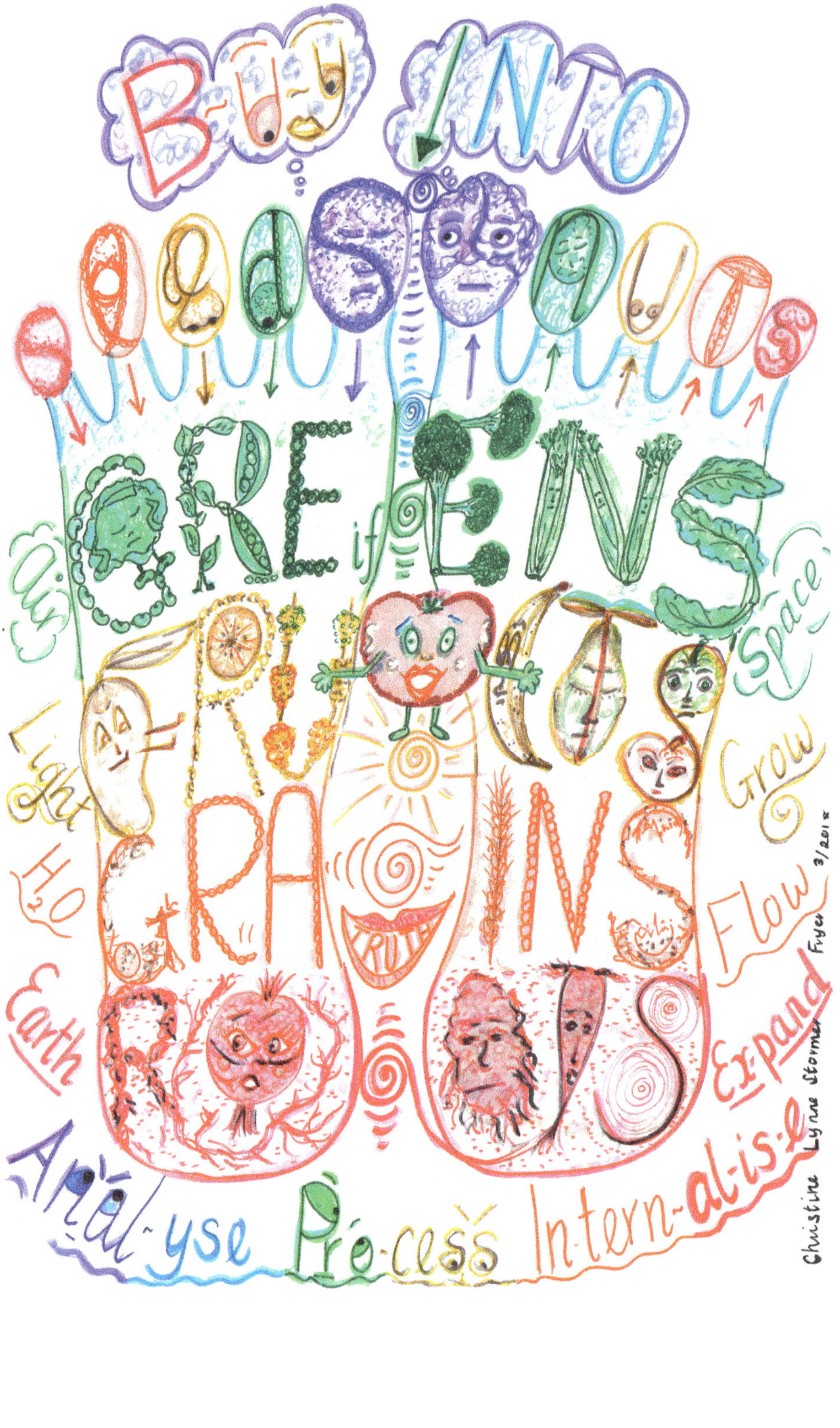

INTO
GREENS
FRUITS
GRAINS
ROOTS
Air
Space
Light
Grow
H2O
Flow
Earth
Expand
Anal-yse Pro-cess Intern-al-is-e
Christine Lynne Stormer Fryer

BUY INTO

Gullible enough to 'buy into' any story or wholeheartedly accept something as true or practical just because it is deemed to be the 'norm'. Accepting a policy or change just because it is 'in line' with personal notions. Acquiring a stake or interest in a business or organisation without knowing much about it. Getting involved, and accepting as valid, any argument or theory. It is no wonder that things go so horribly wrong.

'Buying into' certain seeds and nuts as being healthy is a more sensible option, but only if full of 'nutrients', packed full of 'nu-trends'. The same applies to 'seeds' of thought planted in the 'nut'. The more innovative and unusual, the better. Fed and watered regularly with a consistently high input of healthy energy encourages them to flourish and propagate, guaranteeing a more wholesome and satisfied human being.

'Buying into' eating greens being 'good for you' all depends on the 'e-motional' environment and the type of feelings entertained within the family. Derived from medieval Latin *'vegetabilis'*, meaning 'growing and flourishing', then in Late Latin meaning 'enlivening and quickening'. Air provides the ideal space for one to expand and breathe. Alternatively, allowing feelings to vegetate and stagnate when a 'couch potato' leaves a 'foul stench in the air'.

'Buying into' 'an apple a day keeps the doctor away' is based on the belief that fruit is highly nutritious and 'good for the Soul', but only when seeds come to 'fruition' in prolific ways. Putting plenty of passion and love into life make the 'fruits of the labour' so much more worthwhile. The fruitful and rewarding outcomes are enormously beneficial, satisfying and gratifying, not just for the self but also for family and the 'fruits of the body', the offspring.

'Buying into' 'the rich get richer, the poor get poorer' can 'go against the grain'. Ultimately, it is 'the more put into life, the greater the benefits'. 'Reaping the rewards' and enjoying a 'good harvest' depends on the 'give and take' within relationships. When there is 'not a grain of truth' or an insufficient water supply, it is difficult to trust the 'flow of conversation' that contaminates relationships, leaving a 'bad taste' in the mouth.

'Buying into' 'storms make deeper roots' stems from the ability to go through 'stormy weather' and digging deep within for resourcefulness, derived from family roots. Growing deep roots and recognising that everybody is from the One Divine Source helps in bearing richer and more enriching produce. Thanks to the stability and resources of 'Mother Earth', each new concept can be analysed and processed before being internalised, thereby ensuring the survival and evolution of humanity.

The harvest of tomorrow is determined by the deeds of today!

138 - CHRISTINE LYNNE STORMER-FRYER

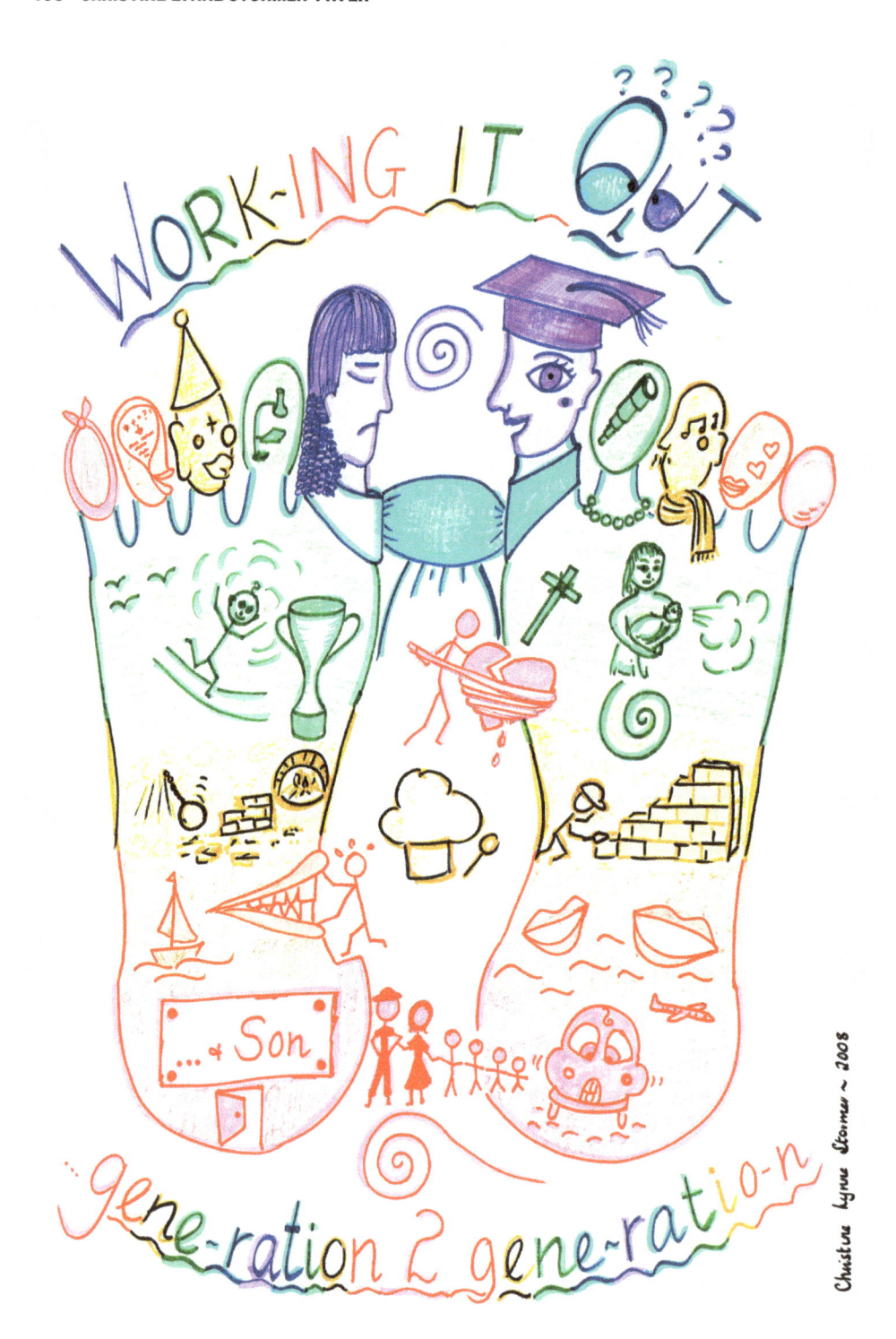

WORKING IT OUT – GENERATION TO GENERATION

Every body has a job to do. Mainly to 'work out' family issues that go back seven generations or more. Trades, traditionally passed from father to son, make sure that this happens. Much insight can be gleaned from the type of occupation chosen, as well as the surname.

For instance 'Baker and Son' provide 'bread', the 'dough', cash, or money, for the 'Baker's dozen', just in case of another 'bun in the oven'. The Baker's 'work is cut out', knowing how to avoid 'sweltering' 'overheated' arguments and 'cooking up' disaster with 'half-baked' notions, as was the penchant of previous family members. Providing 'bread for the table' and 'cakes' catering for 'sweet teeth', bakers serve basic social needs. Having 'worked out' how not to get 'fingers burnt', 'overheated' or 'hot under the collar', some 'sons' chose other occupations to assist in working out additional family issues.

'Butcher and Son' work through 'botched', 'ruined', 'bungled', 'spoilt' events of the past to become 'more sensitive', 'stronger' and 'beefier'. 'Keeping up with the Jones' can be a fixation, even an addiction, of always wanting to own the same expensive items as neighbours and friends to avoid being seen as less important socially. Old English 'Smith' signifies to 'smite' or 'strike' from smelting metal purchased from miners. Casting ideas in a fixed mental mould often led to obstinacy. Being such a common name, Smith was chosen by gypsies and emigrants who wished to maintain secret identities or disappear, never to be found. During colonisation, many Native Americans chose 'Smith' to make it easier to deal with colonists. To avoid discrimination, many Germans anglicised Schmidt or Schmitz.

Whatever occupies the mind, 'occupies' the body. 'Profess-I-on', I admit, own, confess, acknowledge, or recognise the inner Spirit through what is done or not done. Believing that things will not work out is asking for trouble, with endless obstacles proving the point. Believing that things will work out has endless opportunities 'knocking at the door' to make sure this happens.

It is not the job that creates happiness but doing the job well. Each occupation has a purpose that comes with benefits. A role in healthcare is to doctor and nurse childhood wounds, with medicine medicating the pain. A surgeon specialises in operating to fix things that have gone wrong or are out of alignment. Art is the ideal outlet for suppressed 'e-motions'. Entertainment is a chance to act out many roles. Business involves busily trading innermost concerns. Industrial occupations require a lot of hard work, often with minimal return. Manufacturing provides material to fabricate a more worthwhile reality. Entering Law gives the authority to 'bend the law'. Jobs 'in security' are chosen by 'in-secure' Souls to process 'insecurities'. Armed forces are well-equipped to be defensive, compensating for not being able to do so when growing up. As for IT, highly intelligent and evolved Souls find many diverse ways to compute Universal insights.

The benefits of losing a job are great. Generally, the 'heart was not in it' in the first place, with energy zapped through constant complaints of being 'bored' or 'tired'. 'Getting the boot' and being 'kicked up the backside' is a sign to get on be an entrepreneur and 'work out' more relevant issues.

Life is a work in progress with endless possibilities to work things out!

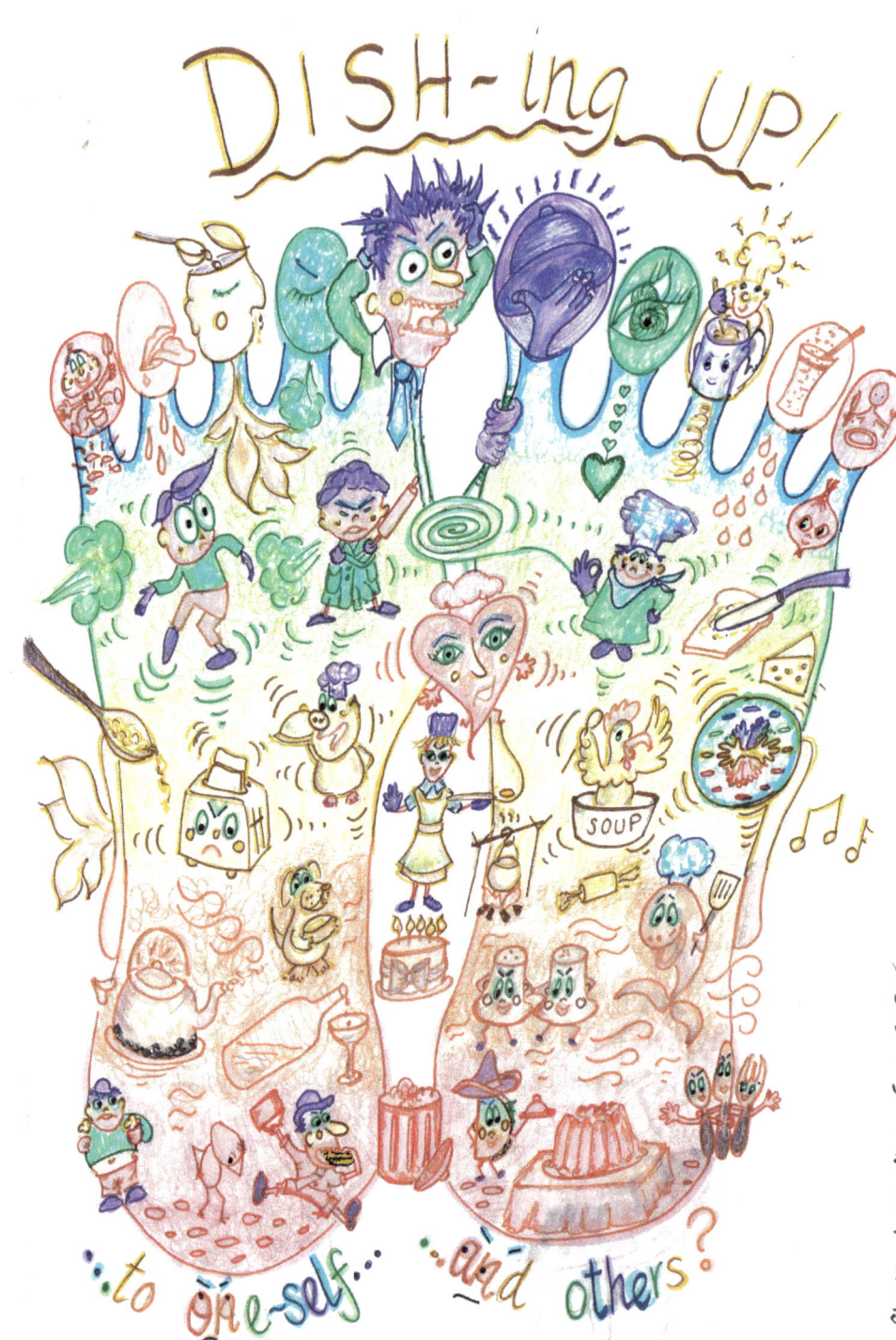

140 - CHRISTINE LYNNE STORMER-FRYER

DISHING UP – TO ONESELF AND OTHERS

The mind thrives on novelty. What was once a source of pleasure can become tedious and boring, with discontent taking over. All the passive idling of the mind generates a great deal of frustration. Not using mental energy to engage in productive tasks leads to a purposeless existence that is either depressing or motivating.

Frustrated and 'fed up to the back teeth' with all the whinging poured ceaselessly into the mind is enough to make it want to 'pull the hair out' and can even make the 'blood boil'. Loads of 'hot air' shoved down and congesting the air pipes is all too much, often bringing 'tears to the eyes' when trying to get to 'know one's onions'.

Bringing up the 'cheese' and vomiting through disgust from being 'cheesed off' with the 'big cheese' is 'not quite the cheese' (the correct thing to do). Nor is 'sneaking away' from constant 'e-motional' onslaught to avoid being 'battered with a rolling pin'. It becomes extremely difficult to 'cook on the front burner'. Instead of 'quarrelling with the bread and butter' of life, giving up a job and being deprived of earning a living, it is far better to 'know which side the bread is buttered on'. Greater appreciation comes when more mindful of and focused on personal actions.

It's time to 'wake up and smell the coffee' and pay attention to what is happening, especially when 'spoon feed' with dollop upon dollop of 'moans and groans' and 'getting the wooden spoon' for losing out. 'Making a pig's ear' out of this dire situation messes things up even further, 'adding fat to the fire'.

Treated as 'toast' and unworthy of further consideration, having been 'given the cold shoulder', makes some 'turn to drink' and 'get toasted'. Failing to 'cater to every whim' really 'takes the cake', making it the right 'time to shut the cake hole' and stop further complaints about things not being 'as easy as duck soup'. Taking appropriate steps to avoid ending up 'in the soup' is so much better.

With 'a little pot soon getting too hot' there is 'no pot to piss in'. The 'stench' of the same old 'non-sense' becomes overbearing. Ragging on about 'living off the smell of an oil rag' feeds the 'poor me' mentality, with 'no leg to stand on'. 'Calling the kettle black' is definitely not the solution.

When 'as mean as a junkyard dog' there is not 'a dog's chance' when a 'dog in the manger' attitude is adopted to engender sympathy. 'Facing the music' for 'venting the spleen' from being 'below the salt' and less socially acceptable is a better option, especially when the truth has been 'peppered' until it is 'down to chilli and beans', infused in absolute poverty.

An aversion to wine stems from being 'full to the brim' with endless 'whining'. As for a 'beer gut', the vain attempt to cover up all the grumbling and mumbling going on inside adds tremendous strain from all that has been poured 'into the back'. It becomes such a pain lugging around so many outdated 'back issues'.

'Always on the run', with knees turning to 'jelly' when running away from relationships, is a cowardly way of scurrying away from the truth. 'Refusing' to deal with reality and 'littering' the body with all the 'trash' 'dished out' and 'dumped' on it, there comes a time to stop 'forking the fingers' and making rude gestures.

A positive attitude is the passport to tomorrow!

142 - CHRISTINE LYNNE STORMER-FRYER

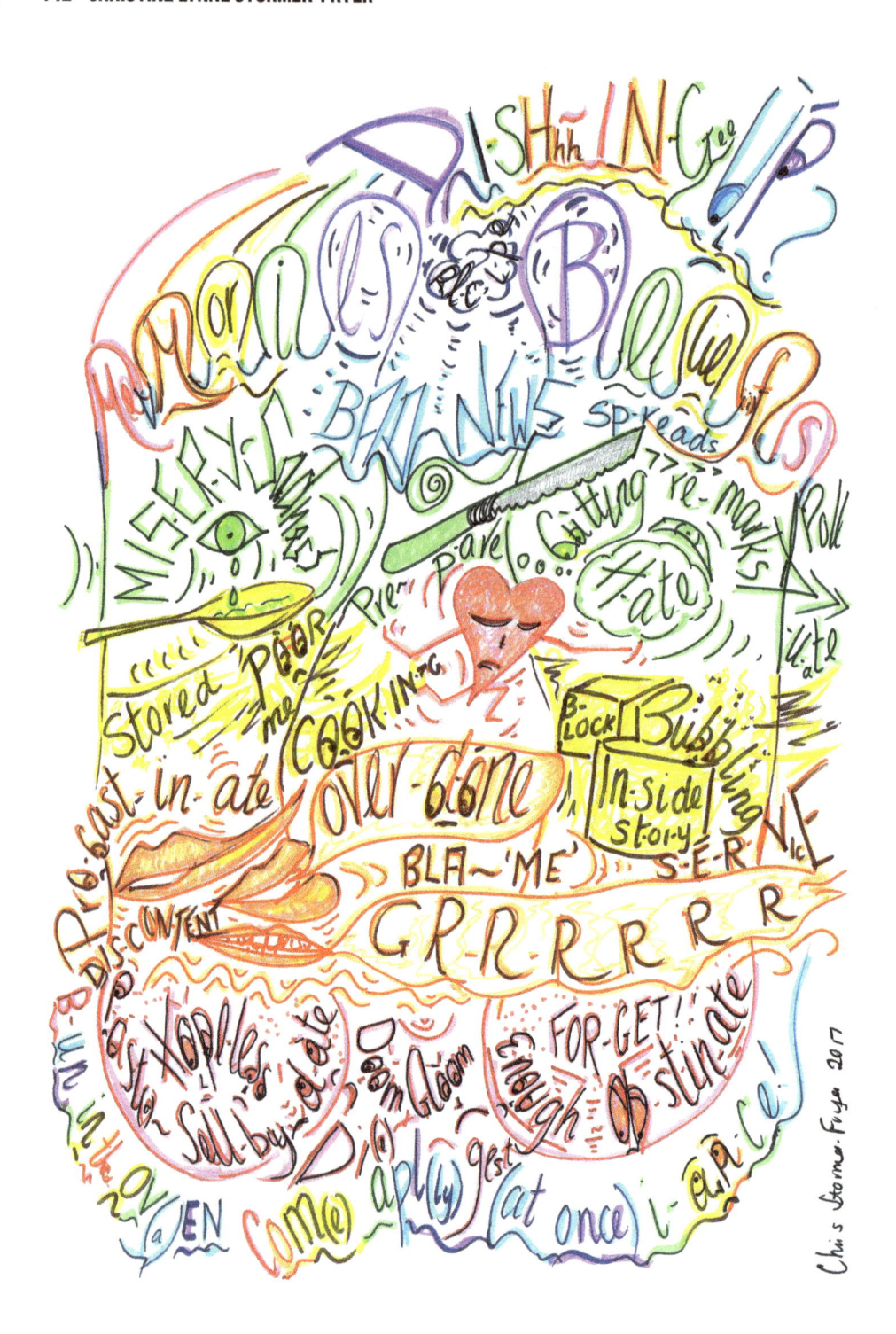

EVEN MORE DISHING UP

When faced with detestable chores, errands and responsibilities, getting into a bad mood and staying there only serves to make matters worse. A bad attitude in no way changes what must be done. It is so much easier and far more pleasant to have a much more serene approach.

It's a 'recipe' for disaster when dishing up the same old disgruntled 'memories' and shovelling foul beliefs down the throat. Doing so is 'bad news', a negative medium, creating and spreading more of what is not needed. 'Uninformed' when not following the news, or 'misinformed' when doing so, masks the fact that drama replaces the lack of excitement in life.

'Happy being miserable', 'misery guts' love to be 'misers' at the best of times. 'Cutting remarks' that 'cut to the core' is to leave mind and body 'cut-up', literally like being 'stabbed in the back'. Breathing out sadness and hostility creates a heavy, often impenetrable, atmosphere while being a 'breath of fresh air' is the perfect 'recipe' for building a solid structure in life.

Committing, or even over-committing, to the happiness of others may sound noble, but serving through sacrifice and self-denial devaluates self-worth. 'Buying into' false expectations is of little or no service to anybody. Sad tales concocted, even after 'cooking the books', only multiplies the already-disastrous situation. With the 'inside story' being a mass of wretched energy in the liver, it keeps 'blocking' the way. The 'recipe' to success is to bite off large chunks of opportunity, chew them over carefully, then 'go the whole hog' and just do it.

Floundering in the grips of procrastination, 'dragging the feet' and blaming others tends to 'overdo' the tragedy. Constantly dishing up regurgitated facts ad nauseam and 'tired of knowing nothing of value' should generate a craving for some personal knowledge and insights.

Obstinately serving up dollops of the same old nonsense well past their 'sell-by date' mixed with heaps of hopelessness drearily dressed in doom and gloom is a classic 'recipe' for indigestion. The body is saying 'enough is enough!'. Rather than giving into 'compliance', cook up a reason to 'come' and 'apply' at 'once' with recipes that tastefully favour a better outcome.

Chores are invariably entwined with gifts, a realisation that comes from adopting a different perspective. Attitude is everything. It is the librarian of the past, speaker of the present, and prophet of the future. More than a mood, an attitude is predominantly a sustained 'e-motion', with a tremendous impact on the matter. Even though the past cannot be changed, or the way others think and behave, attitudes can be altered in an instance.

Innately, everybody loves doing something worthwhile and being of 'service', but nobody likes to be a 'servant'. Consciously serving humanity by 'dishing up' passion, joy and happiness contributes to the overall welfare of humankind.

Ripples of joy become tidal waves of love and compassion.

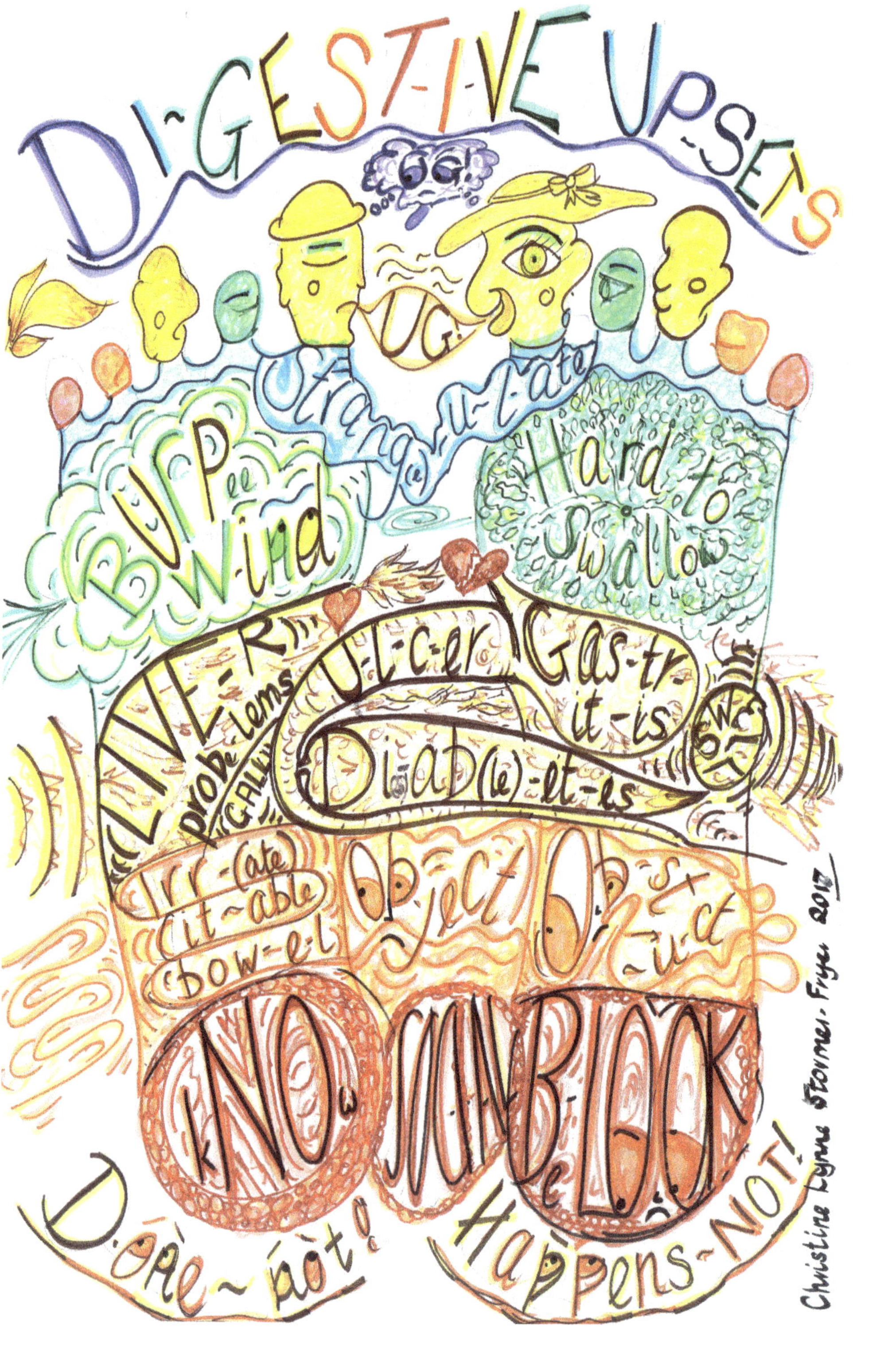
DI-GEST-I-VE UP-SETS
UG!
UG
Strang(e)-u-l-ate
Burp
Wind
Hard to Swallow
LIVE-R
prob-lems
Ul-c-er
Gas-tr-it-is
Dia-b(e)-et-es
Irr-(ate)
it-able
Bow-e-l
Ob-ject
Happens-NOT!
Christine Lynne Stormer-Fryer 2017

DIGESTIVE UPSETS

Challenged with stomaching and processing unpalatable and unacceptable life events leaves a 'bad taste in the mouth'. Taking in a whole load of anxiety, worry, and fear are uncomfortable energies for any body to digest.

With 'nerves on edge', long term dilemmas and indecisiveness make it problematic when it comes to creating new concepts. The body gags on repulsive circumstances that are 'hard to swallow' crushing any chance of making progress. The whole of the digestive tract is 'strangulated' and 'tormented'.

Wind expulsion, such as burping and flatulence, are wonderful ways to 'release 'e-motional' pressure'. Furious at having to unwillingly endure sickening situations makes the stomach flare up into 'gastritis'. Meanwhile, the spleen is struggling, being 'up to its neck' in a desperate 'need to please'.

Feet have no choice but to begrudgingly drag themselves through the burdens of life's challenges imposed upon them by heavy thoughts and weighty 'e-motions'. Depleted of the effervescence of life experiences, with little or no vivacity, makes the liver livid. Meanwhile, the body complains of being constantly exhausted. To rejuvenate the Soul, a passionate approach to everything in life is required.

Being 'irritated' by unrealistic expectations puts the bowels under great pressure. Writhing in pain, the discomfort of twisting the truth makes them squirm uncomfortably, eventually tying themup in knots. Bringing everything to a standstill, by constantly 'objecting' about others taking more than is fair, 'obstructs' the way, making it impossible to rationalise about and assimilate whatever is going on internally.

'Up in arms' and incessantly complaining about all the incredulous 'no ways' over what was 'done or not done' or is still 'happening or not happening' is highly 'irritating', as are all the shocking rules and regulations imposed by 'society'. Internal masses mimicking these external barriers can develop in various ways, one of them being cancer.

The passage of food through the body empathetically symbolises taking in and processing life events. Stacks of memories and beliefs influence how this happens, guiding ongoing notions and, ultimately, a wide range of 'e-motions'.

Digestion is an opportunity to take in life events and enjoy them to the full!

When anxious, 'don't hold your breath', it may never happen!

146 - CHRISTINE LYNNE STORMER-FRYER

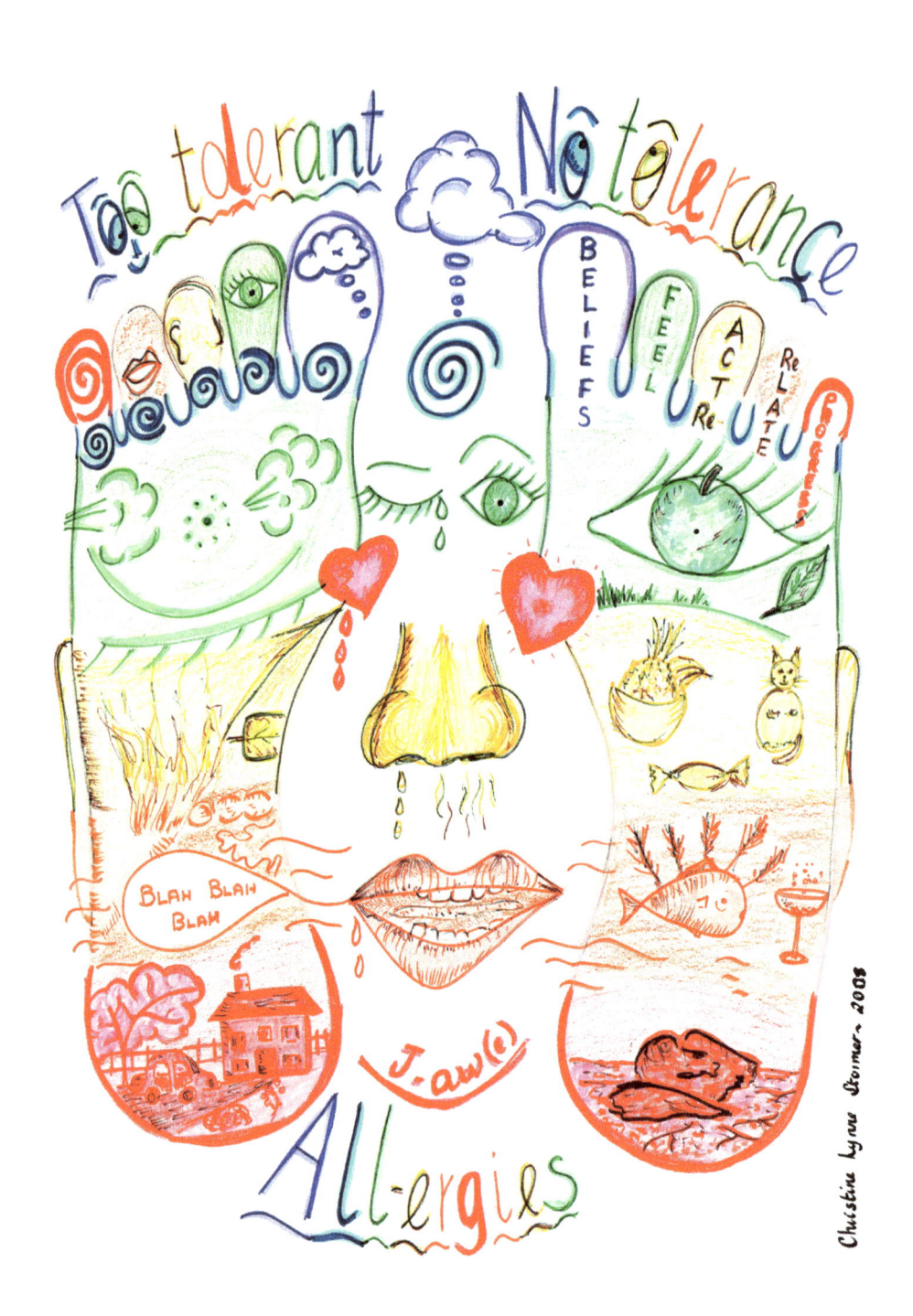

TOO TOLERANT – NO TOLERANCE

Rooted in fear, intolerance camouflages bigotry, prejudice, chauvinism, fanaticism, narrow-mindedness and bias. Focused on lower vibrational energies, it is reflected through appalling attitudes, shocking behaviour, galling conversations, and unfair social structures practised by confused Souls unaware of their true identity or authenticity.

On the other hand, tolerance is the realisation and acceptance of anybody or anything fundamentally different. It is about showing respect for others, not because they are 'right' or 'wrong', but for being human. Being 'too tolerant' can, however, 'get on the nerves', making mind and body react badly. Either way, conflict between individual beliefs and personal perceptions is extremely disconcerting. Irrational issues soon crop up in the tissues to highlight 'th-e-issues.'

Every innovative thought and novel idea is a seed planted in the mind for magnificent co-creations with the Universe. Seeds of despair make the 'head ache', longing to have some encouraging input. 'Bad' reactions' to seeds draw attention to unacceptable 'seedy' circumstances.

The 'walnut-like brain' is often referred to as a 'nut'. Adverse reactions to nuts are spawned when experiencing difficulty in dealing with 'a hard nut to crack'; 'doing one's nut', getting exceptionally angry at not 'getting a-head'; 'being off one's nut', considered stupid, mad or foolish; even 'nuts' about something crazily fanciful. The 'nuts and bolts' of whacky thoughts can 'get on the nerves', causing an intolerance to nuts and seeds.

Gagging on foul expressions make it impossible to 'take in' and fully process all that is going on, especially when 'green with envy' at not being the 'apple of the father's eye'. Revolting notions running from the mind and through the body 'create a stir'. As trapped memories are emancipated, unpleasant 'e-motions' tend to be aroused.

'Buying into' barren ideas for all the 'wrong reasons' and expecting bountiful rewards, without putting in the appropriate energy, is 'fruitless'. 'No stomach' for fruit is a possibility when siblings (the 'fruits of the body') make life difficult or unpleasant, squeezing out all the goodness from life's experiences.

Despite being remarkably small, rain can develop into something vast or formidable. Taking anything with a 'grain of salt' is to doubt its source. The subsequent conflict of interest within relationships makes the assimilation of grains exceptionally tiresome and strenuous. The temptation to resort to mockery such as "blah blah fish paste!" is hoping that there are 'other fish in the sea' to improve the situation.

Intolerances 'too close to home' are numerous. 'Living under the same roof' with irrational 'kin' makes the 's-kin' creep just like the 'creepy crawly' that slithers along the ground or 'creeps up' unexpectedly. 'Dirt thrown in the face' 'rocks the boat', creating a rocky situation.

The 'hi-story' is essential when unearthing the story about being too tolerant or completely intolerant. Only then can everything be calmed down to a 'gentle panic'.

Calmness within spreads outwardly, contributing to a more tolerable environment!

148 - CHRISTINE LYNNE STORMER-FRYER

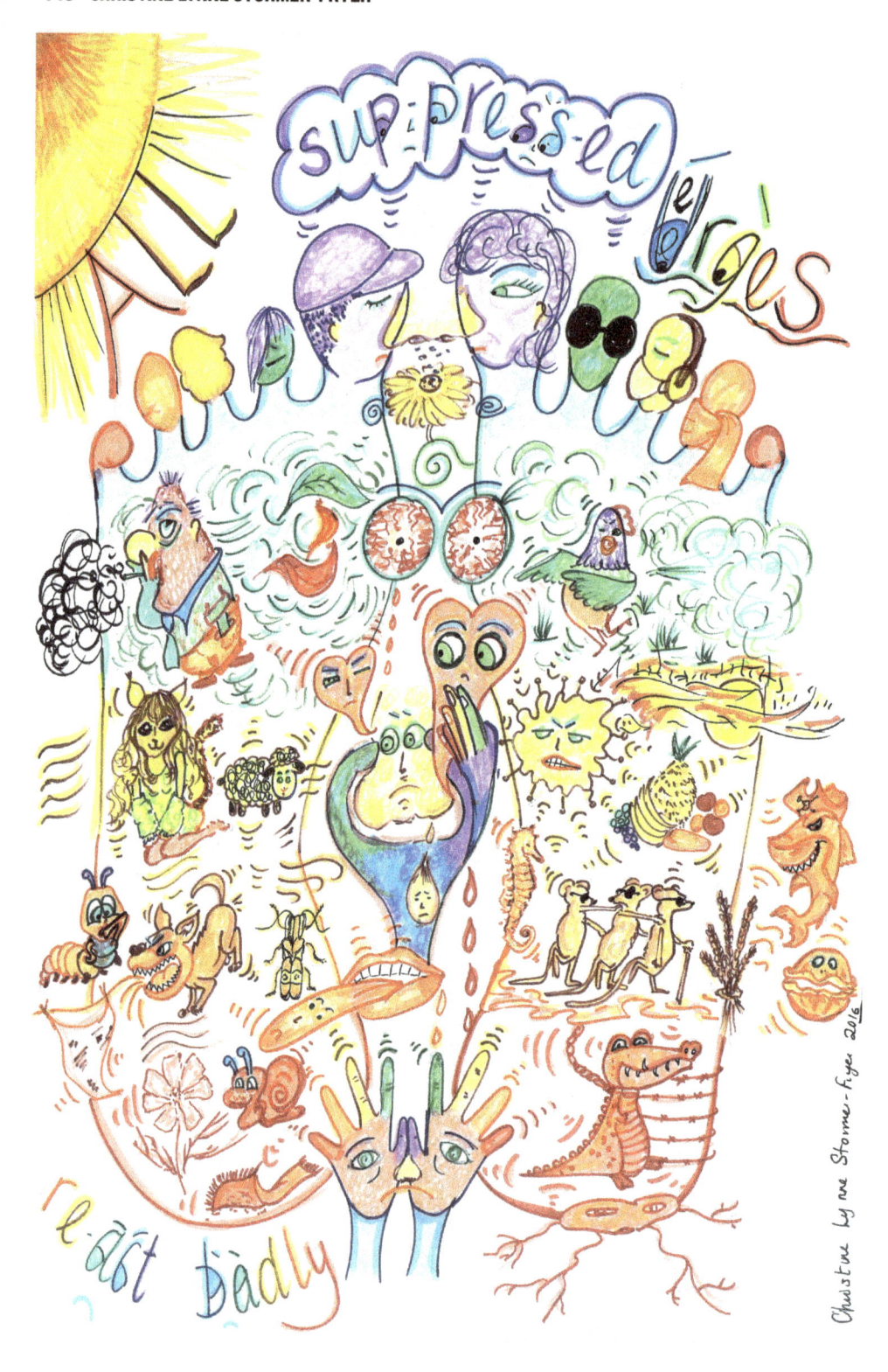

SUPPRESSED URGES

Urges come in all shapes and sizes, be it a strong impulse, a deep inner need, a desperate heartfelt desire, a profound wish, a genuine compulsion, or an absolute longing to be craved and yearned for. The more 'suppressed' yearnings are quashed, crushed, stifled, repressed, restrained, contained, curbed, smothered or concealed, the greater the reaction when a situation becomes unbearable. The mind violently objects, and the body reacts badly.

The external world has an uncanny knack of drawing attention to inner turmoil through 'allergies', which are simply a 'bad' reaction to 'all suppressed urges'. Elements are enlisted to intentionally upset the status quo. Air and wind stir wavering 'e-motions'. Fire agitates flames of injustice bursting into an '-itis', an 'infection'. Water 'rocks the boat' in unstable relationships. Earth-shattering events have the body trembling 'in its boots'.

Plagued by perturbed thoughts, everything comes to 'a head', making it 'ache' to 'get a-head' until at times it feels it may 'explode'. Bottling up all the various urges up, along with the strain of denying self-expression, is a throttling 'noose around the neck', preventing the possibility of 'scarfing' down food too quickly.

Irritated at the despicable scenes being witnessed, the eyes water and even 'see red', with broken blood vessels highlighting areas of deep sadness when innermost pleas are being denied. Putting on 'dark glasses' may reduce the sun's glare but not the glaring truth within. Disturbing 'e-motions' 'ruffle the feathers' and 'go straight to the chest', making the body 'cough up' when the internal environment, sometimes veiled in smoke, becomes overly contaminated.

'Hot and bothered' at denying oneself of coveted opportunities 'gets up the nose', with the occasional 'animated' response. Infuriated at being deprived of the 'fruits of one's labours' badly affects and infects – the body, with an erupting 'out-rage' that makes the 'blood boil'.

Aggravated and 'bugged' when 'led astray' by unwelcome 'sharks' hovering in murky waters, yet having to 'clam up' and 'zip the mouth', generates a sinking feeling, along with a sensation of drowning. Even though a dog's 'bark is worse than its bite', the frightful memory of being constantly 'barked at' can be a long-lasting deterrent.

Peeved at being snapped at for allegedly being 'rash', constantly 'going on and on' about 'dust shoved under the carpet' and opportunities fading fast, slows everything down to 'snail's pace' and soon gets under the 'skin'.

Two forces are constantly at work. The driving force urging action and the restraining force holding everything back. When restrained and stuck in fear, the blame and frustration escalate until things become unbearable. Losing sight of the Soul's innate needs is inevitable when overcome by tangential worries and feeling 'up to the neck in alligators'.

Patience harnesses the dynamic force, keeping the impetus to move 'a-head', regardless of any roadblocks. 'Taking things in one's stride', never giving up hope or letting go, and accepting delays or inconveniences without complaints or getting upset is the key to tolerating and dealing with whatever is 'dished up' en route.

Unearthing what makes mind and body tick takes a lifetime, but it is worth it!

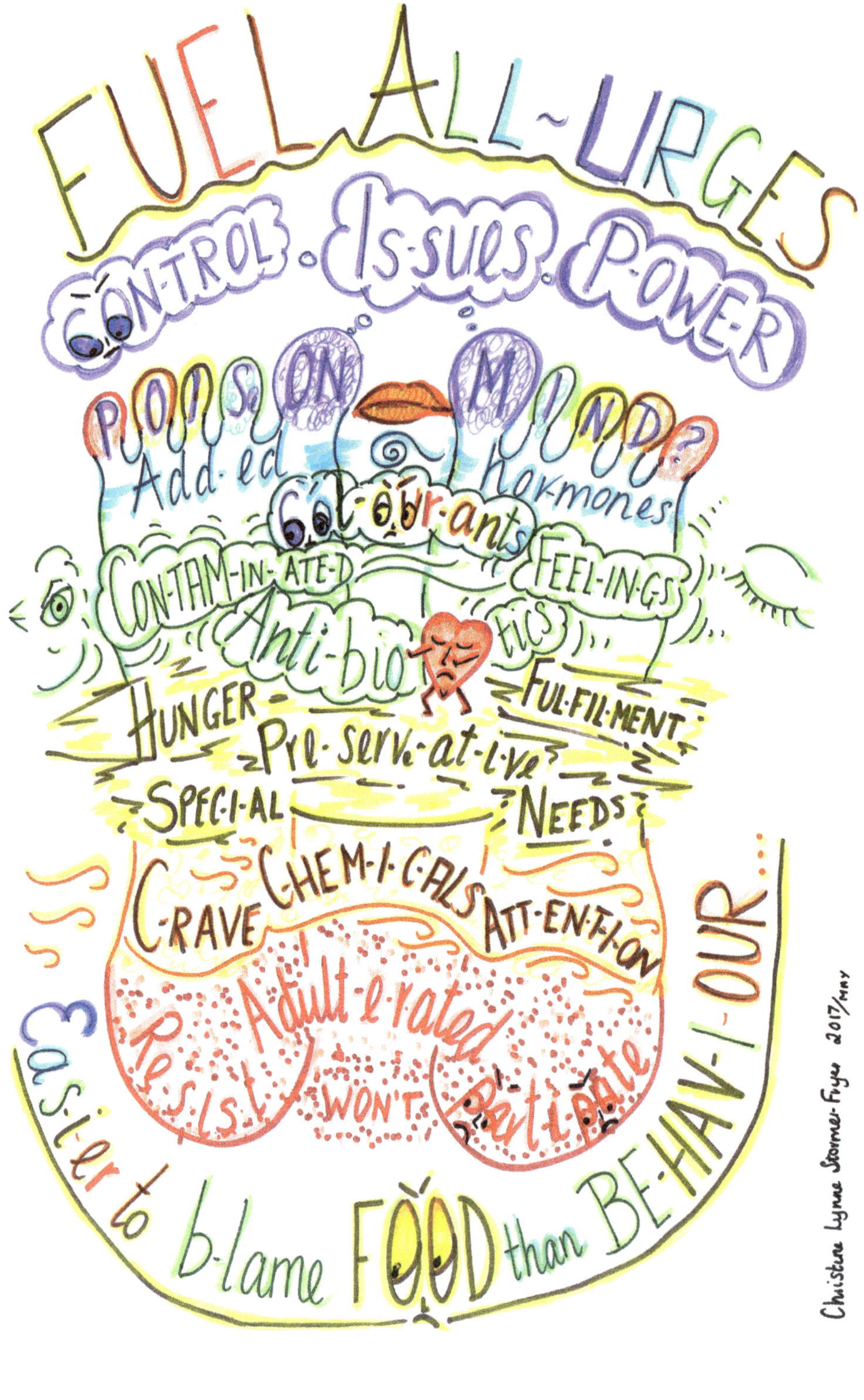

FUEL ALL~URGES
CON-TROL
IS-SUES
P-OWER
POISON
MIND?
Add-ed
hormones
Col-our-ants
CON-TAM-IN-ATE-D
FEEL-IN-GS
Anti-bio-tics
HUNGER
FUL-FIL-MENT
Pre-serv-at-i-ve
SPEC-I-AL
NEEDS
C-RAVE
CHEM-I-CALS
ATT-EN-T-I-ON
Adult-e-rated
Re-s-i-s-t
WON'T
Part-i-pate
Eas-i-er to b-lame FOOD than BE-HAV-I-OUR...
Christine Lynne Stormer-Fryer 2017/MAY

FUEL ALL URGES

According to the 'Law of Attraction', everything is energy, with 'like attracting like'. Invisible thoughts enter the mind to fuel the body, 'urging' it to take action. Fuelled by thoughts, each with its own magnetic frequency, the 'power of the mind' influences and affects all aspects of being human. Lower vibrational toxic notions poison mind and body, whereas innocuous ideas remain harmless.

Fuelling insatiable 'urges' is the unquenchable need to 'control' and be in a position of 'power', especially when feeling extremely insecure from having ignored inner strength and resources residing deep within. The distressed body 'urges' additional hormones to assist, but as the situation becomes increasingly 'out of hand', their effectiveness begins to decline.

Colourants are no substitute for tainted feelings that have lost their colour, corrupted by self-abuse. Anti-biotics are simply 'stepping-stones.' Not dealing with aggressive turbulent 'e-motions' annoys the body and 'gets on its wick'.

Fuelling 'hunger' is a completely 'different kettle of fish'. There are so many different types of hunger to cater to. 'Hunger for happiness' and the opportunity to make things happen. 'Hunger for joy' to be fulfilled when 'en-joy-ing' life to the full. 'Hunger for love' only realised when loving the self. 'Hunger for recognition' satisfied only once personal achievements are self-acknowledged. 'Hunger for peace' attained when at peace within.

An aversion to 'preservatives' is fuelled by an absolute loathing of old garbage 'dished up', with stuff being added to sustain it. Even worse is being pickled and squeezed to derive as much 'juice' as possible'.

Requiring special or additional needs is the Soul 'crying out' for exclusive attention, urging the need to 'dig deep' to get to the 'root of the issue'. The intense desire to be treated as 'special' is a longing to 'stand out' due to something unacceptable that happened that now 'craves attention'.

The 'urge' for chemicals is a desire for acceptable similarities that have not 'adult-e-rated' by 'adult' false 'ratings'. The natural resistance and refusal to participate becomes inevitable when society is rigidly biased and harshly unsympathetic.

'Ranting and raving' gets you nowhere fast. 'Blaming food is so much easier than blaming behaviour'. A habit picked up from a society used to experiencing life externally while refusing to acknowledge the turmoil within. Solutions remain on the periphery for fear of having to confront 'suppressed urges', with no idea what would happen if released.

Yet there is nothing that cannot be overcome with time, persistence, focused thought, and faith. There is always a solution, even for deeply entrenched and suppressed issues.

The grass is always greener when watered!

152 - CHRISTINE LYNNE STORMER-FRYER

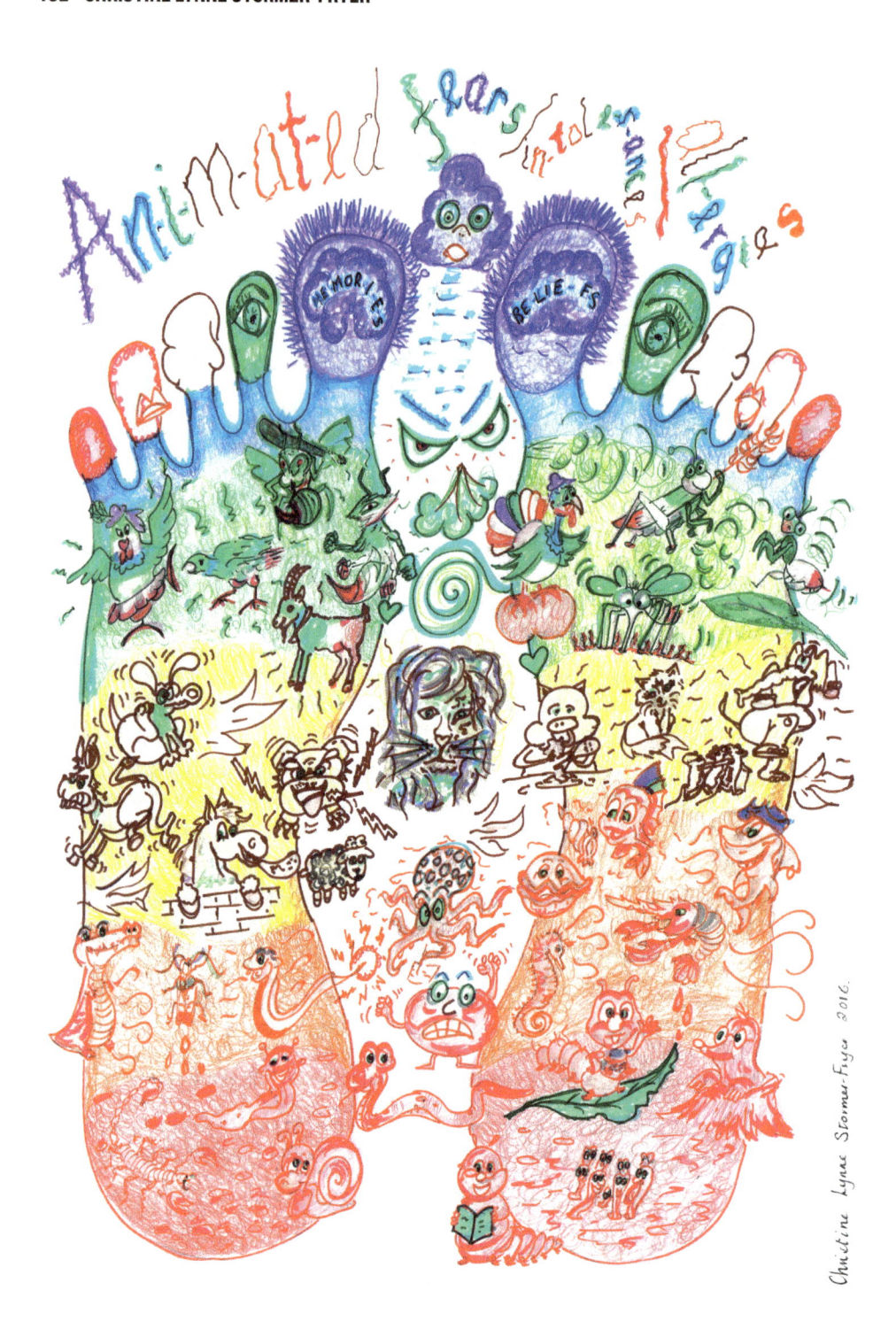

ANIMATED FEARS, INTOLERANCES AND ALLERGIES

Animated fears go back to vicious childhood memories allowed to evolve into terrifying beliefs, a horrific reminder of unacceptable animated or beastly behaviour of specific human beings with animals mirroring this deplorable conduct.

The mind, with its incredible imagination, has no idea what to believe. Is the 'whopper' fed to it real, or is it an intense fear haunting the brain? Acting on impulse, it reacts accordingly, prompted by what happened in the past. Clues as to the story behind the reaction come from the behaviour, and even the name, of specific creatures.

When unexpressed feelings get the 'upper hand', living creatures relying on air for 'motion' flutter in to stir 'e-motions'. It could be a bad reaction to a specific type of bird, or 'birds of a feather' 'flocking together', or a flying insect intent on 'bugging' the bejesus out of one. The mosquito, for one, takes great pleasure in 'sucking blood' to reveal feelings of being 'sucked dry'.

The body retaliates and reacts badly when stopped 'cold turkey' and prevented from doing the same thing again. Or when 'behaving like a dog' or being an absolute 'bitch'. Possibly 'eating like a pig', shovelling food down the throat in the most unpleasant and sloppy manner. Even doing the same old thing for 'donkey's years'. All from the 'horse's mouth'.

Relationships have a creepy way of 'bugging the hell' out of the body. Insects with wings have a dual role when partners get 'hopping mad', with uncalled-for irritation stressed by pesky grasshoppers. Meanwhile, 'locusts' reveal how the products of personal labours are being utterly ruined, leaving a trail of destruction behind.

Fish swimming around in circles or 'against the current', with the possibility of conflict around 'fishy business', could have fingers pointing to the unacceptable behaviour of a Piscean. Intolerance to 'shellfish' comes from being sick of 'selfish' behaviour, or irritated when 'clamming up' as soon as something important needs discussing.

At ground level, basic human behaviour is frequently animated by family and society. There is the scorpion (Scorpio) with its 'sting in its tail'. Others moving at a 'snail's pace' or with 'sluggish' behaviour, getting in the way of progress. In addition, blind moles 'leading the blind'. Just as devious is 'worming the way into another's life'. Or a 'bookworm' glued to the 'make-believe' chapters of life's events.

Animals and insects are extraordinary teachers, with an incredible knack of drawing attention to innermost issues by enacting human behaviour. True blessings from the Divine realm.

Animals help release archetypical energies!

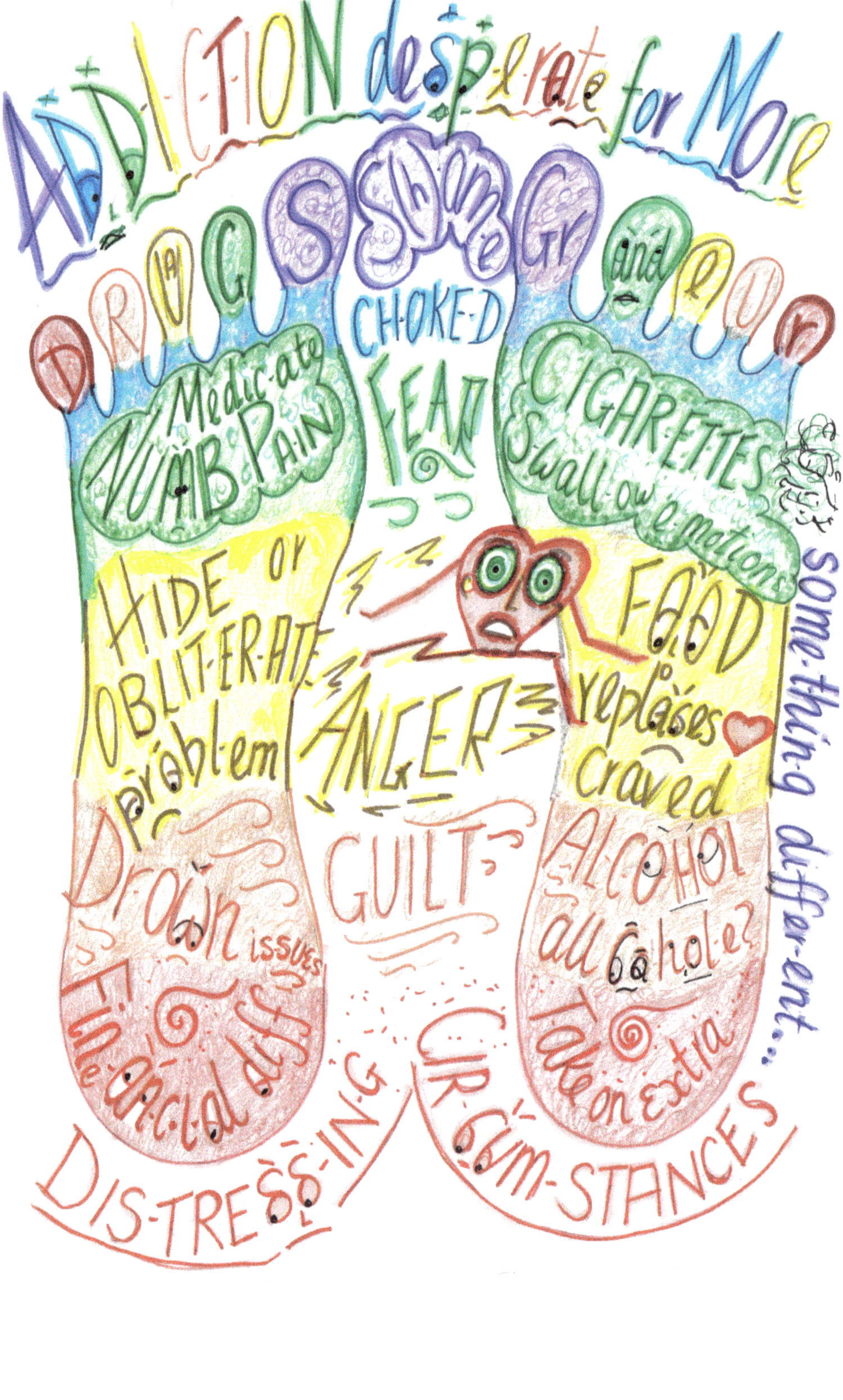
ADDICTION desperate for More
DRUGS
Shame
CHOKED
FEAR
Medicate NUMB PAIN
CIGARETTES Swall-ow emotions
HIDE OR OBLIT-ER-ATE problem
ANGER
FOOD replaces craved
some-thing dif-fer-ent...
GUILT
Drown issues
Financial diff
ALCOHOL all cahol-e?
Take on extra
DIS-TRESS-ING CIR-CUM-STANCES

ADDICTIONS – DESPERATE FOR MORE

Although addiction is considered a brain disorder, addicts are essentially highly-evolved Souls longing for something more, something deeper, and something greater. The roots stem from some form of dissatisfaction coming from the Spiritual dimension. Hence the reason for addiction being so misunderstood.

Every body has their own reasons, although one common aspect is 'isolation'. Feeling alone and awfully misjudged by a bigoted society that poisons the minds of the masses. A feeling of emptiness from not being authentic, yet wishing to detach from the discomfort of not 'fitting in', engenders a desperate search for the 'missing piece of the puzzle'.

Low self-worth, along with a pervasive sense of unhappiness, perpetuates addictive behaviour. Despite society's perception of the detrimental consequences of addictive substances, the repeated exposure to intrinsically rewarding stimuli fills a desperate urge throughout the day. As a form of escapism, it feels good. Easing the distress is a great way to obliterate reality.

The brain appreciates the relief of not having to deal with distressing circumstances, even if it is a form of avoidance. Instilled shame at not buying into adulterated beliefs and ridiculous restraints imposed by a narrow-minded society is vexing. 'Dragging' on 'drugs' takes the drudgery out of life. The mind wanders to other purer dimensions, filled with greater creativity, invariably offering illusions of opulence. Yet many end up 'hanging their heads' in perceived 'shame'.

'Up to the neck' and 'choked' with the drama of 'e-motional' trauma creates a deep desire to 'medicate' and 'numb the pain', or create a smokescreen. Both allow feelings to be 'swallowed', temporarily eradicating the 'fear' of being exposed as a fake.

Desperation for something different ignites an eclectic array of 'e-motions' such as frustration, resentment and anger. To be genuinely loved and completely understood is craved beyond anything else. Food offers a choice of substitutes for those wishing to 'hide' or 'obliterate' the authentic self. It also helps cover up all the 'guilt' and 'anger' emanating from the 'disease to please', and always trying to be 'perfect'.

'Al-c-0-hol' – 'all see the hole' within relationships – effectively drowns communication issues. It is perfect for freeing the entrapped Spirit. The frustration of constantly being 'shot down in flames' when opening the mouth to express more evolved or Spiritual stances on life is enough to 'drive any body to drink'. A way of drowning sorrows through 'Spiritual' relief. 'Having permission' to 'shout the mouth off' in utter frustration, or to 'keep the mouth shut', not bothering to 'waste the breath' is liberating.

As self-worth sinks to an 'all-time low', financial difficulties come to the fore. Hefty expenses entailed in purchasing addictive substances are a clue drawing attention to a desperate desire for appreciation. Social perceptions are the greatest culprits in driving spectacular individuals to despair, with highly opinionated groups of far-from-'polite' 'political' beings operating at a very low frequency, 'rubbing the noses' of the 'fallen' 'in the dirt', further contaminating mass opinions.

Always doing the best possible, regardless of other opinions, is the ideal way to feel fulfilled and personally satisfied. Remaining true to the Spirit within is all that is ultimately required.

Replace all thoughts of emptiness with the energy of completeness to feel fulfilled!

156 - CHRISTINE LYNNE STORMER-FRYER

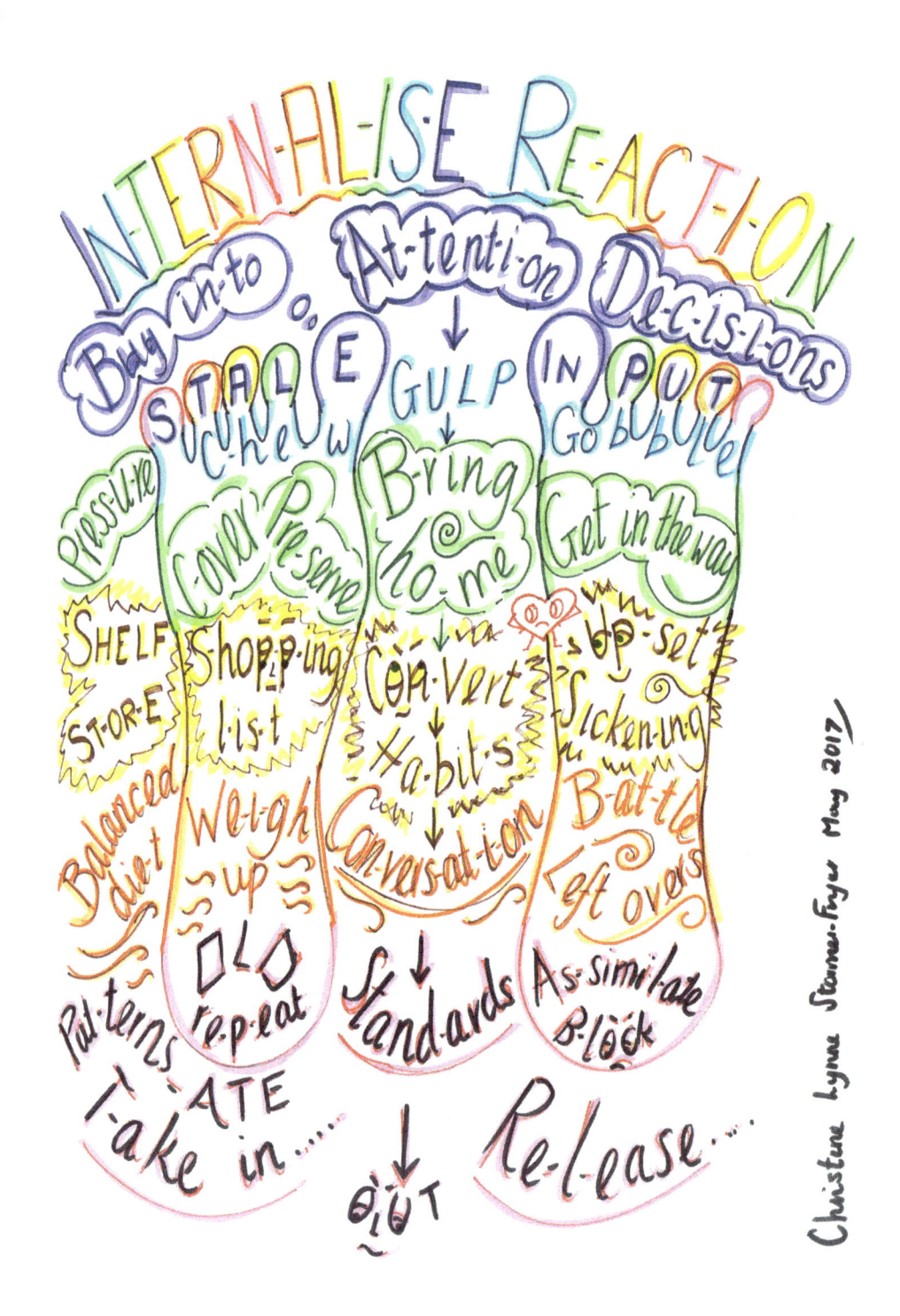

INTERNALISE REACTIONS

Internalisation is the conscious perception of the outer world given consideration within. Many ideals, like religion and Spirituality, are adopted and taken on board from a very early age and recalled when required. Integrated attitudes, incorporated values, adopted standards and assimilated opinions form the 'superego'. Self-moral socialisation starts in childhood, forming a sound basis from which to grow and develop.

Repeatedly 'buying into' stale notions, giving undue 'attention' to previous 'decisions', and expecting different outcomes, is asking for disaster. 'Gulping' with horror and ferociously 'gobbling' down the past, puts 'pressure' on the rest of the body.

With so much going on internally, the mind much prefers taking in and 'chewing' over fresh input. It pays more 'attention' to important matters of substance, making it far more 'decisive' about life in general.

Internalised, hectic 'e-motions' build up like a pressure cooker ready to 'let off steam'. Suppressing and concealing true feelings with additional 'pressure' coming from the side lines (family), numerous unresolved issues constantly get in the way. 'E-motions' in themselves are not bad. Managed in healthy ways, self-esteem is appreciatively boosted.

'Shopping lists' are based on goods labelled according to prior events. Anything considered 'bad' that is internalised and stored generates 'bad' reactions that are even worse when distasteful experiences have gone way past the 'use by date' required for character building.

'Shopping around' for something better is futile and confuses the digested matter. Sick to the stomach with constantly having to process old 'habits', the body craves opportunities to deal with 'new trends' Delightfully fresh 'nu-trients' to be converted into something meaningful and worthwhile.

Staying in a relationship out of fear puts the body under tremendous strain. The repetitive cycle of disempowering behaviour disrupts the 'balance'. 'Conversations' become battlefields. 'Weighing up' disagreeable odds and dealing with revolting 'leftovers' are made worse by not speaking up and verbalising the Soul's truth. A 'balanced diet' of equal 'give and take' is all that is required to equalise matters.

Varying amounts of distress stem from 'internalising' and 'assimilating' stern parental rules. 'Old' worn-out patterns constantly 'repeated' 'block' progress until a family member courageously 'puts a foot down' and 'stands up' to stop 'standards' from 'dropping' any further. The incorporation of cultural traditions and values either complicates or enhances core beliefs.

Everything is relative. The past still plays a vital role in contributing energy to the present with many words ending in 'ATE' – compassionate, deliberate, appreciate, and so on. It is processing this energy beneficially that allow true feelings to surface and then be authentically 'released'.

The roots of all goodness lie in the soil of appreciation!

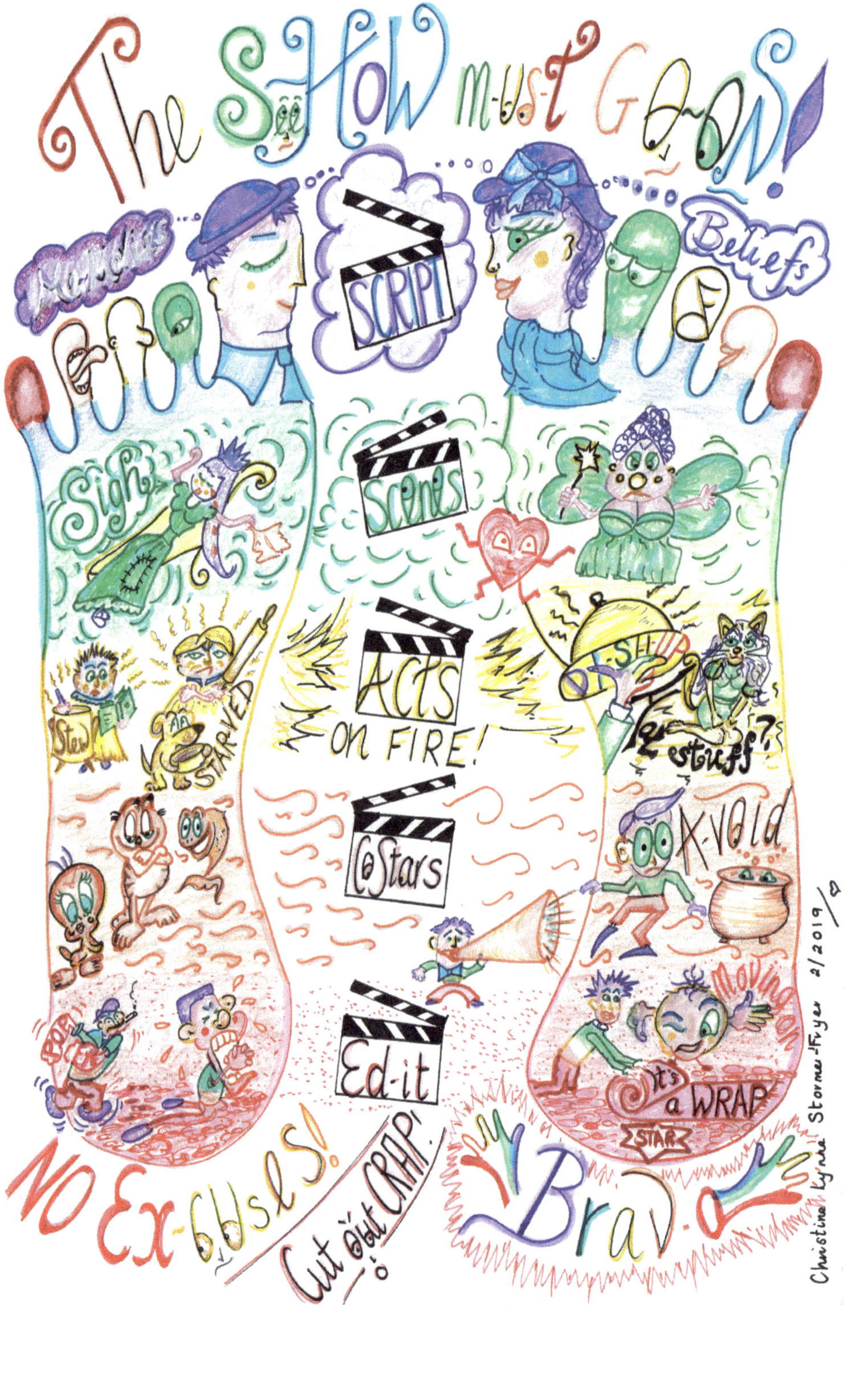
The SHOW must GO-ON!
Beliefs
SCRIPT
Sigh
Scenes
STARVED
Stew
Acts
ON FIRE!
stuffs?
A-void
CoStars
Ed-it
Moving on
It's a WRAP
STAR
NO EX-CUSES!
Cut out CRAP!
Brav-o
Christine Lynne Stormer-Fryer 2/2019

THE SHOW MUST GO ON

Even when floundering in the 'depths of despair', the 'show must go on'. Desperation has been around for as long as humanity has expressed itself. Yet, it is during the darkest moments that it is still possible to reach out from the 'doom and gloom' and find a 'glimmer of hope,' offered by the seeds of light, to emerge from deep sorrow.

Many great artists, gurus and visionaries have laboured through depression and hopelessness. While their lives serve as beacons in the darkness, it is up to individuals to find their own way out. There are no limitations, only self-imposed restraints. Changing restrictive philosophies sets the Spirit free and is incredibly empowering.

Formulating a new 'script' in the mind using 'high-concept' ideas is the first step in creating a masterpiece. Encouraging thoughts inspire and shape personal visions in many expressive ways to get innovative ideas across. The structure serves the 'story', 'hi-story'. As consciousness expands, it soon becomes evident that a great and wonderful world is out there to be discovered. As dormant forces, faculties and talents come alive, inner greatness unfolds.

When it comes to creating 'scenes', many choices come to the fore; to be the 'drama queen' immersed in pathetic self-pity or the 'Fairy Godmother' helping others make wishes come true. Taking deep breaths, knowing it is possible to emerge on the other side of troubled times, offers a whole new outlook, and more tolerant opinions. The heart knows the importance of 'keeping the beat'. How essential it is to look within and keep moving towards the light.

'Acts on fire' either terrify or inspire. 'Stewing' over the past wastes so much time and energy that little is left for the present, especially when there is a 'hard taskmaster'. 'Dishing up' 'passion' and being 'hot stuff' is far more exhilarating for the participants and the audience. All the little molecules wait eagerly for exciting new projects to keep evolving on a regular basis. 'Once off' is just not 'good enough'.

It is tempting to avoid co-stars who are 'not on the same page', along with those acting 'out of character' to 'steal the show'. More reason to always be 'authentic' and 'act the part', selecting the most appropriate and tasteful words in case of having 'to eat them' later.

When 'it's a wrap' and time to 'edit', 'cutting the crap' without 'excuses' is essential. Even with the audience on their feet shouting "Bravo!", suitable changes are still required to move onto the next stage. Formidable inner resources help to address any challenges, with a 'helping hand' from reliable family members and friends. The truest end to life is knowing that life never ends.

Remember you make the world more special just by being in it!

160 - CHRISTINE LYNNE STORMER-FRYER

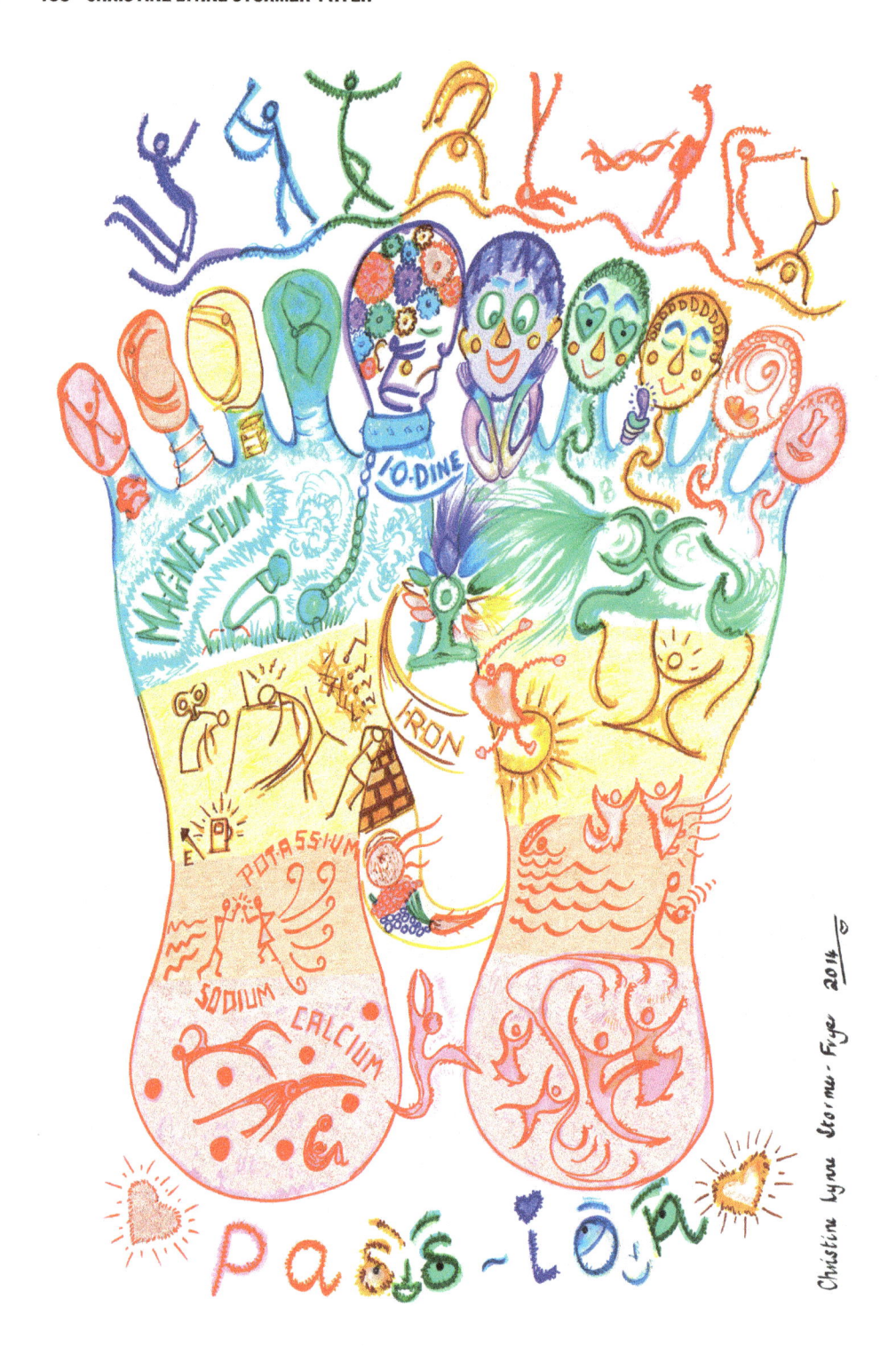

VITAMINS - ENERGY

Vitamins and supplements step in when mind and body need boosting, despite being quite capable of 'standing on their own two feet' and revitalising themselves. Vitality comes from the effervescent essence of life. The more energy and enthusiasm put in, the greater the vitality available. It all depends on which aspects of the body are involved.

Vitamin 'E' (alpha-tocopherol) for instance, is the 'Eager' vitamin, 'enthusiastically' 'extracting' fresh universal input from the 'ethereal' realm. 'Exciting' new concepts and ideas keep all cells animated and 'on their toes', along with Zinc, fondly known as the 'zing mineral', adding a zest for life, 'enhancing' the brain's 'efficiency' in hypothesising.

Vitamin 'A' (retinol), aka the 'adjustment' vitamin, 'augments' the eyes' 'ability' to 'appreciate' all that is seen when looking through a new set of lenses, especially at night when 'anxious' about being 'in the dark ' and having to grope 'around' to find 'answers'. All this 'attributes' to feeling 'at ease' within one's own skin and less vulnerable, making 'keeping the nose clean' more 'attainable'. Iodine is the 'I mineral' 'immersed' in the 'I'. 'Adjusting' misleading 'illusions', it makes sure that 'I' is seen to make a good 'impression'. Both are responsible for 'illustrating' 'individuality' in an 'illustrious' way to 'improve' personal 'image'.

Vitamin 'B1' (thiamine 1) likes to 'Be One of a kind', while vitamin B2 (riboflavin) is more of a 'Be True to yourself' vitamin, and Vitamin B12 (cobalamin) tends to 'be perfect' in every way. All the B vitamins are friendship vitamins, all about 'b-eing' authentic. 'B'eing water-soluble, they are responsible for 'going with the flow' by 'just b-eing', either being a 'co-factor' and catalyst with the courage to inspire, or a visionary 'precursor' showing the way.

Then there is magnificent magnesium 'managing' the state of the nerves, 'manifesting' 'marvellous' outcomes, and 'maintaining' a 'magnificent' state of 'b-eing'. Along with 'sodium', the heart's incredible 'magnitude' becomes increasingly 'significant' as it effortlessly 'sends' out love and joy to 'sustain' all cells and 'support' all the body's 'movements'.

Vitamin D, the 'doing' vitamin, likes 'making hay while the sun shines'. Warming the heart and strengthening the body 'does' a lot to make a world of 'difference'. No fishy business required. With 'iron', the 'inspirational' mineral, 'ironing' out the creases to 'smooth things over', it also 'ignites' the flames of passion, 'injecting' enthusiasm and strength throughout the whole.

Vitamin C, considered the camaraderie vitamin, 'consistently' 'contributes' towards the inner strength of teeth, encouraging them to be 'conclusive' when deciding what to 'chew' over and what to 'censure'. It also provides the 'capacity' and 'capability' to 'stand out from the crowd'. Its partner, potassium, as the performing mineral 'proffers' energy of ongoing 'perceptions', vital for 'playing 'authentic roles with 'passion' ensuring that the 'charisma' is 'puffed' up with 'pride'.

Vitamin K, the 'kindness' vitamin, uses 'knowledge' obtained from life experiences to 'kerb' combustible 'e-motions'. 'Keeping' up to date with the latest trends goes 'hand in hand' with calcium, the 'come and see mum' mineral. 'Comforting' and 'co-operative', it 'calms' 'concerns' by 'constructing' a strong and 'cheerful' inner 'core'.

All energies interweave and fit together like a perfect puzzle to constantly revitalise the whole!

162 - CHRISTINE LYNNE STORMER-FRYER

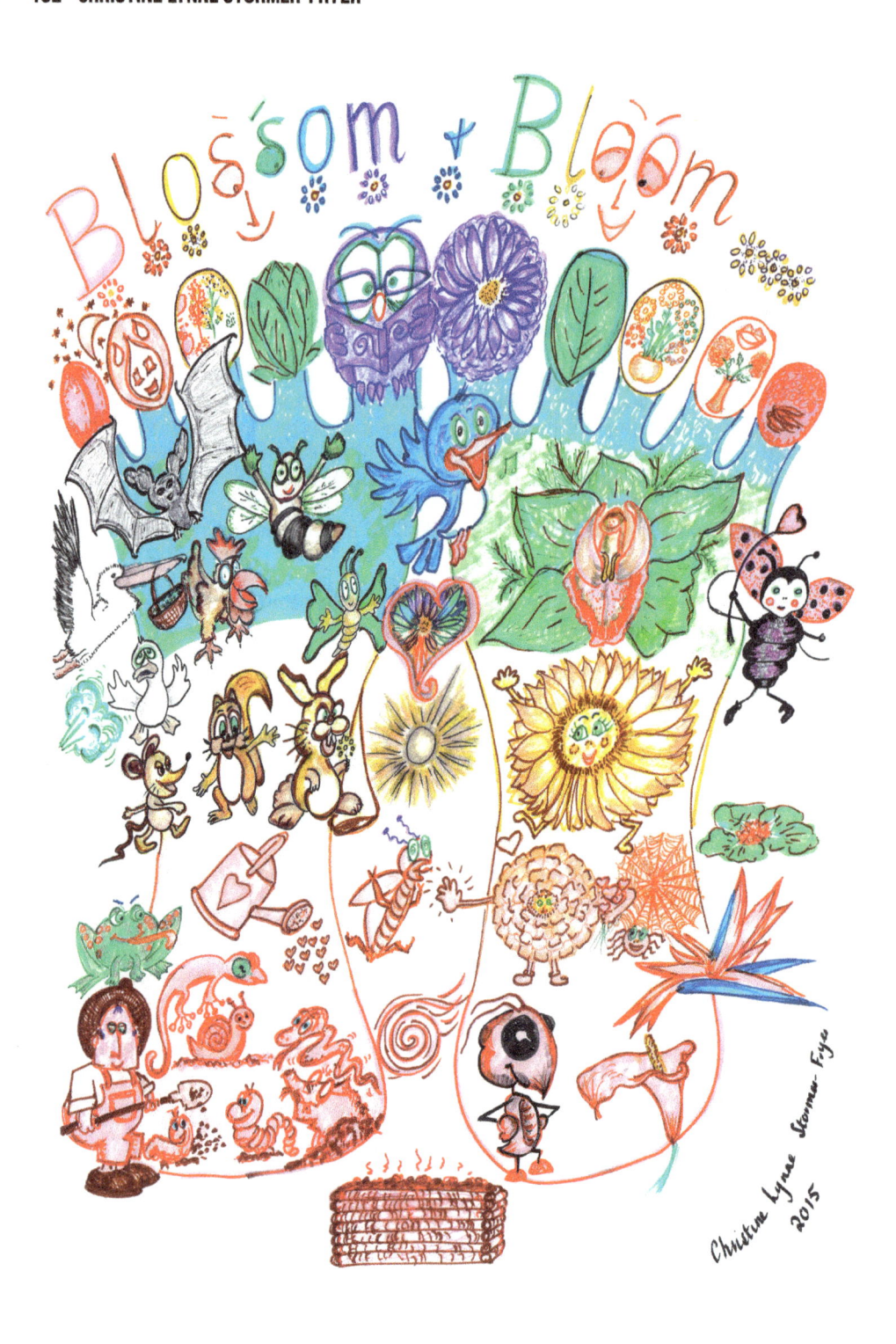

BLOSSOM AND BLOOM

The very best blooms come from the very best seeds. Thoughts are the seeds that encourage the body to flourish when cultivated well. Family and social situations provide ideal grounding and soil conditions, no matter how disadvantageous the circumstances may seem. Meaningful communications determine the availability of water. The healthier the relationships, the better the supply. Abundant sunshine encourages active growth for enduring progress. Plenty of air and space guarantee a favourable emotional environment, with ongoing love and encouragement being vital.

Every moment is ideal for opening up to blossom and bloom. Having taken root, there are endless opportunities to become established and extend the heart's energies. Even when conditions do not seem ideal, it is a matter of embracing and making the most of what is available. Times of vulnerability are inevitable, but hope springs eternal when having faith in Divine Timing.

The effervescent ingredient required is 'desire'. Just as each flower has its own shape, colour and dimensions as it moves through many life stages, so too do humans when reconnecting with the Soul's essence. Every moment of every stage has its own essential beauty. In time, blossoms drop their petals, wilt, and even fold back on themselves, having made the most of enriching the environment with their glorious display.

As moments come and go with every sunrise and sunset, and with each 'hello' and 'goodbye', gratitude for the pulsating ebb and flow of being alive thrills and enlivens the heart. So much so that in days gone by, men would 'go gathering orange blossoms' and look for a wife. A phrase referring to the bride's 'innocence' – 'inner sense'.

Second toes and balls of feet, like petals, rely on air and space to enlarge the Spirit and show their true colours. Using the sun's rays to photosynthesise light energy into chemical energy, flowers know how to energise themselves. The fiery third toes and passionate upper halves of both insteps also reveal the body's amazing ability to process life force energies.

Moisture from dew maintains a vital energy exchange. A process stimulated by the fourth toes and lower halves of both insteps. The flower provides inner resources and pollen to generate budding new beginnings. In the body, it is the ovaries that create new concepts, stimulated by a fertile mind.

Companion planting is all about establishing mutually beneficial communities. An organic way to protect whatever is being cultivated while enhancing individual performances. Monocultures and being planted in rows en masse are not the way to go. Bunched together makes them easy targets for pests, with the subsequent uneasiness spreading rapidly through the ranks.

Taller specimens provide shade and protection for those with a tendency to bolt. Effectively repelling unwelcome bugs are the strongly scented leaves of herbs, while others attract beneficial species.

So it is within human relations. Using the assets of one to benefit another means that every body has a chance to 'blossom and bloom', even if only for a brief while. Yet the beautiful memory lasts forever.

Every flower is the Soul blossoming in nature!

Know Length of Feet!

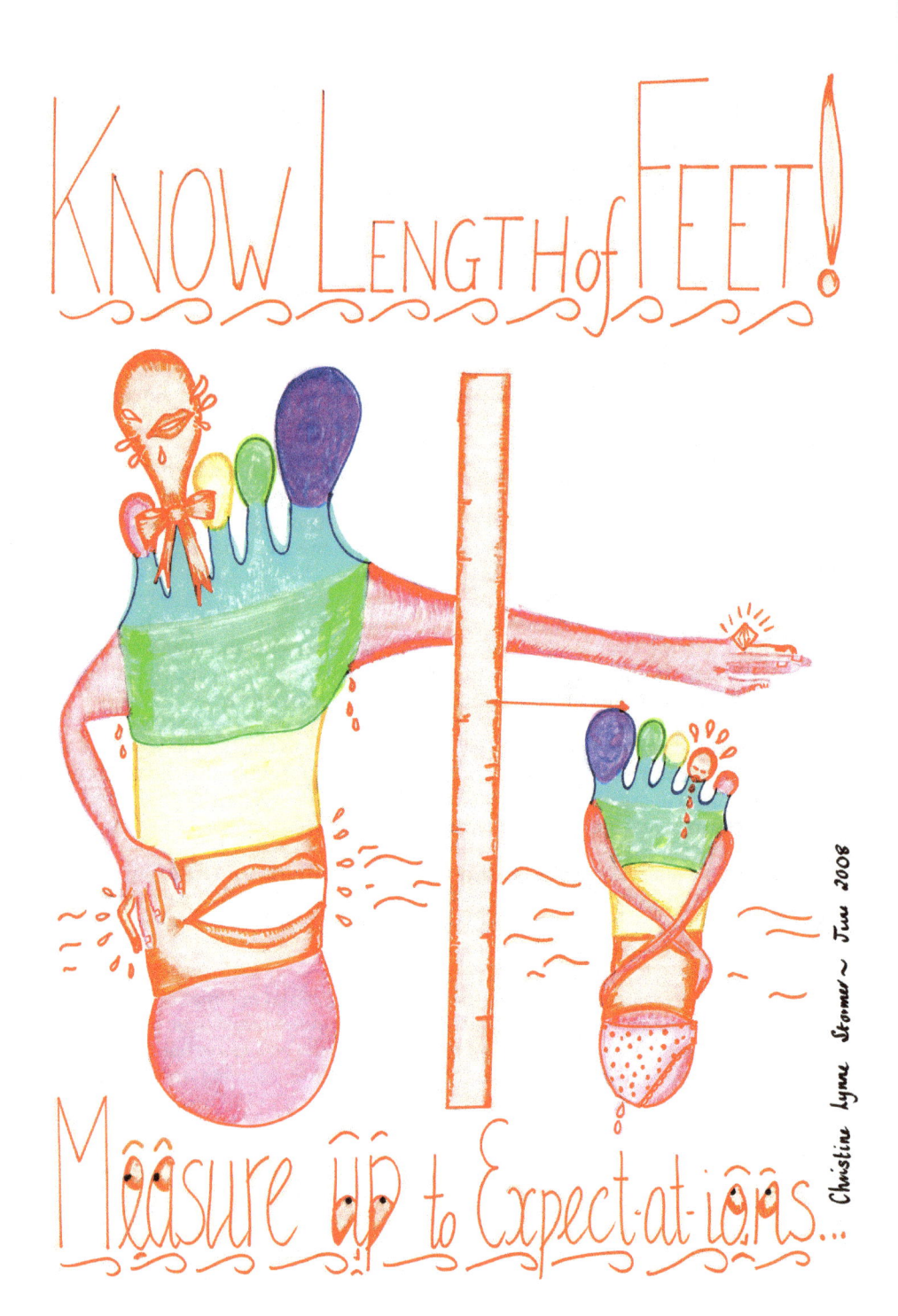

Measure up to Expect-at-ions...

KNOW THE LENGTH OF THE FEET - MEASURE UP TO EXPECTATIONS

'Measuring up' and feeling good enough can be challenging in such a 'goal-oriented society'. Constantly comparing and worrying becomes a destructive habit. Yet worrying does not empty today of its sorrow but of its strength, giving small things big shadows.

Stress in itself does not concern the mind and upset the body. It is inability to 'cope' and 'not making the grade' that triggers 'dis-tress', building up explosively inside until it erupts, creating absolute havoc, internally and externally.

Set expectations invariably lead to disappointment. Living a life to achieve so-called 'perfection' is to live in a state of constant fear. Believing in 'perfection' in a non-perfect world is absolutely pointless. Some perfectionists do not speak for fear of saying the incorrect thing. Others do nothing for fear of doing wrong. A holdover from childhood, 'perfectionism' is the confusing ideal inherited from demanding parents.

The road to 'perfection' is a linear one, fraught with rigidity. Making a mistake and not 'cutting the mustard' when unable to reach or surpass a desired standard is an essential part of experimenting and experiencing. 'Perfection' and 'striving for excellence' are completely different. The 'perfect' life only exists when a better one is no longer craved.

It is human nature to keep 'measuring up' against others and comparing, conveniently forgetting that everyone is a 'one-off'. Looking for faults is meaningless. Nobody is better, and nobody is worse. Everybody is incomparable. Each has a specific role to play and is accordingly equipped to 'step into those shoes'. Acknowledging and embracing special qualities is to appreciate gifts from above.

Drowning in a 'sea of expectations' and unable to 'live up' to them is painful and humiliating, creating a sense of inferiority over not being able to 'crack it' or 'meet with approval'. The pressure of having to 'be up to snuff' and 'make the grade' is nerve-racking for the colon. The utter devastation of having to perform uncharacteristically puts huge pressure on the intestines. Irritated beyond words, its petulance becomes evident when afflicted with the 'irritable bowel syndrome'.

It takes courage to be self-referential and 'measure up to personal standards'. Valuing uniqueness and focusing on the goodness within, and in others, brings out best in every body.

Without expectations, life becomes liberating and exhilarating. Expecting the best in life is to 'expect the unexpected'. Unpredicted twists and astonishing turns, filled with endless surprises and possibilities, enrich the experience. Ultimately, every need is met.

The measure of love is loving without measure!

166 - CHRISTINE LYNNE STORMER-FRYER

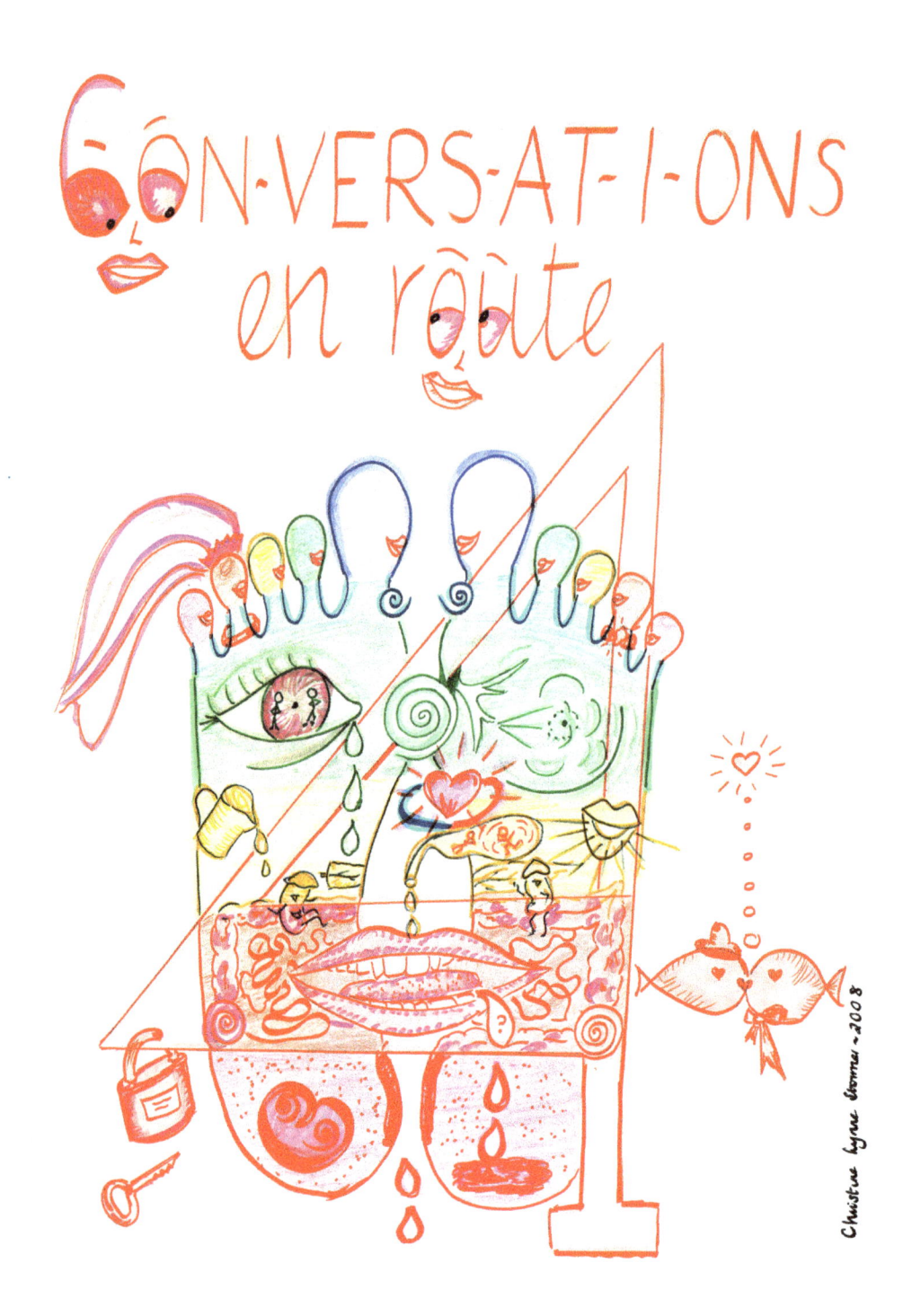

CONVERSATIONS EN ROUTE

Throughout life's journey, conversations en route invariably influence the next step. They also determine the choices of directions taken.

Fourth toes pick up the brain's interpretation of these exchanges, with the number 4 being responsible for decoding the connection between everything, especially when persistence and endurance are required. The impact of the spoken word profoundly affects the lower digestive system and lower-middle back, reflected onto the tops and bottoms of both feet from the waistlines of the feet to the start of the heels.

With so much more lying beneath what is said, irritating conversations that 'go against the grain' infuriate the brain. Unspoken nuances, such as a fraction of a frown, a flicker of an eyelid or a nonchalant shrug of the shoulders, subtly affect the context, eventually 'getting on the nerves'. Bringing a 'smile to the dial' are a twinkle in the eye, a glimmer of a grin, or a delightful change in the tone of voice, all of which uplift the Spirit.

Using clever put-downs, amusing meaningless insults, intentional misunderstanding, zippy wise-cracks, flirtatious zingers, and fun puns in a verbal war of wit may be amusing to some but 'taken the wrong way' can be insulting and offensive to others. The secret to appearing 'smart' is to stay quiet and allow others to do the talking. People invariably find their own conversations far more interesting anyway. Involved in matters of the heart, placing a ring on the fourth finger embodies commitment within a relationship based on trust.

Everybody has a lot to say but do not always know how to say it. Words get stuck in the throat when overcome by fear. Not wishing to participate is asphyxiating. Gagging the throat hinders exchanges between the outer and inner worlds as well as between the upper and lower bodies, both physically and Spiritually.

Eyes get 'e-motionally' involved, 'seeing what they believe, but not always believing what they see'. Personal identity, defined through dialogue, depends on 'which way the wind blows', swaying opinions, no matter how ludicrous.

The art of conversation is the art of hearing as well as being heard. Essential to socialisation is relating to others by finding 'common ground'. Conversations then become an opportunity to expand personal horizons through the 'give and take' of information. When the co-operative principles are not adhered to, situations rapidly deteriorate, bringing the conversation, and possibly the liaison, to a standstill or even to an end.

Intestines are not amused. Constantly stretched and re-stretched, swaying between dysfunction to passion, puts tremendous strain on the innards. It takes re-inventing the true meaning of conversation to make them settle down.

The best conversations are remembered not for their content but for the exquisite feelings evoked.

All conversations should be magnetic experiences!

168 - CHRISTINE LYNNE STORMER-FRYER

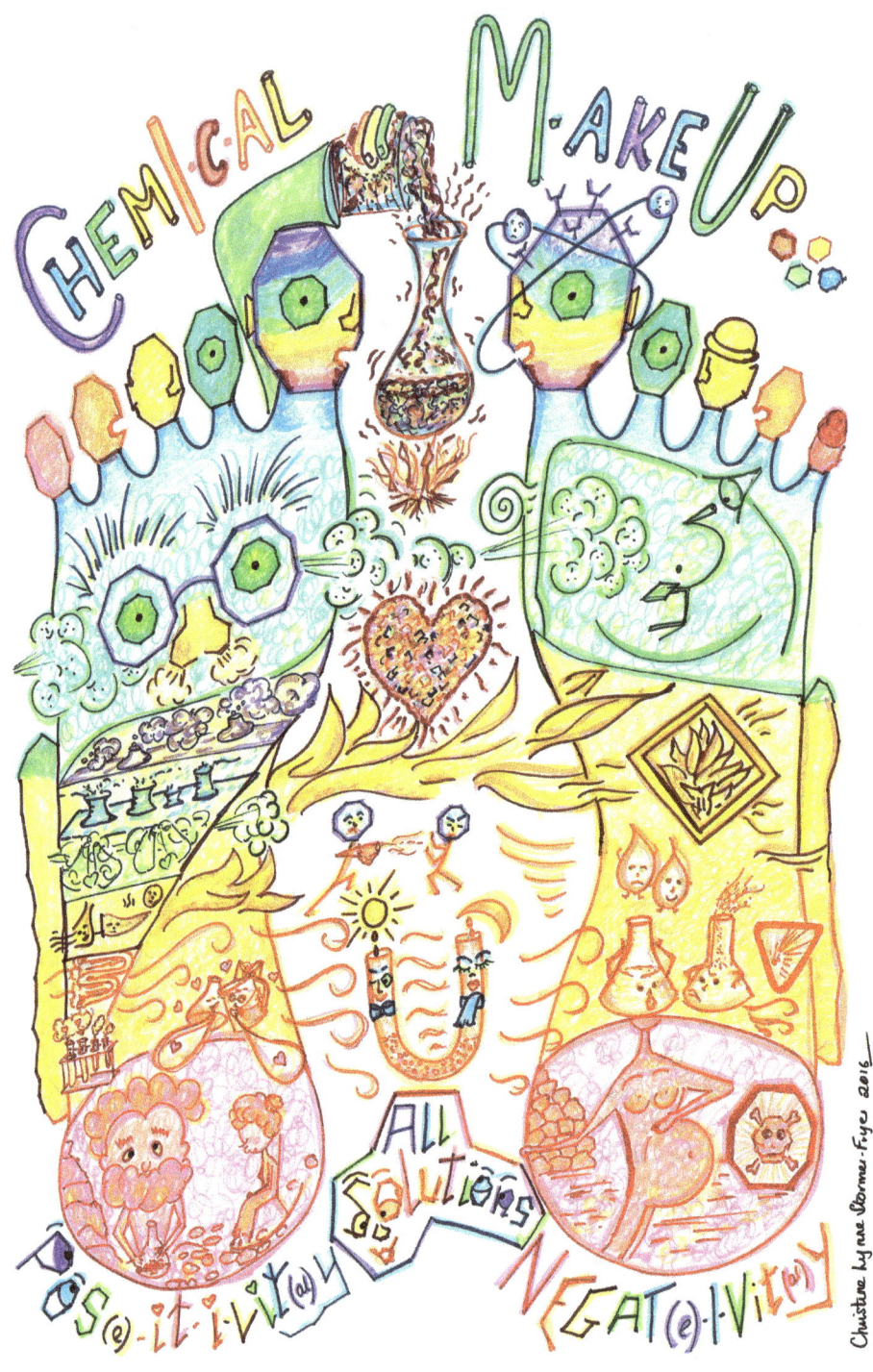

CHEMICAL MAKE-UP

Chemistry between two individuals evokes complex 'e-motional' reactions and mystical changes. Neither is random, nor a fluke, with hormones romancing the senses being the first step towards ongoing attraction. Strong chemistry makes for a wild ride of love. The sudden rush of 'e-motions' can be scary. Suppressed issues erupt, offering opportunities to become a fuller version of oneself.

Magnetic qualities, such as reciprocal candour, mutual interests, personality similarities and physical attraction, draw people together. Captivated and infatuated without any apparent rhyme or reason, even after only exchanging a couple of words.

The allure is a fascinating amalgamation of every aspect of 'being human'. With chemistry being so highly 'e-motive', the 'windows to the Soul' are drawn in, with love entering and leaving by the eyes. Yet egotistical feelings, such as jealousy, contempt, judgement and doubt, invariably jostle for attention, being solely responsible for bad reactions when evoked.

The lessons of love are many. A multitude of qualities that evolve en route, whether hidden, desired or lacking, 'come to light'. Even when others choose not to continue along the same path, valuable insights are derived as chemical reactions have already taken place.

Complications arise from each human being a complex compilation of components. Opposites *do* attract, provided there is some form of common interest. Speaking the same language with tell-tale smiles, along with pleasant sounds of silence, creates a deep understanding. Meaningful conversations reinforce this inter-connectedness.

Long-lasting, loving relationships require sticking together and dealing with inevitable challenges. Intense feelings are invariably triggered. Some positive, others not so pleasant. Once solutions to each issue are found, the bond is strengthened and enhanced. With no body being 'perfect', every body is capable of repelling and attracting. Respect is the key ingredient in forming 'healthy' relationships. Greater 'chemical bonds' with atoms held together are formed with trust, openness and dependability.

Everybody has the chemical ('c-h-e-m-i-c-al' – 'See he/her $_{in}$ m$_{e\ then}$ I see all') makeup of every thought ever entertained, every 'e-motion' ever felt, every action and reaction ever experienced, and every conversation ever exchanged, mixed with fragments of ancestral energies, all put into a giant test tube, shaken until well mixed, and then dispensed into human form.

The world of chemical reactions is the stage on which scene after scene is perpetually played. The actors are the elements, while Earth provides the ideal surface, with water ensuring the flow.

A chemical reaction is touching the arm and setting the heart alight with love!

170 - CHRISTINE LYNNE STORMER-FRYER

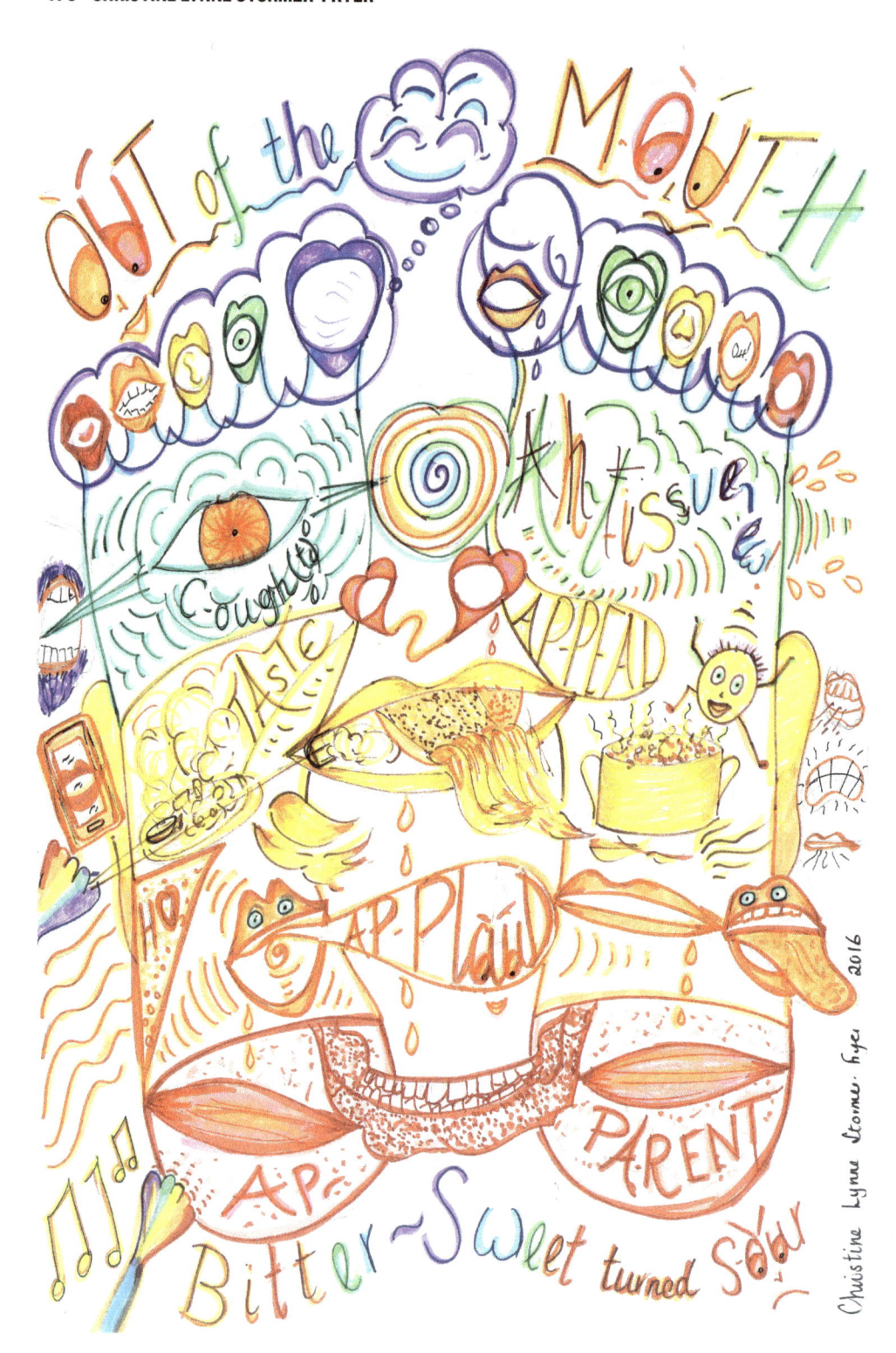

OUT OF THE MOUTH

'Out of the mouths of babes' comes honesty, until adulterated 'words are put into the mouth'. As the organ of communication and avenue of expression and creativity, words formed in the mouth are meant to make personal needs and inner desires known.

Instead, the mouth is often used to criticise, demand or manipulate and occasionally to praise. 'Tell-tale' signs are the set of lips and jaws instantly conveying the mood. Whether a new idea, innovative concept or some form of nourishment being 'taken in', the mouth always shows its approval or disapproval. Having chewed things over and swished the various aspects of life around its vestibule, it is prone to 'giving a mouthful' and saying exactly what is 'on the mind'.

Seething and fuming, with 'smoke going down the throat', the body quickly dispenses with these raging irritants, 'coughing' them out the mouth. The lungs are particularly intolerant and cannot wait to expel noxious 'e-motions' that take up precious space and smoulder inside. Forced to 'cough up' something after a period of evasion, or to surrender the lead of a game, can be humiliating. But not as humbling as 'puking' when 'sick to the stomach' after having 'to rinse the mouth out with soap and water'.

'Shooting the mouth off' instead of 'putting money where the mouth is' is in 'bad taste'. In cahoots with the nose, the mouth finds a 'discerning taste' more appealing, especially when laced with a 'taste of imminent success'. As 'taste buds are teased' the 'mouth waters' in delightful anticipation.

As an outlet for innermost feelings, 'laughing on the wrong side of the mouth' (showing chagrin or embarrassment), or 'laughing out the other side of the mouth' (shifting from happiness to vexation) are quite different from 'keeping the mouth shut' or keeping a secret.

It is quite 'ap-parent' that many 'bitter-sweet' words have been deceptively shoved into and then entertained in the mouth, leaving a 'sour' taste that often eats away at the lining ulcerating its cavity, or smelling foul with 'halitosis'.

'Many mouths to feed' is quite a responsibility. Having to earn enough to do so can leave many 'down-in-the-mouth'. 'Making a wry mouth' is justified when stupidly 'placing the head in the lion's mouth' and being utterly reckless. To 'shoot the mouth off' and speak about sensitive issues without discretion is so irritating. Bragging boastfully makes the intestines cringe with embarrassment. Words of reassurance and encouragement are always welcome to soothe things over.

It is quite 'appalling' how often 'words are taken out of the mouth'. 'Leaving a bad taste' is 'putting the foot in it' and making a huge blunder. 'Talking out of both sides of the mouth' while trying to please everybody is bound to eventually 'set the teeth on edge'. When floundering in doubt, it is so much more effective to just smile.

Constantly communicating with inner and outer worlds through speech, eating, and kissing, the mouth uses every experience as an opportunity to understand how to satisfy heartfelt desires.

Being the master of the mouth prevents being a slave to its words!

172 - CHRISTINE LYNNE STORMER-FRYER

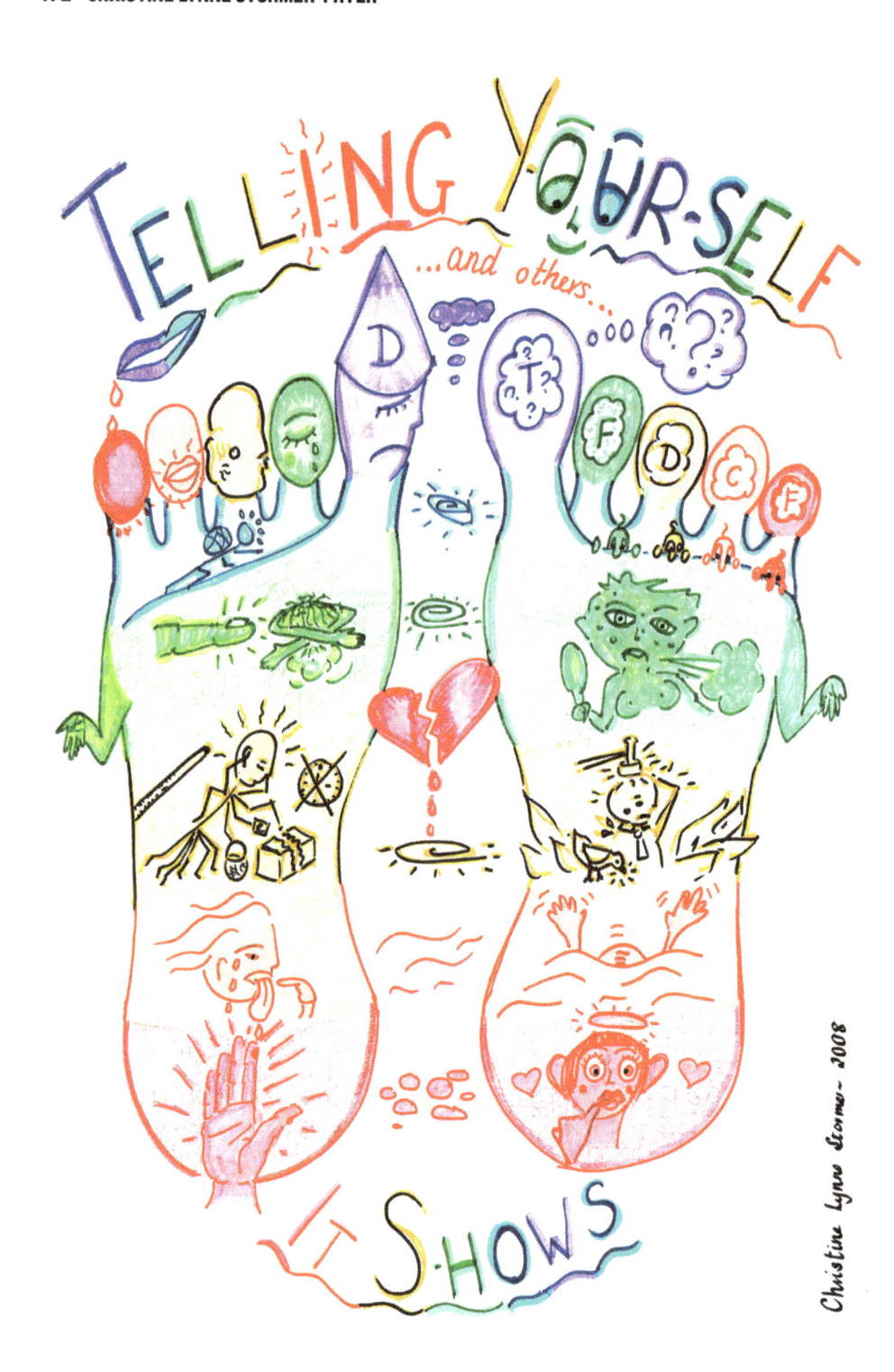

TELLING YOUR-SELF AND OTHERS – IT SHOWS

The unspoken word is exceptionally empowering, especially when told to oneself. Throughout waking hours, self-talk is natural. However, spending a lot of the time entertaining 'non-sense' ultimately affects the quality of life.

The innate tendency is to 'personalise' everything and 'take the blame', 'magnifying' situations by throwing everything completely out of proportion, by focusing on the negative, or, 'catastrophising' the situation by expecting the worse without reason or logic, or 'polarising' with labels of 'bad or good' or 'black or white' with no in-between.

Negative self-talk can be terrifying. It is a form of self-torture. Formulating what to say and how to say it by repeatedly replaying the same old gremlins of the past generates cringe-worthy thoughts that torment the Soul. Being so extremely anxious and needlessly worried can eventually lead down a dark tunnel to a deep hole of depression.

Typical self-talk agendas include over-thinking, over-generalising, and over-reacting. Convictions about being stupid or incapable are intensified through a fear of being the subject of gossip. Torturous thoughts twist the mind and distort the feet, showing just how much bowing and bending is required when attempting to try and please everybody. Terror, insecurity and bewilderment rigidify the whole, making change seem impossible.

Beliefs that 'life is one long battle' and an 'uphill' journey of 'doom and gloom' is a lot for the shoulders to bear. Weighed down by overwhelming responsibilities mentally thrust upon them is hurtful, with prickly feelings of disgruntlement often extending down the arms.

Memories of always being 'in the wrong' as a child and constantly being belittled by 'Peter Pointer', the accusing index finger, are reinforced by mirrors serving as 'ugly' reminders. Mentally rummaging over the resentment and frustration of being 'ruled by an iron rod' in a strict and often cruel way can impose tremendous pressure on personal undertakings, and how they are executed. 'Stopped' by ridiculous rules and regulations and attempting to be the 'Angel' of the family by succumbing to society's demands, cripples the Soul and dampens the Spirit.

It's a back-breaking slog to keep 'bending over backwards' 'to put out fires' and 'fight the way through life', which strains the back and upsets digestion, making it extremely difficult to process life. Piling one pitiful conversation onto another about feeling abandoned and deserted, with a 'nobody cares' attitude creeping into the scenario, along with 'all that others think about is themselves', in an overwhelming wave of self-pity unsettles the intestines. Having a 'gut's full' results in 'hanging onto the SH1T' and getting constipated, or 'running' as fast as possible to get away from all the crap.

Freeing the mind of drama and feeding it with an abundance of positive self-talk enhances not only personal performance and well-being but also attracts delightful like-minded Souls into its orbit.

Self-talk is the ideal channel for behaviour change!

174 - CHRISTINE LYNNE STORMER-FRYER

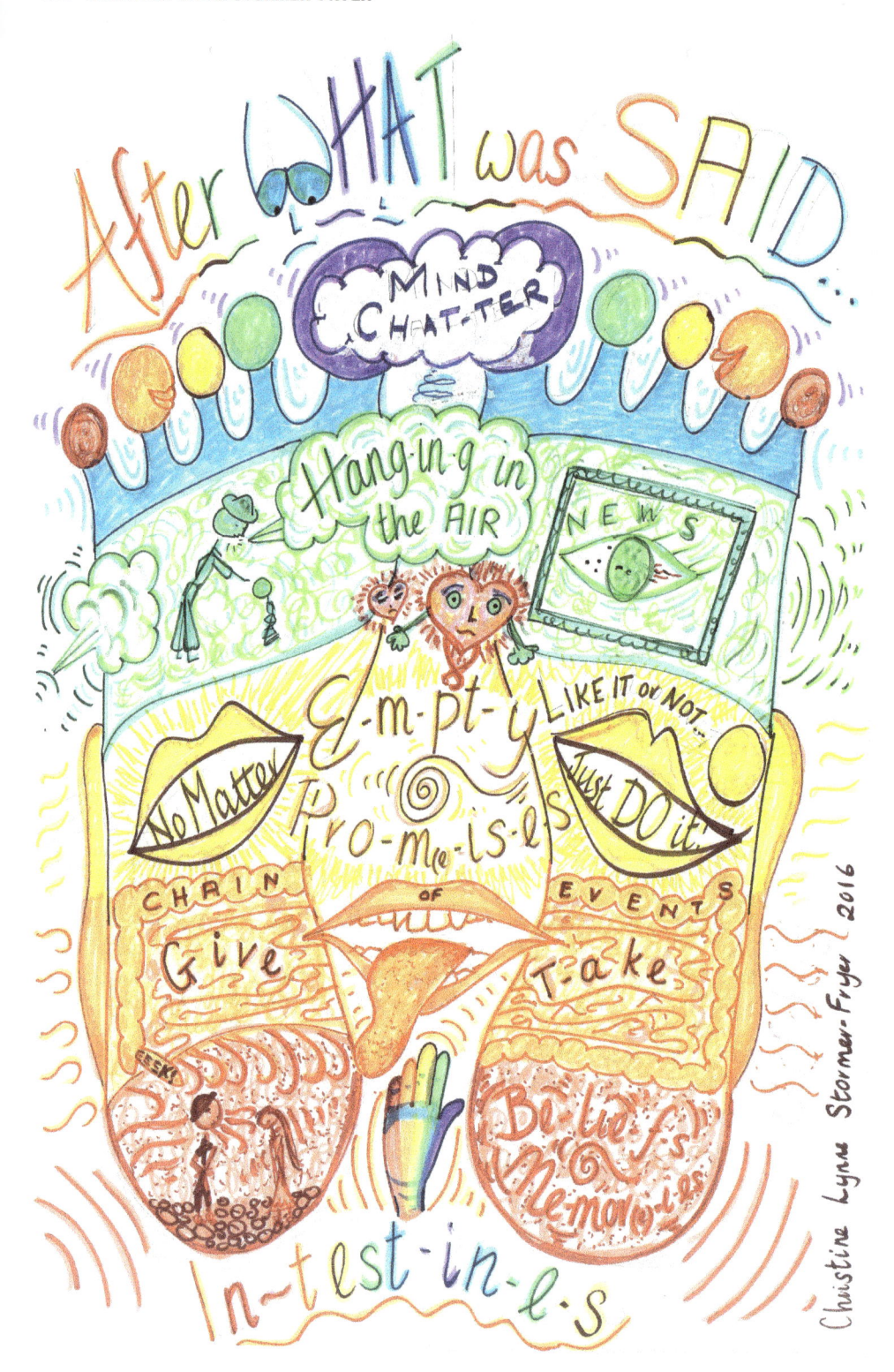

AFTER WHAT WAS SAID – IN-TEST-IN-ES

The moment a thought comes to mind, the aura changes. Once dismissed, the notion dissipates into thin air, with the stratosphere shifting higher energies above and bodies of water and the soil below.

Every word uttered, every expression articulated, every breath experienced, and every feeling felt fill the air, influencing the surrounding atmosphere. The richness of breath-taking decisions, heartfelt 'e-motions' and profound feelings reverberate throughout, fuelling the sustenance of life.

Jumping from one notion to another, the monkey mind constantly analyses relationships, going over 'what was said', deliberating about how to handle situations, and worrying anything and everything. All notions scramble for attention in a massive whirlwind of mind chatter. It 'takes guts' to disengage and still the mind, but it pays dividends in the long run.

'Airing views', especially when 'full of hot air', often leaves unresolved issues 'hanging in the air'. Incomplete feelings filled with uncertainty and annoyance contaminate the environment with the body left gasping for air. This is not helped by distressing NEWS spewing out misleading reports about disasters happening **N**orth **E**ast **W**est and **S**outh to exacerbate the situation. Long deep breaths of fresh air assist in clearing the lungs and liberating the Spirit.

Not being of any importance has little or no effect on the matter, but when things matter, significant changes take place in the matter, depending on how much it matters. The brain minds the matter, and the matter reflects how much the brain matters.

Promises are easy to make, but not so easy to keep. An 'empty promise' is worthless, making it hard to trust again. Once betrayed, it takes time for trust to be regained. Like it or not, taking action and 'just doing it' makes all the difference.

A series of chain events, life is an ongoing sequence of 'give and take', testing the energy in the 'in-test-in-es.' 'Giving' kindness without conditions, expectations or boundaries, and 'taking' back what is worthwhile during verbal exchanges. It is not always what is said that hurts, but what is not said. A 'dead-end' relationship exasperates the appendix until it bursts in an attempt to find another way out.

Lingering in the subconscious are memories of what happened or didn't happen. A lot of 'hearsay' is passed from one generation to the next. 'Bought into' 'beliefs' powerfully determine expectations and impact mass consciousness.

It is what cannot be said that often carries the greatest value. Kind words can be short and easy to speak, but their echoes are truly endless.

Nobody passes through life without leaving tracks!

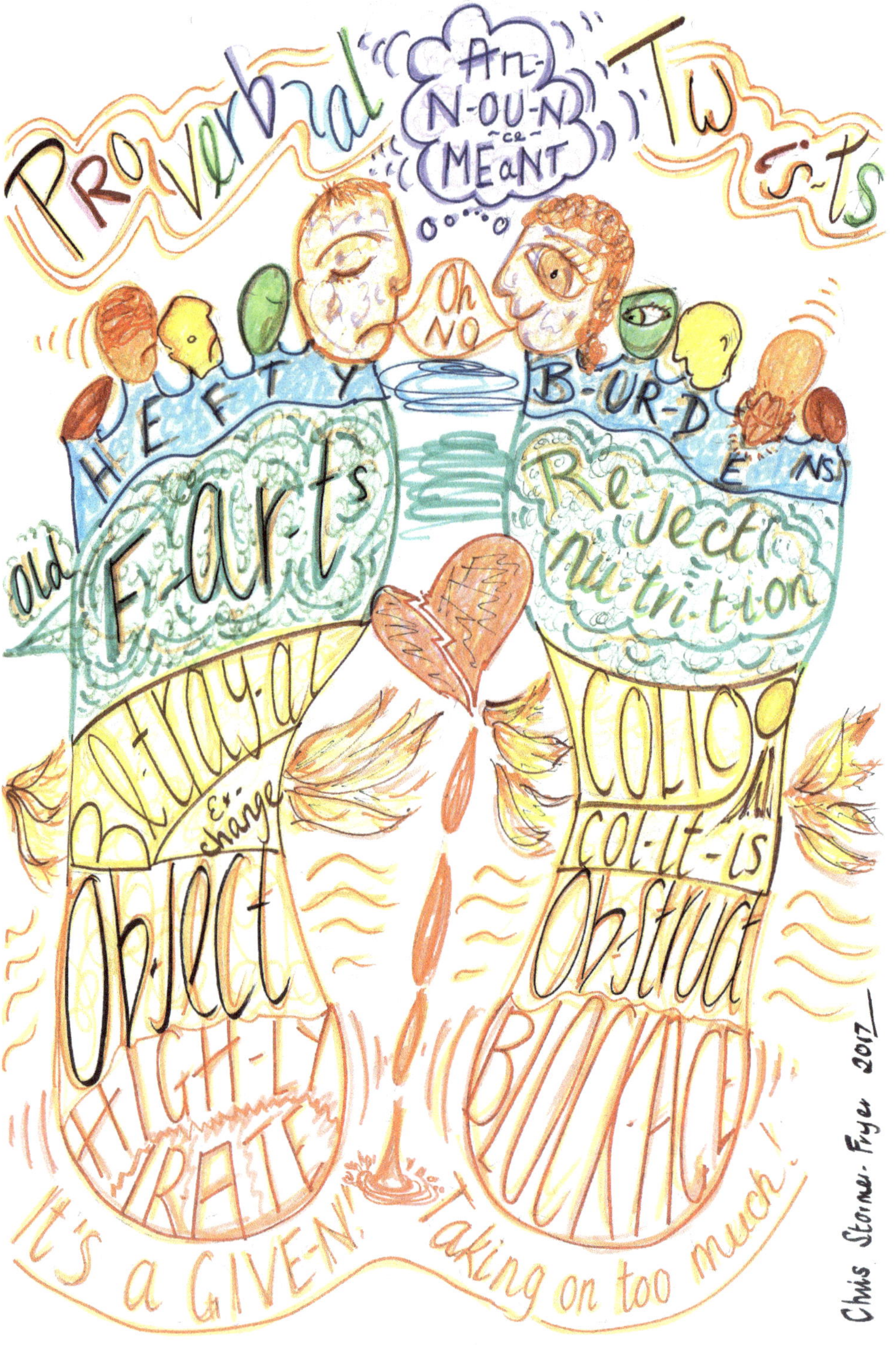
Proverbial Twists
An-N-OU-N-ce MEaNT
Oh NO
HEFTY
B-UR-D-E-NS
old F-ar-ts
Re-ject nu-tri-tion
Ex-change
Object
COL-IT-IS
Obstruct
It's a GIVE-N!
Taking on too much!
Chris Stormer-Fryer 2017

PROVERBIAL TWISTS

Proverbs are popular and generally well-known sayings that express common beliefs. Either disempowering or empowering, these 'pronouncements' have an impact on the emotional state with a cumulative effect on the subconscious.

Constant 'a-noun-c-ments' of "Oh no", with disaster perceived at every 'twist or turn' within relationships, plonks 'hefty burdens' onto the shoulders. Expected to take on the additional 'responsibility' and 'respond appropriately' is a real strain.

'Old farts' tend to flatulate frequently, with sudden expulsions of stale wind from the anus ridding the body of tedious 'e-motions'. Feeling too 'e-motionally' confused to embrace the 'new', and even refusing to 'try it on' for size, is to 'reject 'new trends' in the form of 'nu-trients'.

Miffed by 'betrayal' having 'be'en a 'tray' to 'all' is a 'blow' to the 'e-go', especially when entertaining high moral standards. Having personal trust and confidence violated enrages the already 'livid' liver, further infuriated at any attempt to try and 'change' an 'ex'. It only 'adds extra fuel to the fire'.

Griping on and on about all that happened or did not happen and 'bellyaching' about injustices cramps the stomach's style with 'colic'. Infuriated about not being in control of events before they come our way inflames the colon into a state of 'colitis'.

Constantly 'objecting', and always protesting and complaining at the least little thing, 'obstructs' and 'gets in the way' of any form of progress, leading to the temptation to intentionally distort and twist the truth to shift the blame. Contorting the interpretation of words wilfully falsifies the facts. It may be through a 'twist of fate' or a 'twist in the tale' that there is often a sharp turn of events that come with an element of suspense and surprise.

'Getting the knickers in a twist' about a trivial or unimportant matter after having the 'arm twisted', or being 'twisted around little finger', effortlessly 'twists things up', mercilessly creating confusion and uncertainty.

Taking a 'stab in the dark' when feeling threatened makes it tempting to 'twist the truth', or even 'twist the knife', but this only serves to exacerbate or amplify the wrongdoing. Enticed into 'twisting words' when 'bitter and twisted' over of past traumas has the intestines squirming in shame. It can even have them 'tying themselves up in knots' should there be a 'twist in the wind', leaving them in a problematic situation. 'Taking on too much' to compensate eventually acts as a 'blockade'.

Each living creature is dependent on other living things to survive. Earth is the web that connects everything through a spinning kaleidoscope of relations, revealing that life is not about acting true to the face, but also remaining true behind the back.

Undoing the shackles of the past is to live fully in the present!

178 - CHRISTINE LYNNE STORMER-FRYER

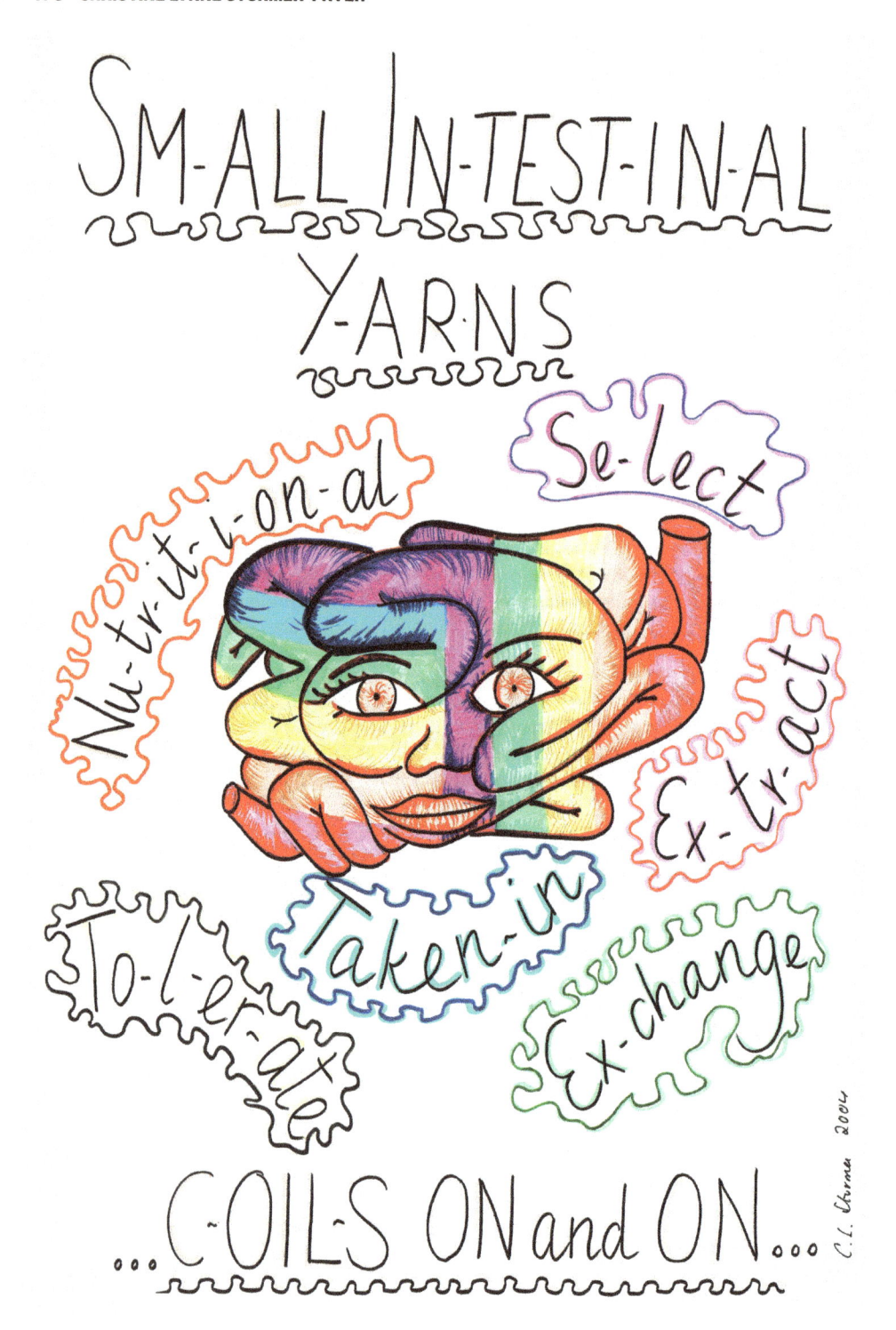

Sm·all In·test·in·al Y·arns

Nu·tr·it·i·on·al
Se·lect
Ex·tr·act
Tak·en·in
Ex·change
To·l·er·ate

...C·OIL·S ON and ON...

C.L. Ukuma 2004

SMALL INTESTINAL YARNS

Coiling on and on, the small intestines sort out relevant concepts and significant 'e-motions' for Spiritual nourishment, but only after the stomach has rummaged through them to pick out the most nutritious parts. In cahoots with the heart meridian, it is the small intestine's mission to ensure that every cell thrives, beneficially transforming the new intake.

Taking in and digesting the energy of all that is happening, the small intestine selects and absorbs anything relevant and useful, while dismissing anything surplus to personal requirements, to ensure a healthy exchange within relationships. As poignant feelings are stirred, a certain amount of confusion and complexity may be involved.

With a steady heart and a composed mind 'going hand-in-hand', the small intestine relies upon them to create the ideal 'e-motional' and intellectual foundations for all alternatives to be considered. With equal measure of both, essential compromises can be made, making it so much easier to sort out the new input.

Intense distrust upsets this fine balance. The exaggerated analysis of everything stems from extreme possessiveness, selfishness or jealousy. The desire to have it all, along with a righteous belief that others are clueless, makes it impossible to accept, assimilate or understand life's lessons. Disgruntled by the internal state of affairs the mouth cannot but help state its displeasure making it even more difficult to take in what is really going on.

Uneasiness within relationships due to a lack of self-worth agitates the intestines enough to go into 'a flustering dither'. As peristalsis mercilessly speeds up the anxiety to get away from it all, it urges the contents to pass through at such an incredible speed that there is little or no time for absorption. The deprived body ends up being an uptight and nervous bag of bones. Depression or unhappiness slow peristalsis down until the sluggish villi barely move. With stuff hanging around for far too long, more than required is 'taken on', burdening the system.

Extremely pernickety, picky, fussy or finicky behaviour, not just in the choice of foods but also in relationships, comes from a deep intolerance of memories transformed into intense beliefs. This prevents certain interactions from being tolerated, no matter how beneficial. It all depends on how much is taken from relationships, and the type of contribution made in return, to nourish the Soul. To ensure that no time is unnecessarily wasted, the small intestine passes on all the physiological and psychological residues to the large intestines.

The small intestine delights in going to great lengths to serve and nourish mind and body, encouraging relationships to flourish.

What is communicated today lays the foundation for relationships tomorrow!

Colonic Chronicles

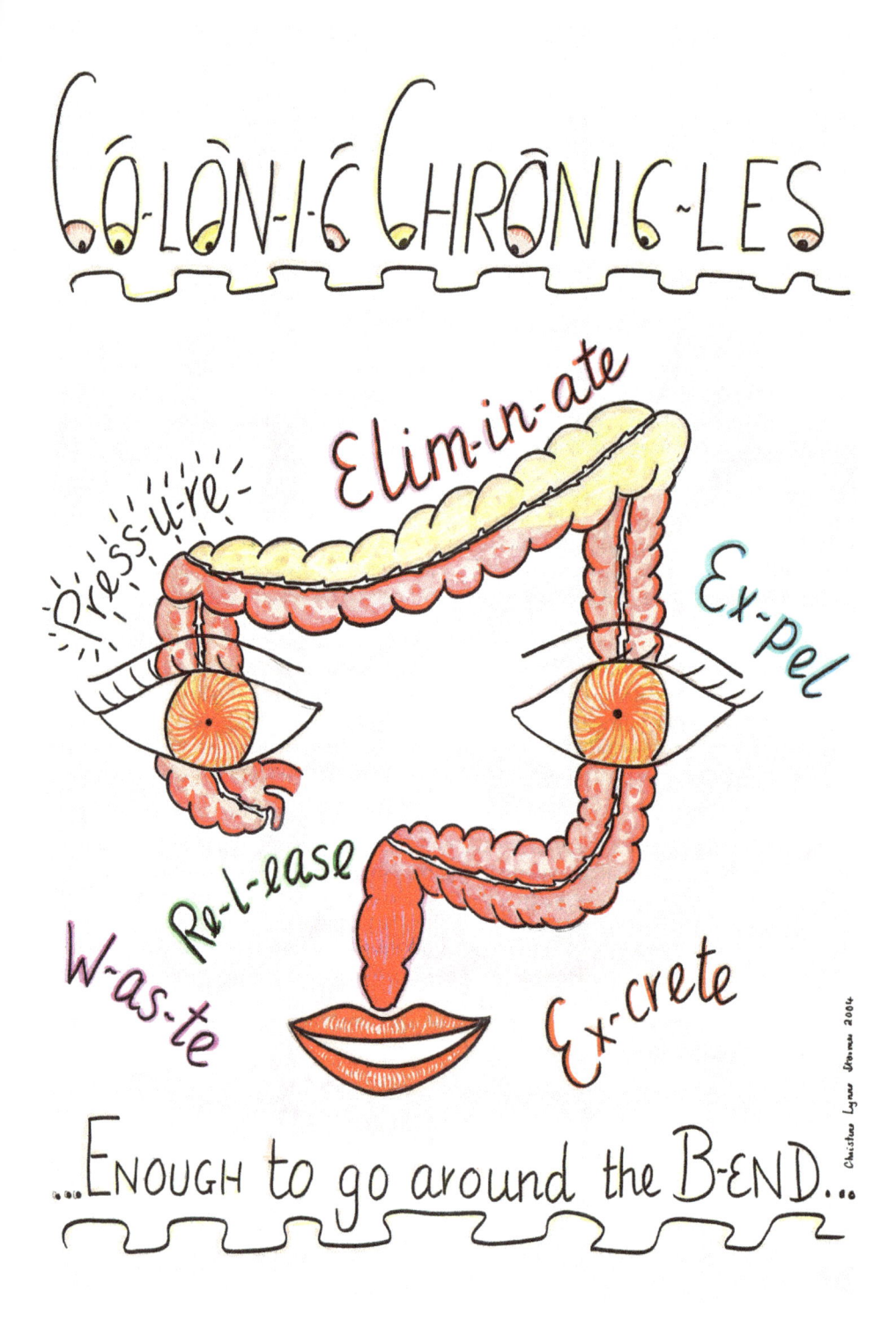

Press-u-re

Elim-in-ate

Ex-pel

W-as-te

Re-l-ease

Ex-crete

...Enough to go around the B-END...

COLONIC CHRONICLES – ENOUGH TO GO AROUND THE BEND

To the colon, it does not matter whether it is referred to as the 'large intestine' or the 'bowel system', as long as it can get on with the job of eliminating whatever is considered by the mind to be superfluous, useless or undesirable.

Affected deeply by profound feelings, clinging onto the old and resisting change is a form of self-poisoning. Hanging onto sadness, stubbornness, rigidity and regret saps the body of its strength, as does an endless thirst for material objects

The colon's worst enemies are dehydration due to an unquenchable desire for meaningful communication, and a sedentary lifestyle with little initiative to get things moving. Another enemy is rapidly gulping meals down with no time to make worthwhile decisions, as is a boring job with nothing to ignite the passion, 'pass-i-on'. Even a toxic environment where belittling is the 'norm'. Perhaps low-nutrient foods with no 'new trends' or sufficient rough edges to soothe the way. Even unsuitable dairy products, products of mother's nurturing (siblings) who leave a 'bad taste in the mouth'.

Dreading failure, it groans, gripes and grumbles when under too much pressure, often expected to perform against its will. Depression, irritability, discouragement, distrust and apathy make it hard to let go. With things 'piling up', the pressure and backlog become too overwhelming to get on and do anything worthwhile. The colon already has many parts to attend to. At its entrance is a sphincter muscle, the ileocecal valve, which goes by many names, including Tulp's, Tulpius and Bauhin's valve. Regardless of what it is called, its role is to prevent processed substances back-tracking into the small intestines.

The lungs and colon complement one another. Lungs bring in new life forces, while the colon lets go after everything has been appropriately dealt with. The ascending colon picks up and relays ancestral and past remnants before passing them onto the transverse colon. Here the 'stuff' is transported from the past to the present across the 'waistline' ('waste line') before being despatched onto the ascending colon. Lingering family paraphernalia joins in here before being relayed through the sigmoid colon in which deep dark secrets are buried, even unbeknown even to the self. It is then onto the rectum (anus) for final release and relief.

Symbolising the realm of the dead with materials that cannot be brought back to life, the colon also represents the 'unconscious shadow side'. The home of anything not brought out into the open. Producing Vitamins 'A', the 'adjustment' vitamin, and 'K', the 'knowledgeable' vitamin, the colon is the generator of change and evolution.

Generosity is a much-appreciated asset to the colon!

182 - CHRISTINE LYNNE STORMER-FRYER

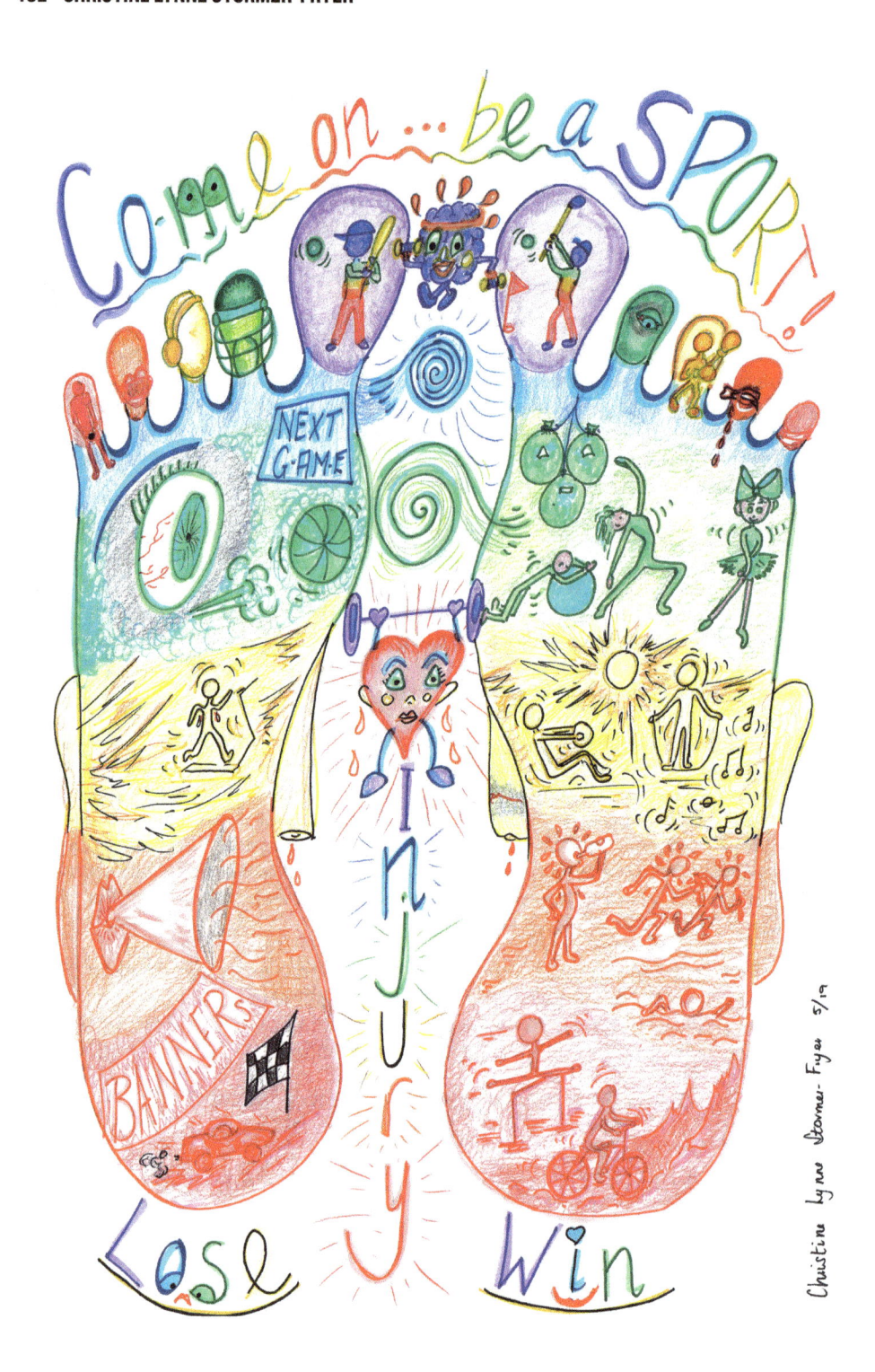

COME ON - BE A SPORT

Life is a game made up of zillions of interlocking pieces joined together to form a vast puzzle. Everybody is a team member in this game called 'life', encouraged to 'be a sport' and accept challenging situations with aplomb and dignity. Jogging the memory are various pastimes. Playing 'mind games' and 'going on power trips' serve the ego's agenda, but it is 'not cricket', especially when GOLF was commonly believed to be an acronym for 'Gentleman Only, Ladies Forbidden' but is now a well-known joke with the name apparently stemming from an old word for 'club'. Like it or not, life is a full-on game for every body!

Many 'twists and turns' make life a 'merry-go-round' that can 'spin out of control' at times. 'Juggling' five balls namely, work, family, health, friends and Spirit, and trying to 'keep all the balls in the air' before the 'bubble bursts' takes talent. If dropped, work is a rubber ball that bounces back. The others are made of glass, easily damaged and even shattered, but rarely the same again.

Life is not a spectator's sport. Watching from the stands and not getting involved in things that really matter is a game of pretending to be human. It is not about 'holding good cards' but in playing those held in the hand well. Being a 'sore loser' is 'one in the eye' and a form of self-rebuke. Broken red blood vessels highlight the sadness from eyes being 'scratched out' or unable 'to look another in the eye'. It is an absolute 'balls-up', making it difficult to keep the 'eye on the ball'.

The strain of 'leading a merry dance' and ending up 'running around in circles' is exhausting, 'wearing the body out' long before its time. Far from 'feeling swell', it may require 'biting the bullet' and enduring intense hardship through a series of painful operations to 'be a sport'. It may require an 'ace up the sleeve' to participate enthusiastically in the 'next game'.

Going to the gym can be a pro-active way of 'working things out'. 'Running others down' and telling them to 'take a running jump' in the mind while running on a treadmill is preferable to 'boxing the living daylights' out of opponents. 'Skipping' is likely to be better than 'getting hopping mad', while 'lifting weights' to take a 'weight off the mind' and developing a 'six-pack' to 'take the punches' protects the ego from attack.

Held prisoner by a sense of incompetence, with no goal and no purpose, deprives the game of life of excitement and meaning. To get the adrenaline pumping, 'sport' is viewed on the 'goggle box' or from a distance at matches. As the 'competitive streak' rears its ugly head, spectators make more of a spectacle of themselves by getting 'all worked up' and shouting, or even yelling, at a box.

Unseen aspects of oneself are triggered by other players, generally when undermining self-worth through comparisons. This is not fully participating in the true game of life. The only option left is being caught up in the rat race of modern-day living.

Sports injuries do not happen by accident. They are a plea from the Soul to opt out rather than 'give in' to social pressure and abide by rigid boundaries reinforced through out-dated rules. Sport has become so disciplined, competitive and structured that all the fun has been taken out of it.

Participating or not, the game of life goes on, with an open invitation to jump in at any time and choose a suitable position. Each Soul determines what to play and how to play it. It is only over when the Soul decides to quit. The secret is to play a meaningful part and enjoy the ride.

Life is not a race but a journey to be savoured each step of the way!

184 - CHRISTINE LYNNE STORMER-FRYER

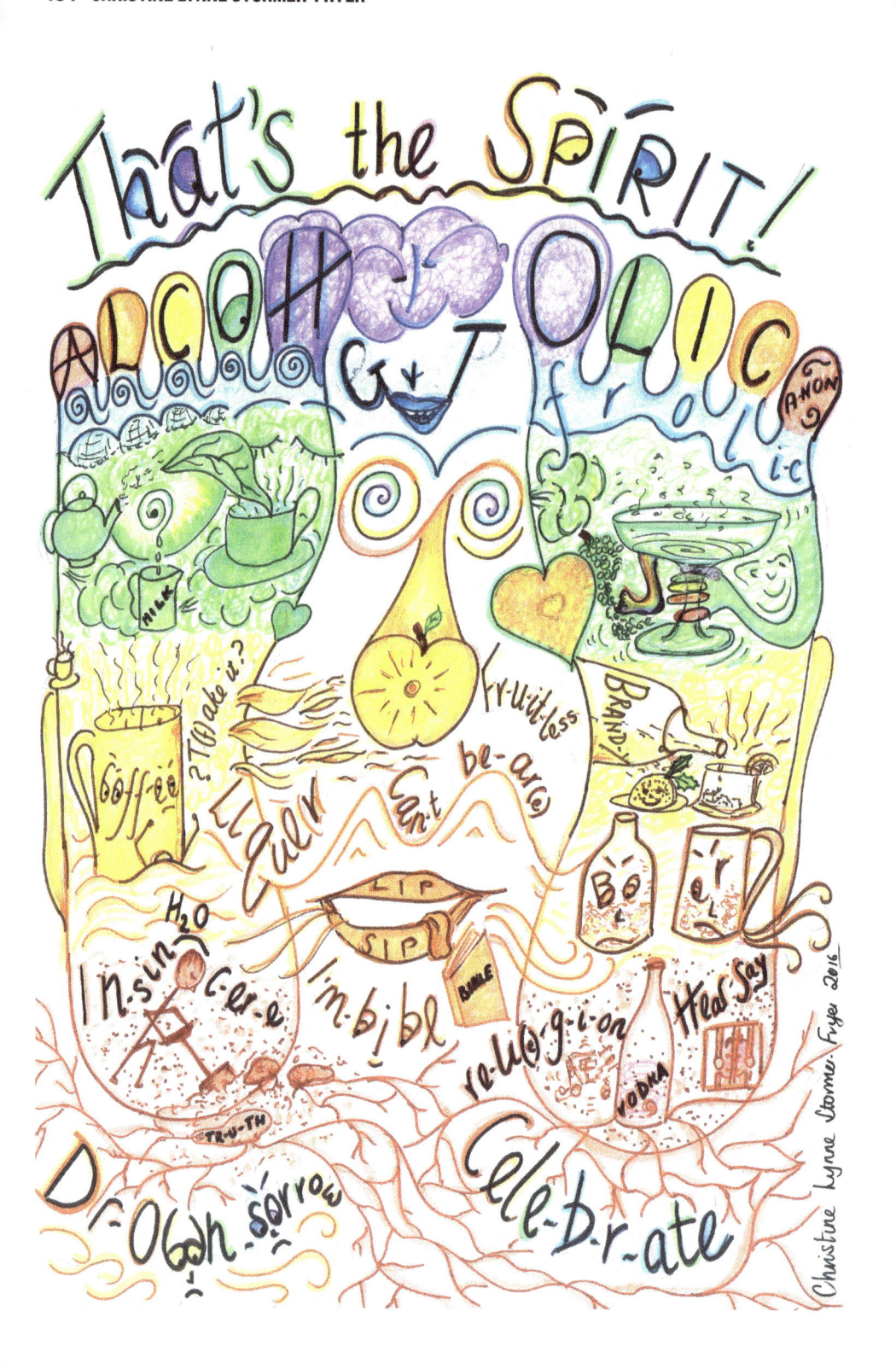

THAT'S THE SPIRIT – DROWN SORROWS OR CELEBRATE

Cheerfully buoyant, the Spirit expands beyond the physical. It is an invisible force that overrides the density of humanity, travelling through every atom of the body and bringing it to life.

It takes courage and perseverance to incarnate, with powerful Spiritual experiences shaking up the entire thought process. In doing so, mere beliefs are replaced with the wisdom to understand the power of love. 'That's the Spirit!'

Accessed via 'e-motions', the Spirit prevents the body from becoming completely senseless. A Spiritual being is conscious at all times with the guru, 'Gee U aRe U', within awakening potential. Reaching back to the roots in pursuit of Spirituality invariably begins as a search for the true meaning of life. Certain religions are intolerant of this quest, for fear of it generating different conclusions. Yet, deep down every body is unified through Spirit.

The mishmash of misleading beliefs comatose the mind, with many staying Spiritually asleep. Others suffer from Spiritual amnesia. Seeking an outlet in alcohol is a way of liberating the bottled-up Spirit. It is not good nor bad, it just *is*. Certain sectors of society forbid the consumption of alcohol, concerned that, once liberated, the free Spirits will challenge the rigidity of antiquated beliefs.

'Out-rage-ous' behaviour among certain Asian immigrants after imbibing Spirits has prompted the ambiguous belief that a missing enzyme is the cause. A strict religious upbringing, along with suppressing the indignation at 'having the wings clipped', are more likely to be the culprits. Unshackling a crushed spirit through alcohol allows curbed 'rage' to come out in 'out-rage-ous' ways. The alcohol simply highlights whether it is being imbibed to 'drown sorrows', to 'cope with challenging situations', or to 'celebrate' life. The labelling beliefs are bound to have a huge influence.

Alcohol is made from the purification of provoked forms of nourishment.' Abusing', 'abnormally using', it draws attention to areas of 'Spirit-less-ness' needing some spunk. 'Gin' helps one to 'grin and bear it'. 'Wine', made from grapes resembling the lung's alveoli, helps deal with 'whining' in the family if red, or whinging about distraught feelings if white. 'Brandy', 'burnt wine', is allied to the 'fruits of one's labour', made mainly from fruit. Distilled from grains or potatoes, 'vodka', originally from Russia and Poland, is associated with communications that go 'against the grain', otherwise used to avoid 'getting to the root' of issues.

Once 'Spirited' and full of Spirit, not just from alcohol but the essence of life, makes it so much easier to face life's challenges. The power of the Spiritual self is limitless in co-creating reality, with worthwhile decisions continually refreshing the Spirit and recognising the miracles of life. The human race is making a massive Spiritual leap, evolving from the microcosm and smallness of ideas to the macrocosm and the expansive awareness of all that is.

Being too Spiritual is of no Earthly use to any body!

186 - CHRISTINE LYNNE STORMER-FRYER

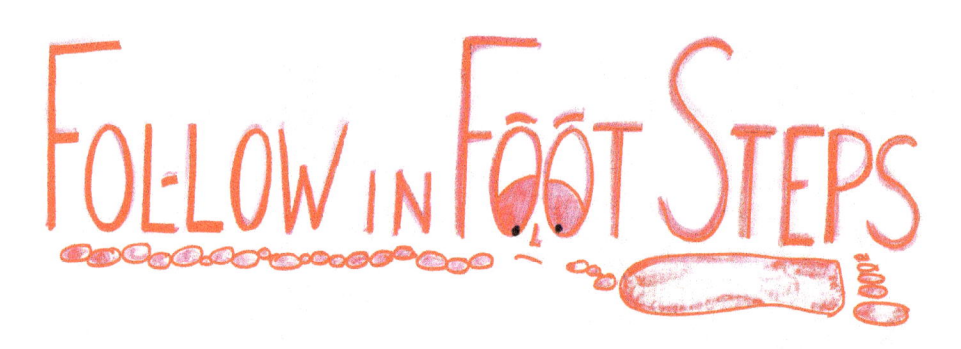

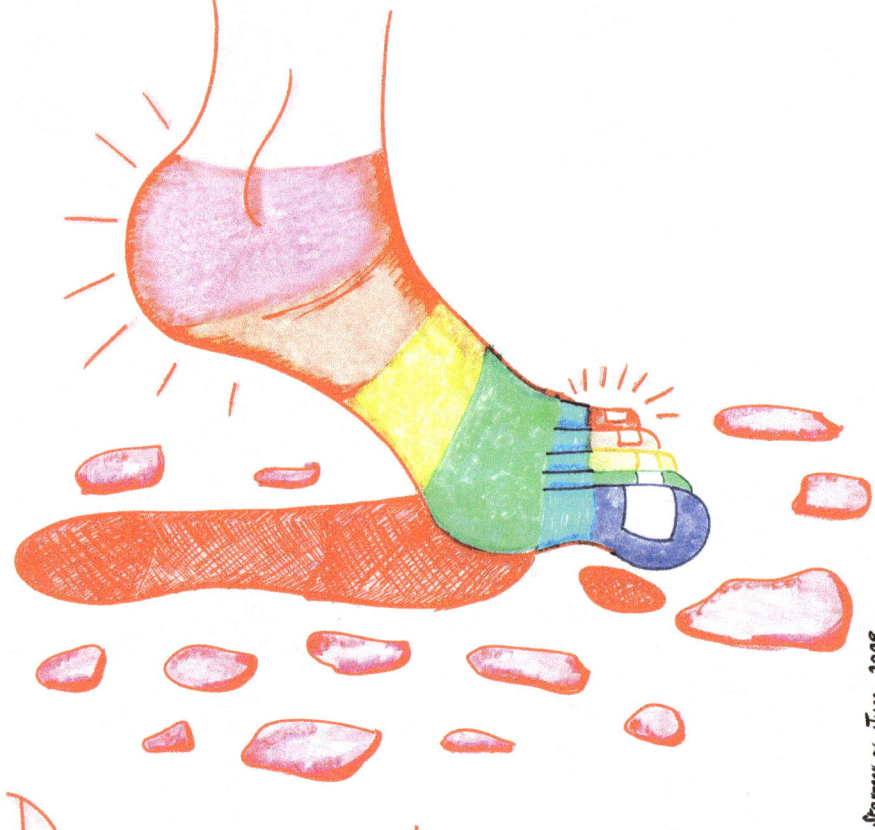

Follow in Footsteps

Dis-appoint-ed...

Christine Lynne Stormer ~ June 2008

FOLLOWING IN ANOTHER'S FOOTSTEPS

Admittedly, it is easier to 'follow in another's footsteps' along tried and tested pathways of life. However, emulating what has been done before by following the same well-worn tracks invariably leads to disappointment.

It has already been done many times before, so 'what's the point'? Continuing the tradition of behaving or working in the exactly 'same old' way' gets so boring. Not only is it monotonous, but it is generally devoid of passion and enthusiasm.

'Setting foot on Earth' is the ideal opportunity to evolve and introduce innovative ways to 'make a world of difference'. To 'follow the heart's desire' as well as 'follow the nose' is to pursue a lifestyle that delights the Soul.

The excitement of the unknown, the anticipation of wandering into uncharted lands, and the thrill of 'what next' all have the heart beating with happiness and the Soul bursting with joy. The rewards are immeasurable.

Being a visionary or a leader can be daunting. Having a strong, clear and distinct picture of the future of how things might be different, even better, imagining what does not yet exist, seeing something long before it becomes a reality, is an open invitation to criticism, especially among pessimists.

Being an entrepreneur requires taking risks. It involves massive leaps of faith, but it is so worth it. It also gives others the courage to 'follow their dreams' in extraordinary ways.

Having unfeasible expectations and trying to force the outcome, instead of trusting in Universal Guidance, invariably leads to disillusionment. The range of 'e-motions', from feeling slightly let down to depressed or even angry, are tough but necessary feelings to endure.

The gift of being disappointed is to prevent getting stuck in a realm of how things should have been when totally 'off track'. It is the way the frustration is handled that matters. What happens subsequently relies on it.

True leaders tend to be visionaries who size up situations and lead by example. Speakers of words and doers of deeds, with enormous amounts of energy to energise those being guided towards a more harmonious state of being. Leadership is the incredible ability to share clear visions and outrageous dreams to others.

Great leaders lead others into believing in themselves so that they too can become great!

188 - CHRISTINE LYNNE STORMER-FRYER

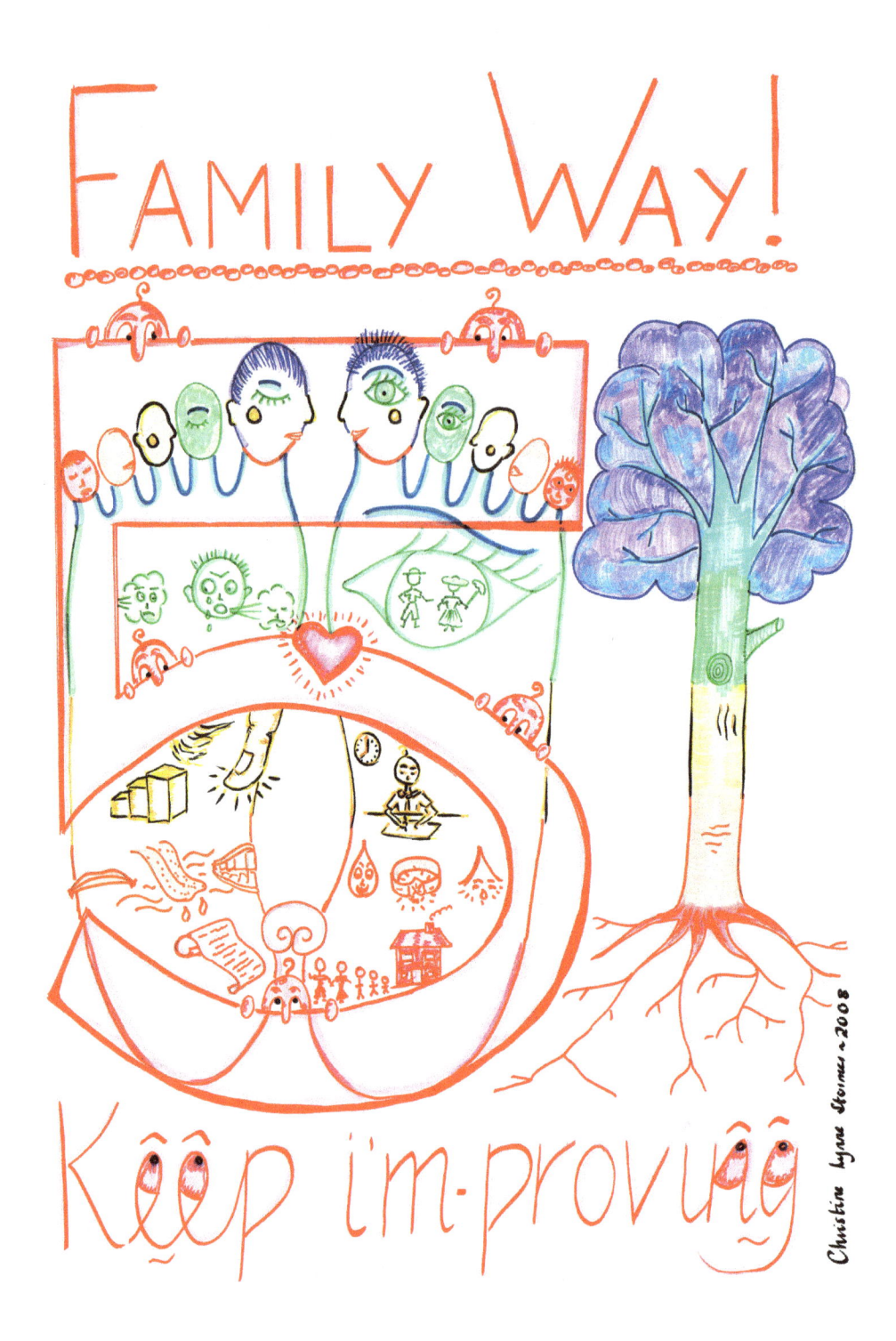

FAMILY WAY – KEEP IMPROVING

'5' is the number symbolising being human. Four limbs and a head move the Spirit throughout life, while the six senses provide insight and guidance. Related to freedom, independence, adventure, curiosity, experience, and intelligence, 'five' is a combination of the female number 'two' and the male number 'three'.

'Five' ensures that humanity survives and thrives within all family groups and tribes worldwide. It embodies the coming together of Heaven and Earth through peace and harmony. The 'five' Olympic rings, symbolising five continents, is an international emblem.

Amulets used as magical protection against the evil eye have no little finger, which generally represents 'family', but has two thumbs signifying the highway to Spirituality. The Luther Rose also has 'five' symbols, as do the cross of faith, the heart full of love, the white rose of peace, the heavenly joy of blue skies, and the yellow circle of eternity.

Related to individual Spiritual journeys, 'five' is a reminder to stay positive. Whatever happens is a gift in the form of the 'pre-sent'. A brilliant chance to 'improve', 'I'm proof', and increase vibrational energy through travel, escapades and movement.

Along with the highs, 'five' also conveys uncertainty and volatility, accompanied by many radical changes. Drawing attention to the incredible wonders of the world, 'five' beckons an appreciation of the order within the chaos.

A free-Spirited creative number of manifestation, 'five' relies on the 'five' elements of earth, water, fire, air and ether to evolve. All are essential components in initiating and maintaining innovative concepts and making a valuable contribution towards the betterment of humankind.

From the Latin *familia*, a 'family' is a group of 'familiar' Souls – whether blood-related or offering some form of 'familiarity'. Families are meant to provide the roots to stand tall and strong, with an element of predictability, structure and stability – the means to acquire the social skills required to operate in the big, wide world of ambiguity.

The primary function of the family is to supply a framework to keep generating refreshing new energy by first letting go of old, now wasted, energies to make space for new beginnings. A substantial skeleton of an eclectic selection of 'bones' eager to 'be one of a kind', offer all the support required. Meanwhile, the muscular system provides the flexibility to expand and move 'a-head' with ease. The reproductive system affords space to create and bring through new concepts, ensuring the advancement of humankind.

Some of the best journeys are in the mind and Spirit!

190 - CHRISTINE LYNNE STORMER-FRYER

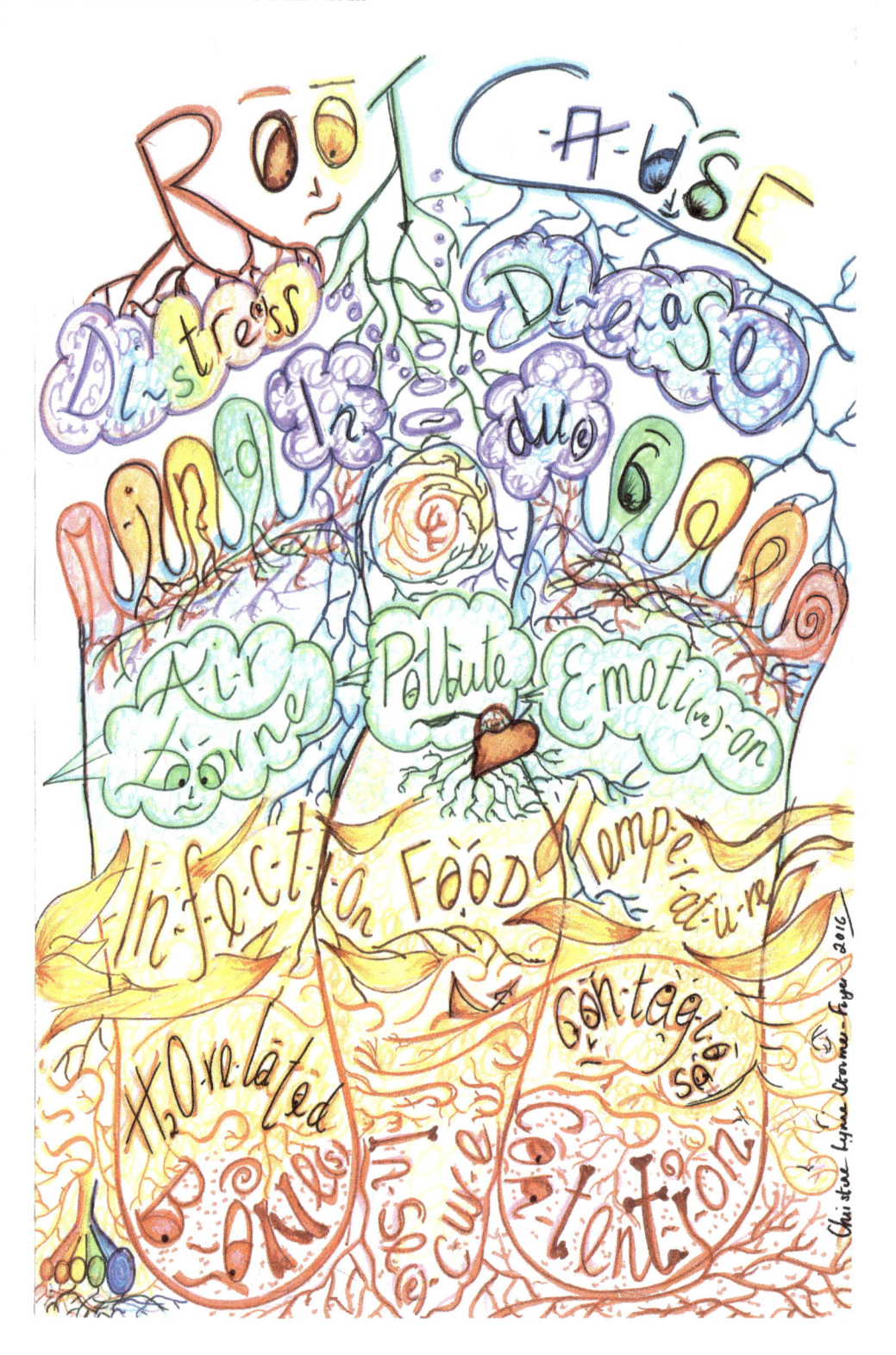

ROOT CAUSE OF DISTRESS AND DIS-EASE

Every body is a piece of a larger puzzle, each with its own unique and complex network deeply connected to well-spread ancestral roots. Under-standing the endurance of cultural trials and tribulations gives a slight inkling of why certain roles have been taken on in the ongoing drama called 'life'.

Constantly in touch with Spiritual and family roots, the unconscious and subconscious minds form the roots of life in the base chakra, where pain, anger, shame and guilt reside with far-reaching effects. Revolving around personal legacies, unsettling issues go back seven generations or more. Whether it is the position in the family or society, fitting in or not fitting in, the colour of the skin, or religious and Spiritual beliefs, all issues ultimately stem from deep-rooted fear.

Horrendous thoughts make grooves of despondency and hopelessness on the mind, breeding a host of destructive elements. Overthinking and obsessing about matters beyond reach brings on mind-induced mental disorders, made worse by an intense desire to control everything and everybody when utterly out of control. Stigmatised and being discriminated against stagnates the mind, contributing to depression, bipolar disorder, dementia, schizophrenia and so on, all of which deplete the body of energy.

The stimulation of sensory organs provides an essential source of information for conscious experiences. By regulating and balancing vital energy flowing throughout, everything comes together. Ongoing distress interferes with the ability to perform well, with the uneasiness causing 'bad' reactions.

Unsettling 'e-motions' once air-borne, pollute the atmosphere with grief and sadness often 'taking the breath away' and making it hard to breathe. The heart is kept well informed to determine what lives inside. Its discontent or content is then spread throughout by the bloodline, providing either an unstable or stable environment for the Spirit.

The subsequent temperament affects the body's temperature. Getting too heated and furious leads to irritability, fever and inflammatory conditions. 'Flying off the handle' at the slightest thing makes it extremely difficult to digest life. Invariably, fingers point accusingly to food, yet reactions to this type of intake merely highlight what is having to be processed on a daily basis.

From roots to fruits, there is a lot of 'food for thought' as senses are constantly 'fed' a whole range of stimuli. Intense reactions occur when vexing memories ignite stored frustration and anger, until flaring up into a full-blown 'infection' to reveal what 'it is' such as 'men-in-g-it-is' from mental agitation; 'bronch-it-is' from 'e-motional' rage; 'gas-tr-it-is' from anger at stomaching life, and so on.

Anything related to water is connected to the flow of conversation and its impact on relationships, internally and externally. Contamination happens when adulterated with filth and deceit. It is then considered contagious, with 'waves of disillusionment' spreading rapidly.

'Getting under the 's-kin' are highly irrational and irritating 'bones of contention' that have 'got way out of hand'. Coming from the same family tree, all related 'kin' carry a similar genetic code determined by the roots. Clinging to the drama of the past is disastrous. Far better is 'turning a new page', refusing to 'repeat history', and starting afresh. Establishing a 'den of peace' is empowering. Once well-rooted, it is so much easier to stay strong and adapt to every situation.

To become rooted in the physical body, the physical body needs to feel accepted!

192 - CHRISTINE LYNNE STORMER-FRYER

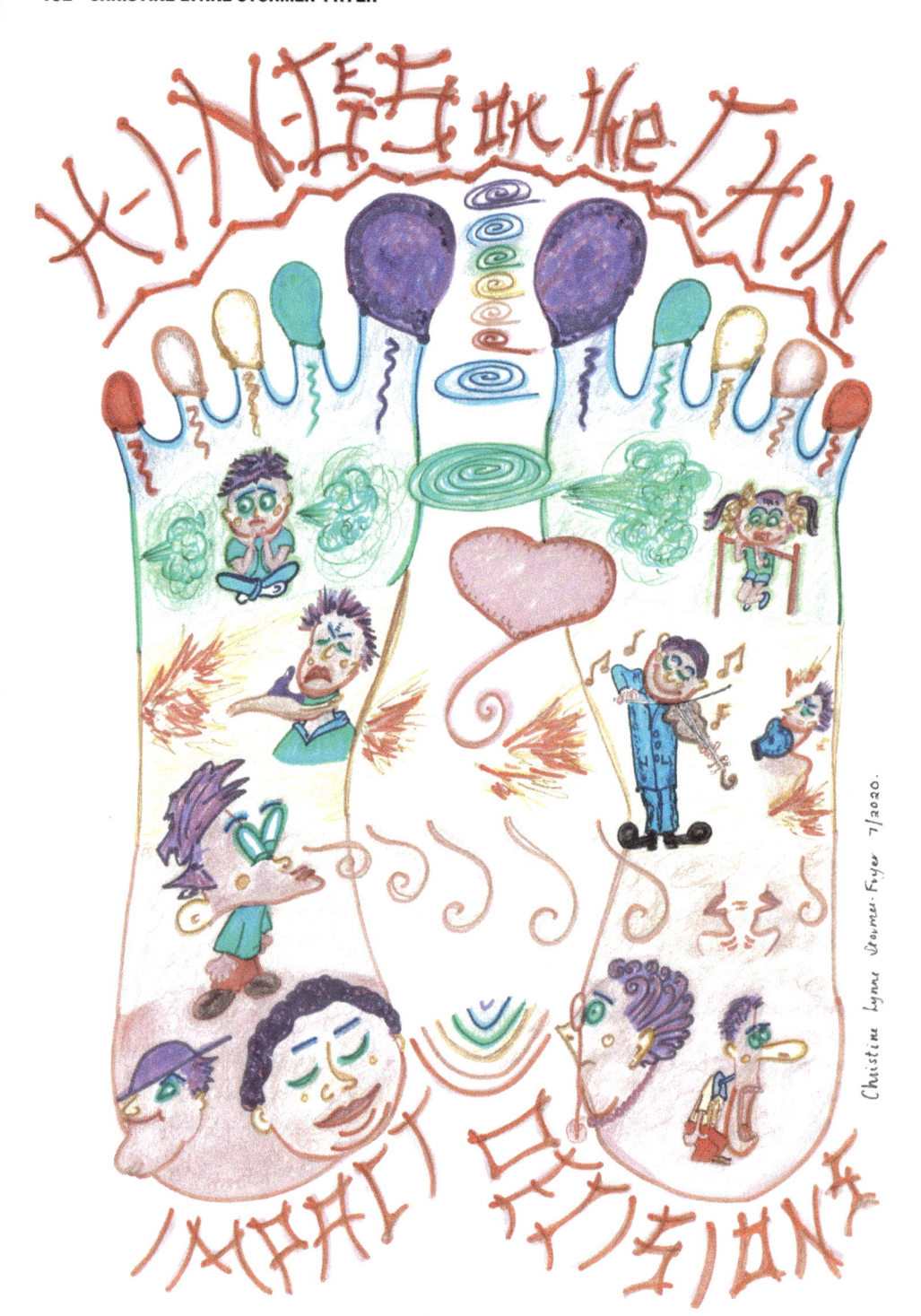

HINGES ON THE CHIN

The human chin, also known as the 'mental eminence', 'protuberance', 'osseum' or 'tuber symphyseos', is best known for its 'chin-wagging' gossiping about others, generally 'behind their backs', or going on and on idly at great length about something that the 'mind is set on'. The resultant tension engendered by extreme obstinacy and the utter refusal to 'change the mind' can 'lock the jaw'. Shutting the mouth up indefinitely brings all the 'chin music' talk and chatter to a temporary halt.

The chin being in control of one of the 'en-trances of the mind' into the body, clenches with uncertainty, anxiety and fear, trapping Spiritual energy within the jaw. Bridging the gap between the head and the torso, it takes a lot of rigid 'shoulds' and 'should nots' and 'thy musts' taken 'on the chin' to avoid reacting badly.

With so much 'give' and 'take' required to 'transform', a 'chin up' of encouragement helps to improve the mood when sad or discouraged. With raised Spirits, a 'brave face' can be put on. An affectionate 'chuck beneath the chin' offers further encouragement.

It is admirable watching gymnasts 'lung-e' at the bar to 'chin the self', pulling the whole body up to chin level by bending the elbows. All well and good when doing this is the Soul's passion, but forced to be constantly 'poised' and courageously perform against the will, 'egged on' to hold 'the chin up' and never give up, can be seriously injurious. The Soul invariably ends up begging to be set free from the rigorous regime. Reluctantly having to practice day in and day out can take its toll later in life.

Being 'up to the chin' with so much going on or feeling completely overwhelmed is to feel a sense of drowning, invariably in self-pity or sorrow. A cue to raise a violin to the chin and play a sad, sympathetic symphony.

With there being so many 'Chins' in China, having 'more chins than a Chinese phone book' is a phrase not always appreciated by the 'Chins' or those with multiple rolls of fat around the neck. With the jawbone lacking definition, a double chin or second chin is a way of covering up basic insecurities. Being 'two-faced' is often the only way to survive when holding back.

Approaching an opponent with the 'chin thrust out' is an aggressive act that lacks caution and makes the 'chin' vulnerable. 'Sticking the chin out' to show resolve, determination and fortitude can be risky and dangerous in certain situations. A challenging display of smugness, confidence, pride or confrontation, it is often a dare to attack, not just physically but also mentally. In certain parts of Italy, the 'chin flick' is an obscene gesture of not caring less.

The 'cleft chin' with a dimple is an often-inherited feature, a bony peculiarity, with the two halves of the jawbone not fusing, symbolising a possible rift in the family being 'a blow to the chin' in the long-distant past, with the memory of being 'led by the chin' lingering on.

A morphological characteristic of homo sapiens, well-developed chins have evolved greatly throughout the generations, possibly due to the willingness to 'stick the chin out' and 'speak the mind'.

Consider the impact decisions have on generations to come!

194 - CHRISTINE LYNNE STORMER-FRYER

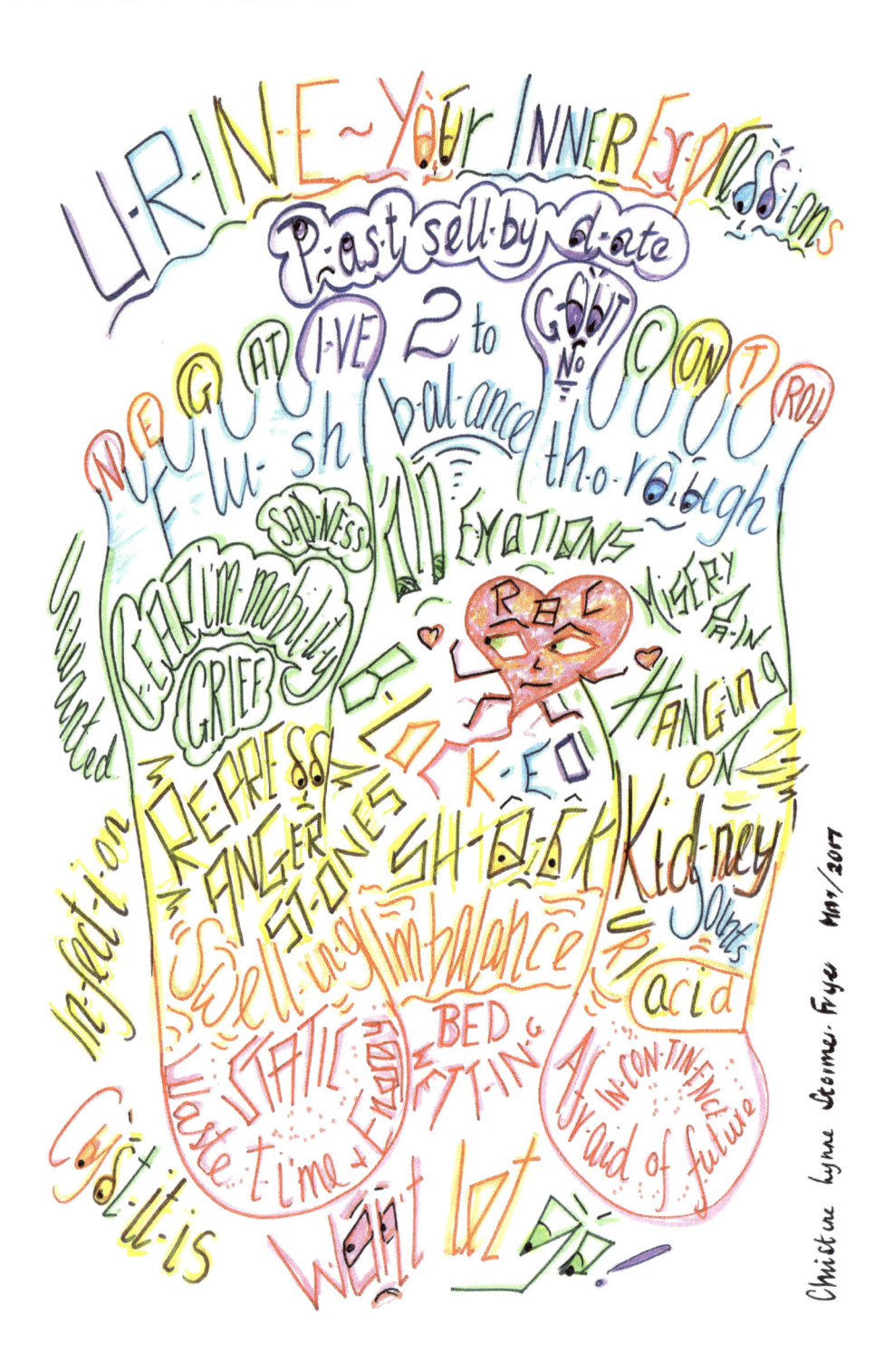

URINE – YOUR INNER EXPRESSIONS

Urine has been considered a medicine, beauty aid, and fountain of youth for aeons. Life begins bathed in amniotic fluid, consisting primarily of urine, with substantial amounts ingested while in the womb. Its phenomenal healing powers remain widely unknown due to the stigma attached to it. The novel coronavirus (COVID-19) brainwashed the masses into 'washing their hands of it' knowing of its Spiritual benefits.

With urine having so many healing properties, why does the body excrete it? Urine removes key ingredients that are not required at specific points in time. The excess water is full of vitamins, minerals, enzymes, salts, and so many other elements such as vital antibiotics, urea and uric acid. Being so sterile after secretion, it also has an antiseptic effect.

Urine holds records of the blood's condition, so when reapplied the body knows exactly what to do with it, whether it is a drop on the tongue, bathed in, wiped on the skin, or physically consumed. Its greatest potency is, interestingly, in the early morning.

It is an ideal way to let go of worked-through thoughts and 'e-motions' for equilibrium to be maintained. Detrimental to personal well-being is the need to be in absolute control when completely 'out of control'. The intense urge to 'hang onto' energy well 'past its sell-by date'. Subsequent reabsorption of these exceptionally 'negative' aspects increases mind and body toxicity.

A build-up acidity and bitterness often manifest as 'gout'. The refusal to 'g-et out' of one's own way has the big toe swelling and rigidifying and becoming excruciatingly painful. It makes it almost impossible to walk with such a huge mental stumbling block of obstinacy obstructing the way.

Terrified and precluded from 'flushing out the rough' old 'e-motions', kidneys become immobilised with fear, frequently losing control. The red blood cells take on the sadness, grief, 'miser-y' and hurt, distributing these wretched energies throughout.

Shock is especially debilitating to kidneys. Extreme anxiety, picked up from the adrenal glands above, convey a lack of courage in following through with personal convictions to put innovative notions into action. Repressed anger flares up with the indignation, ultimately infecting the urine. Sediments of resentment, particularly towards family and society, gather to form kidney stones, replicating ongoing disappointment that constantly gets in the way.

Static urine gathers in the bladder when hanging on needlessly from feeling 'pissed off' with an intimate partner. 'Taking the piss' and being cruelly mocked as a 'sissy' infuriates this small muscular sac, resulting in 'cystitis'.

Many references to the healing capacity of urine can be found in various religions around the world. Aristocratic French women bathed in urine to beautify their skin in the seventeenth century. It was also customary to soak stockings in urine and wrap them around the neck for sore throats. In Mexico, farmers prepared poultices with a child's urine mixed with charred corn for broken bones. Urine has also been used for whitening teeth and healing wounds.

It takes courage to let go of old familiar energies to make way for the unknown!

196 - CHRISTINE LYNNE STORMER-FRYER

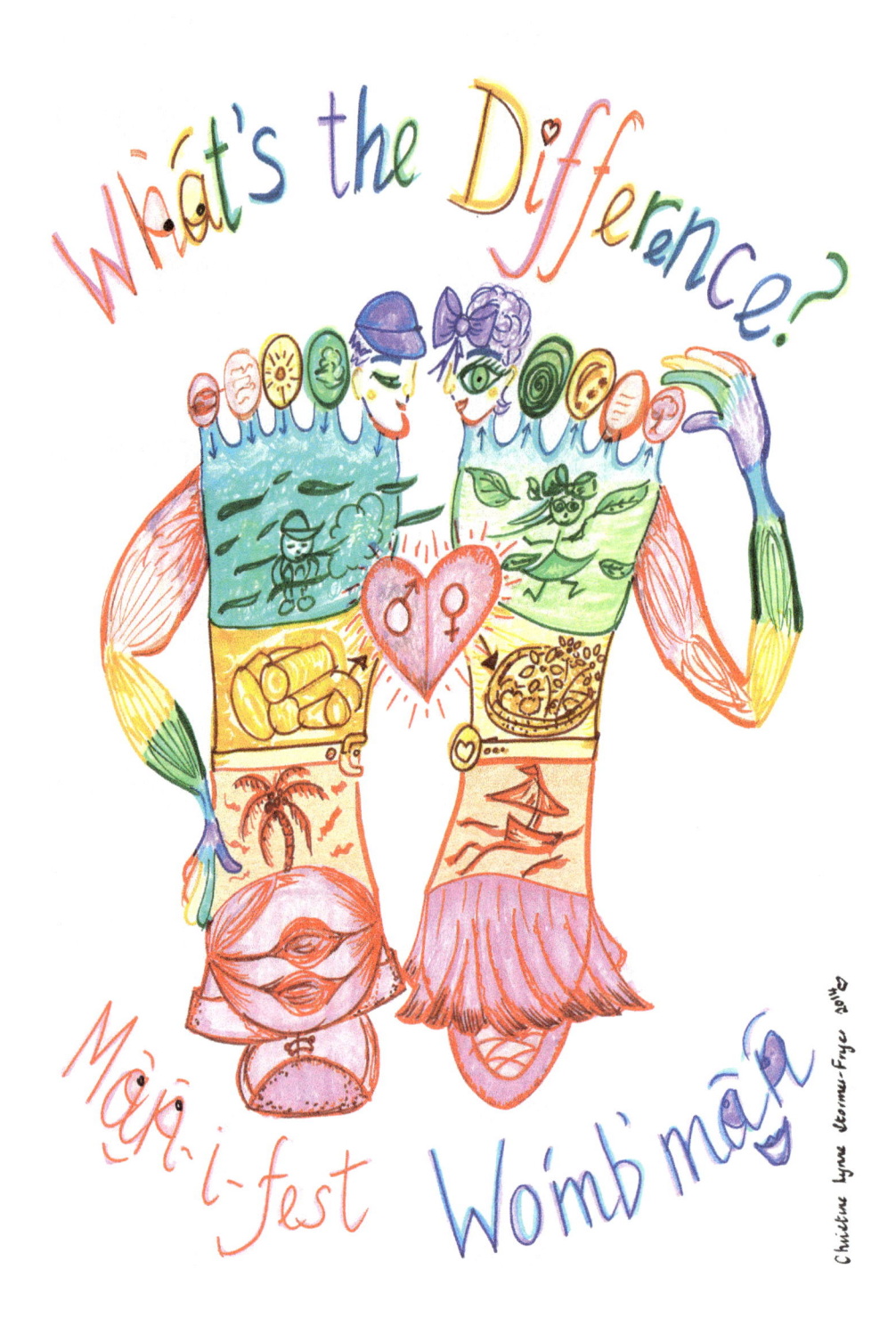

WHAT'S THE DIFFERENCE? MAN-I-FEST/WOMB-MAN

Each side of the body is subtly different. Akin to father is the right side, representing the logical, factual, structured, and self-absorbed masculine aspects of the personality. Akin to mother is the left side, resonating to the more intuitive, feeling, open and generous feminine qualities. Together the two provide a much-needed balance, with the key to wholeness being the ability to maintain harmony between the two extremes.

Never 'alone' every body is 'all-one'. The roles of male and female were intentionally separated for aeons by society, but now gender roles are merging, with the creative force of feminine energy blending with the active force of masculine energy. As labels fade, the rising equality is often accompanied by confusion due to deep scars on the genetic subconscious mind left by the patriarchal world.

The male source of energy is 'Father Sun', reverberating with the bygone era. As 'light is thrown onto situations', past events become increasingly exposed and significantly more visible. Unearthing explanations and information assists in making life more understandable. The 'bigger picture' becomes more apparent when seen in many 'different lights'.

Related to masculinity are the solid bodily organs like the lungs and the liver. Both retain and store processed energy derived from previous events. Contained air, once past its 'expiration date' is forced out of the lungs and 'ex-haled', carrying with it the remnants of uncertain feelings, contributing to the nature of the surrounding atmosphere.

Constantly evaluating broken-down residues of what happened or did not happen, the liver stockpiles this energy for future use, sometimes hoarding it for longer than necessary. Having experienced the fullness of life, male energies are encouraged to 'give' and pass on knowledge and wisdom, but only after relieving mind and body of all the worked-through and rougher aspects of life. 'Contracted' to let go and 'excrete' past remnants so that no further time or energy is wasted.

'Mother Moon' uses 'Father Sun's' rays to unveil and resolve past mysteries. Filled with global memories, the 'dead of night' is ideal for illuminating the way to enlightenment. As lungs expand to 'take in' and 'in-hale', 'breaths of fresh air' are lovingly 'well-come-d' into the body. The passive movements of 'in-halation' complement the active male force of 'ex-halation', encouraging a constant adjustment of 'e-motional' presence and pressure within.

The willingness to receive and process insights from the past 'takes guts'. Feminine energies possess the ideal tools, equipment and materials to process anything that has been ingested. By beneficially utilising the new intake, an excellent foundation is laid for a more fulfilling and worthwhile future.

It involves living fully in the 'pre-sent' and being prepared to evolve. Progress requires 'change', and women are renown for 'changing their minds'. In so doing, the muscles can effortlessly expand to embrace the fullness and true meaning of life.

Gender equality means progress for all!

198 - CHRISTINE LYNNE STORMER-FRYER

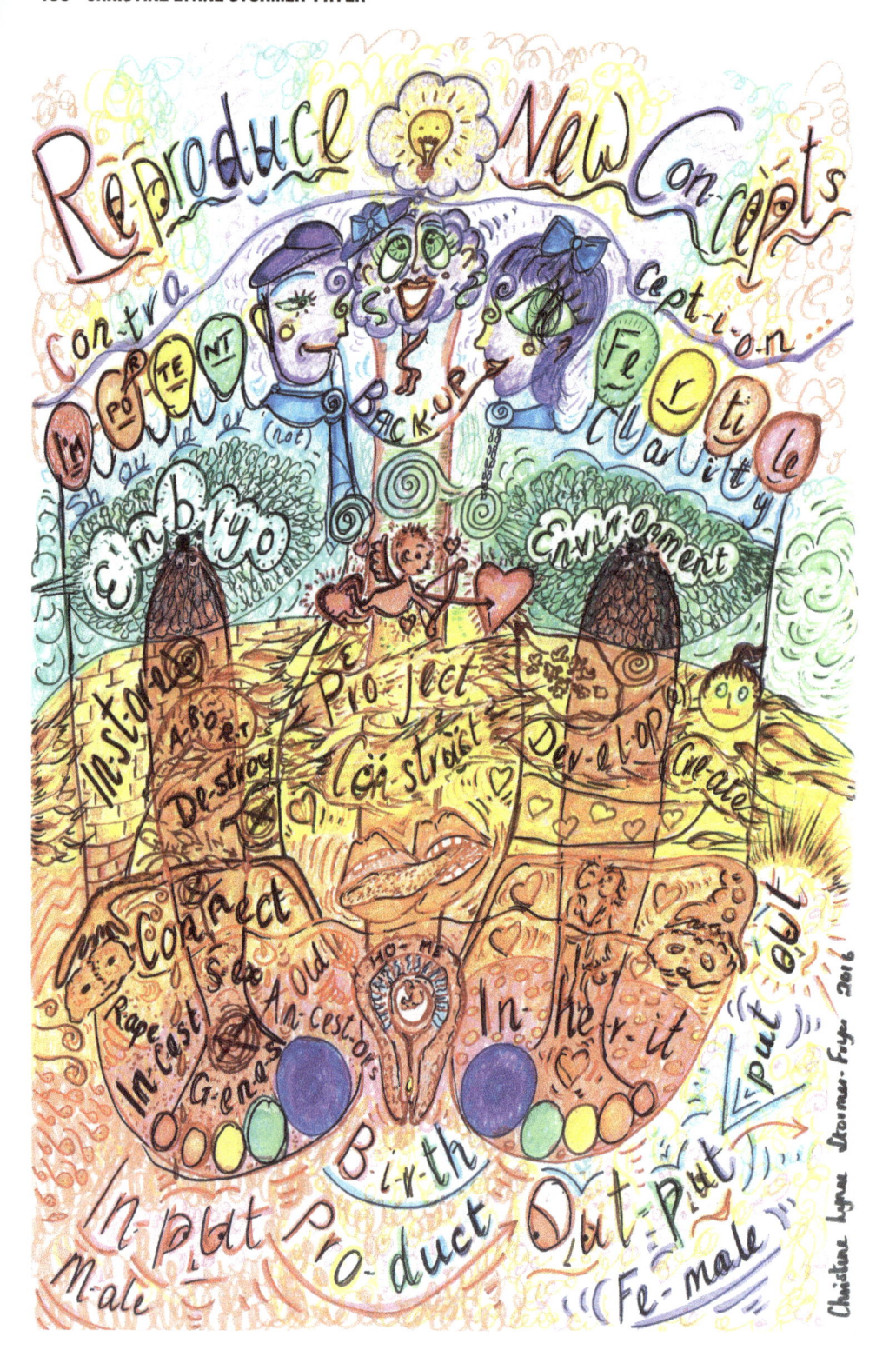

REPRODUCE NEW CONCEPTS

Tapping into magical Universal forces, everything is created twice. Firstly, in the imagination and then in reality. Creativity is 'intelligence having fun', conceptualising something in the 'mind's eye' that does not yet exist. It provides the freedom to dream and the joy of not knowing it all. It is mental energy creating reality through ongoing experiences.

Contraception is contrary to creativity, deliberately preventing a woman from becoming pregnant. Constant interception and interference with the imagination is another story. It puts a stop to any new projects, often referred to as a 'baby'. Yet it takes a lot to stop a fertile imagination once passionately activated.

Backed-up by intuitive self-talk, the inner tutor and 'in-sight' offer the courage to follow the heart. Lips joined through conversations or kissing get the 'juices flowing', often bringing together the lower parts of the anatomy to reproduce what has been done many times before. The difference is 'passion', 'pass-i-on', to generate unique innovations.

The power to create comes not from the intellect but from feelings. The creative mind loves to play with objects that tease and stretch its imagination. New concepts growing in the womb are related to concepts emerging in the mind. Both rely on heady 'im-portant' feelings rather than on weak 'im-potent' notions. Not feeling 'im-portant' enough to 'kick out the old' makes it hard to 'import' and entertain new way-out conceptions.

Whether imagined or real, concepts require a loving 'e-motional' environment that is well-nurtured by 'keeping a-breast' of the times. A heart filled with 'heart-felt' energy is the ideal target for Cupid to aim and shoot his arrows to inject fervent desire. Once inspired to leap into action, all that creativity requires is perseverance and the courage to take risks. A big plus is the willingness to 'look stupid' and take 'failure' as a valuable life lesson. It all depends on what is 'in store', especially from the male sperm bank that counts on substantial, worthwhile, and valuable contributions being made.

A history of constantly aborting projects that are not working out as expected is to risk destroying and 'mis-carrying' when unable to carry on. The greatest culprit in preventing new ways of constructing and building a new life is the 'dis-ease to please', being excessively obsessive, and constantly creating obstacles.

Nothing happens without the Soul's consent or invitation. Like magnets, situations are attracted to reveal what is really going on inside. 'Rape' happens when it is a crime for a woman to allow a man to force her into undesirable acts that she does not wish to perform. Society's refusal to address the real issue is a deterrent in processing heavy burdens born within due to outside pressure.

When it comes to issues regarding 's-ex' ('see the 'ex'), the needless need to prove self-worth through misplaced desirability, stretching back many generations, becomes increasingly evident. It is possible to have 'sex' with anybody, but it's only possible to 'make love' with a loved one.

The 'womb' is every body's first home. It relies on the 'in-put' to determine the 'out-put', in the hope of not being 'put-out'. With the generosity of the genes passed on from ancestors, old energies are constantly being replaced by the new incoming generation. With no 'in-her-ent' uneasiness, every birth gives rise to welcoming a 're-generation' for human evolvement. Filled with mystic superstition, life and death are the two most creative processes.

The magic of creation is using death for rebirth!

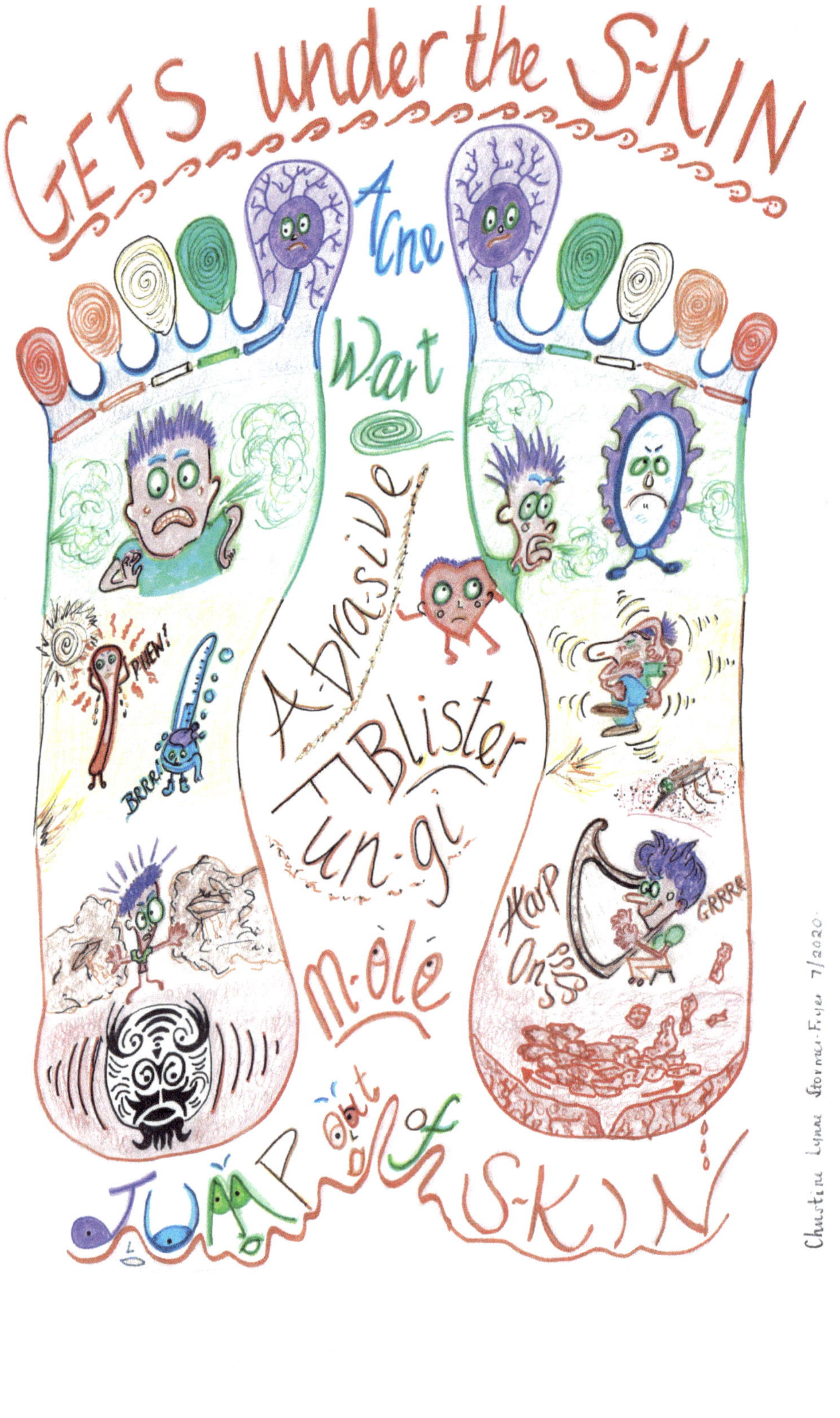
GETS under the S-KIN
Acne
Wart
A-bra-sive
Blister
Fun-gi
PHEW!
BRRR!
Harp On
GRRRR
M-olé
JUMP out of S-KIN
Christine Lynne Stormer-Fryer 7/2020

GETS UNDER THE SKIN

By holding everything together, the skin defines physical characteristics. It safeguards individuality while honouring the profound need to stay connected through the sensation of touch. Intimately connected to nerves, it mirrors issues in its 't-issues', influencing social interactions as well as internal psychical self-interactions.

Acutely aware of the external environment, it brings to the surface anything internally annoying. Hairs on the skin are the antennae that, like radars, keep the skin well informed, 'standing on end' when horrified or frightened. Extremely sensitive Souls are 'thin-skinned', touchy and more vulnerable, whereas more insensitive Souls have thicker, tougher skin, sometimes like that of a rhinoceros. 'Making the skin creep' are all the psychological, 'e-motional' and Spiritual concerns that 'bug' the mind, making it 'react badly'.

'Corns', like mini-shields, prevent notions from being 'stamped out'. 'Birthmarks' mean different things to various cultures. Essentially blemishes from previous lifetimes, attention is drawn to something significant. Its situation and appearance give vital clues as to the 'hi-story' behind it. Interestingly, 'cuts' and 'scars' can appear from nowhere. Indicative of some form of trauma or being 'cut up' about something, often a sign of 'hi-story' repeating itself.

Like a mirror, skin 'reflects' colourful 'e-motions', frequently changing colours on the feet. 'Flaking' when treading tentatively or 'unsure of one's footing'. 'Weeping' from wailing and bemoaning one's fate. 'Swelling' to attract attention and get more space when overwhelmed. 'Blistering' when 'rubbed up the wrong way'. 'Peeling' to expose what is going on 'beneath the surface' or to shed less 'appealing' aspects of life for Spiritual transformation.

Changes in 'temperature' mimic changes of 'temperament', 'blowing hot and cold' from one extreme to another. 'Hot under the collar' one minute, then having 'cold feet' the next. Other warning signs include being 'infected' when inflamed and furious. 'Lumpy' with 'pockets of discontent'. 'Moles' due to making 'mountains out of molehills'. 'Freckles' and 'black marks' revealing previous lifetime hurts. 'Warts' as protrusions of self-hate. 'Cracks' from 'cracking up' when 'pulled apart' and divided. 'Callouses' becoming a form of protection from hard-heartedness. 'Bruises' when 'knocking the self'. 'Fungi' from the parasitic behaviour of taking advantage of others. 'Herpes' ('shingles') when 'harping on' and 'getting on the nerves'. 'Abrasions' from abrasive, uncompromising or argumentative behaviour. 'Rashes' when too impulsive, hasty or careless.

'Acne' is 'actually' extreme exasperation. Not liking oneself upsets the skin, causing it to erupt to highlight areas of torment and conflict. On the face, it reveals the fury of at all that is being 'faced'. On the neck, it highlights 'getting it in the neck'. On the back, it draws attention to all that is going on 'behind the back'.

Religious beliefs and ethnic customs determine the amount of flesh exposed, along with tribal markings, and so on. Some find folklore scary enough to 'jump out of the skin'. When used by social conditioning to conceal innermost thoughts and heartfelt 'e-motions', it essentially numbs the Spiritual connection. Separating yet connecting inner and outer worlds, the whole arena of life is experienced through this semipermeable membrane, with an ongoing interchange between the two.

Skin reflects 'kin'!

202 - CHRISTINE LYNNE STORMER-FRYER

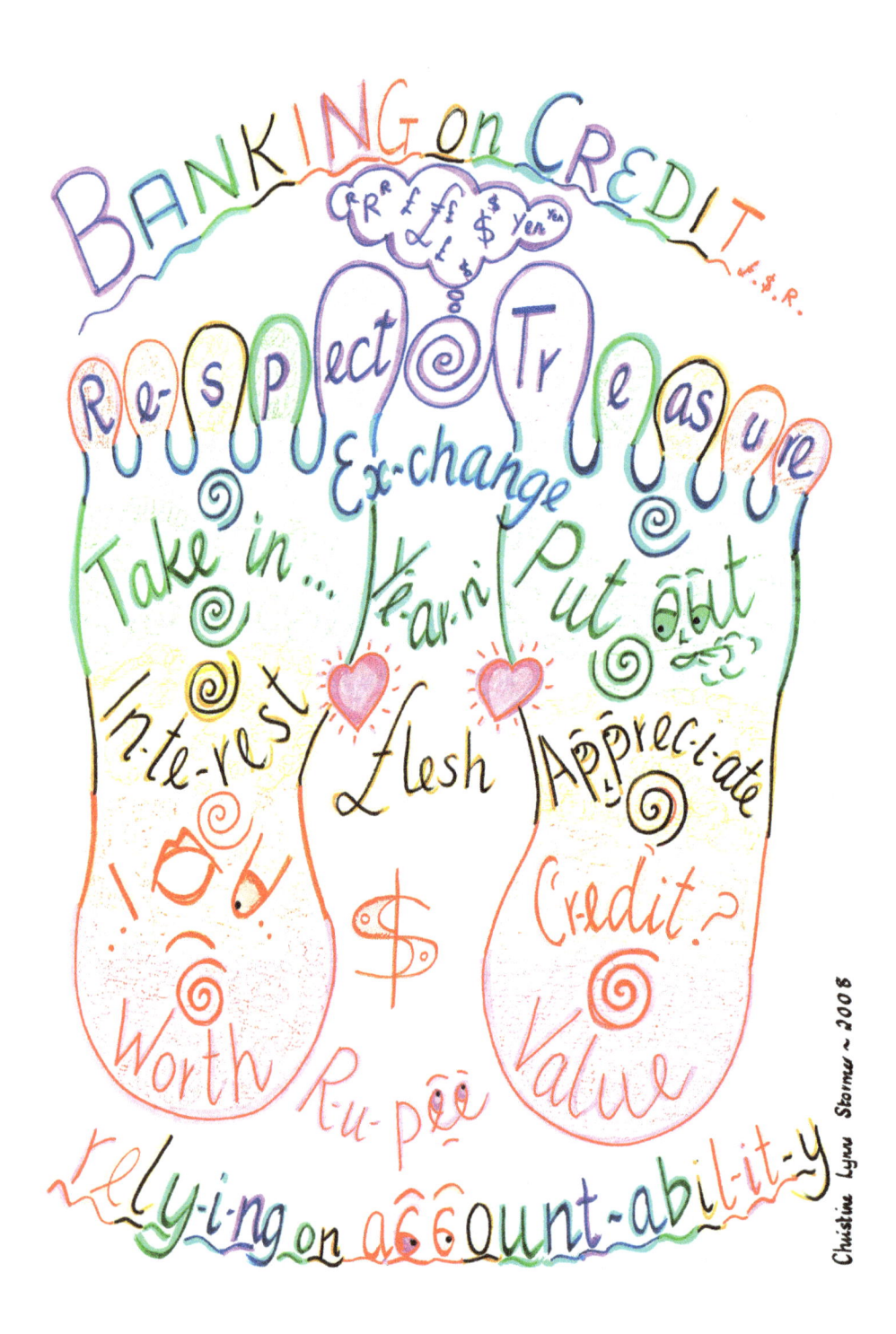

BANKING ON CREDIT

'Banking on credit' takes a substantial amount of trust. 'Counting on' the future is easier when 'banking' benefits in the present. 'Saving' precious energy ensures there is plenty in 'reserve' when required. Believing certain Spiritual statements to be true and 'taking them to the bank' builds up a 'bank of valuable knowledge and wisdom'. It sometimes takes time for the 'penny to drop', but it is preferable to 'having more money than sense'.

A 'penny for the thoughts' could be a real 'eye-opener'. It all depends on the energy spent on investing in personal ideas, dreams, and visions. Withdrawing energy from limiting notions frees up space to build up a valuable repository of innovative perceptions with the power to make the inner economy thrive.

After 'taking everything into account' and 'making allowances', 'respect' for extraordinary concepts can always be 'treasured'. Utilising the wealth of novel ideas is well 'worth' the high rating. Adding value and paying dividends in the long run engenders and boosts much-appreciated self-esteem, even when accepted at 'face value'.

The 'exchange rate' between the outer and inner worlds, as well as conversions between the head and the remainder of the body, relies on the 'value' placed on current thoughts, as well as the type of currency 'on offer'. Also, whether the 'amount' of effort required to get them 'out there' is actually 'worth it'. Common notions are 'a dime a dozen', wasting 'precious time and energy' with a possibility of ending up being 'strapped for cash'. 'Keeping an eye' on the in-house fluctuating 'inflation rate' is essential for ongoing stability.

'Feeling like a million dollars' does not 'cost an arm and a leg'. All that is required is an affable, charismatic and interesting personality with a passion for making a beneficial difference. Bargaining on high-quality goods and wishing to reduce prices may save a 'penny or two', but it only serves to deflate and devalue self-worth. With little left to 'put out' there, the heart anxiously 'pounds' with a 'yen' for greater 'appreciation'.

The best 'interest' comes from valuing kind deeds and generous gestures, with time being 'saved' through constant curiosity and a desire to evolve. In debt with a stack of IOUs takes far more than 'a pound of flesh'. It depletes and exhausts the inner resources. Meanwhile, 'being a credit' and a source of admiration, 'giving credit where it is due' rather than 'stealing another's thunder' enhances the coffers admirably. No matter what, when 'in for a penny, in for a pound', once committed, it is worthwhile to keep on going.

'Betting the bottom dollar' and being certain enough to 'put money where the mouth is' could end up being 'fraudulent' with so much 'money laundering' going on. 'Money talks', with unnecessary comparisons of who is more highly regarded within the relationship, upsets the chemical balance. 'Robbing Peter to pay Paul' is simply a disguise when 'money is being poured down the drain'. On the 'other side of the coin' are many other options.

Whether 'filthy rich' or having to 'slog' for rewards (as 'rupee' as 'wrought silver' could imply), or 'dirt poor', constantly 'spending a penny' or 'pinching pennies' to 'pay the way', is degrading. Being 'tight-arsed' with a firm 'hold on the purse strings' is a sure way of turning 'red in the face'. For 'what it is worth', relying on one's own accountability is so valuable that it brings in abundance, making life copiously worthwhile.

Money is a form of potential empowering energy that generates change!

204 - CHRISTINE LYNNE STORMER-FRYER

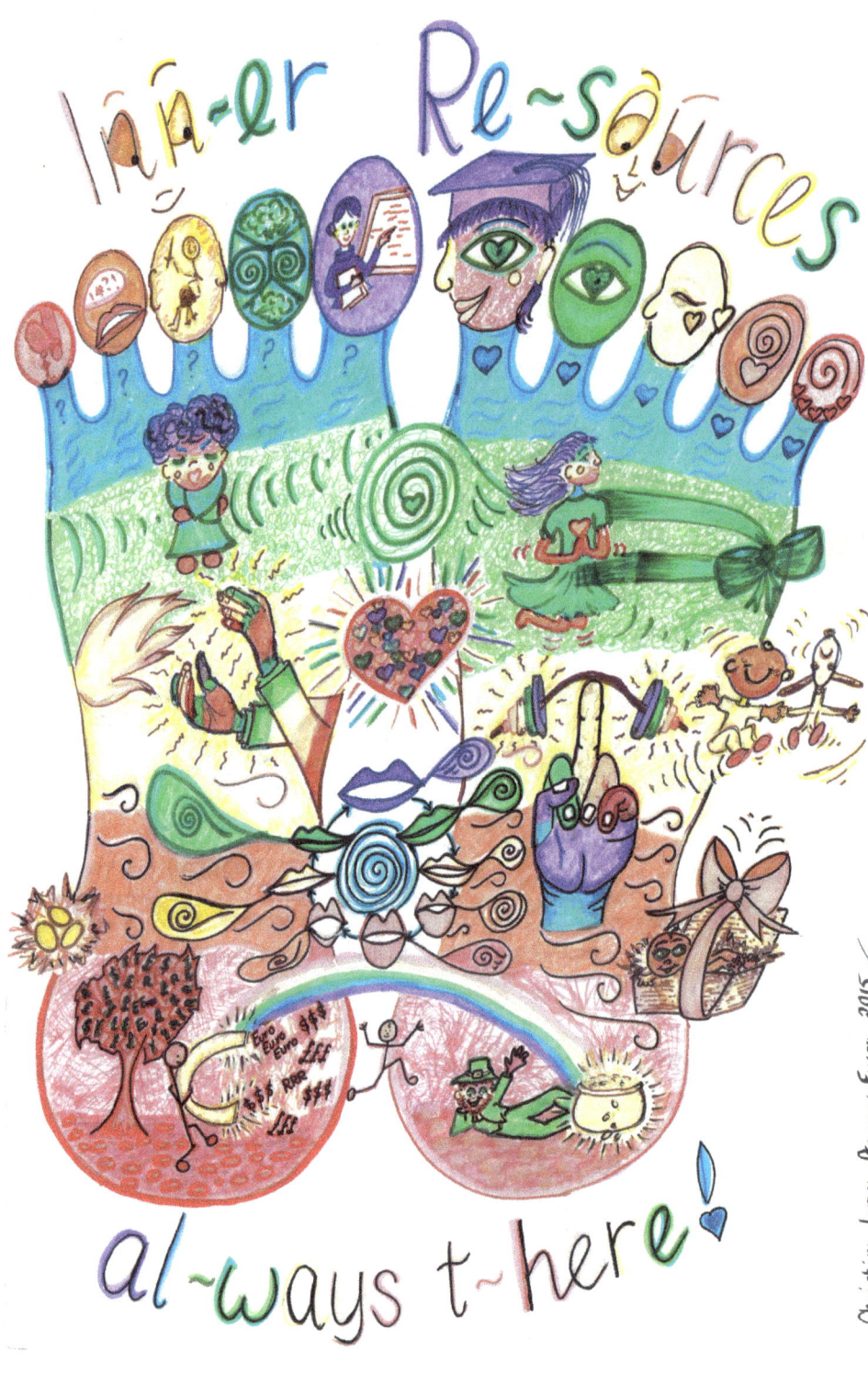

INNER RESOURCES

When lost in uncharted territory, a map is typically looked at to figure out how to get to the chosen destination, which is all very well if there is a map and a known destination. It is comforting to know that everybody is venturing into the unknown covering ground that even our ancestors were not aware of.

Without a map, one's instinct kicks in. Although it can be initially scary with a niggling feeling of fear hovering in the background, trusting in Universal support provides all the guidance required. It is essential, however, to first find the trust within. While this is intellectually possible, it sometimes takes a little longer to believe it in the heart.

The journey of self-discovery is only conceivable when it begins with self-love. Accepting the inner child and the dynamic, authentic self. During times of constant change and growth, being gentle on and taking loving care of oneself is essential. Honouring the vibrant Spirit within assists in adapting to change. Mind and body love it, knowing that once it has caught its breath, overcoming obstacles is the Soul's forte. Surviving numerous trials and tribulations, each breakthrough brings with it a greater appreciation of the hidden reserves stored within.

Many complex roles are played throughout the journey of self-empowerment. As pressure mounts, with doubt escalating around the ability to carry on, a deep strength emerges. The capacity to cope far outstrips the capacity to feel nervous. Even as raw 'e-motions' are nourished when facing conflict, chaos and confusion, it is important to remain on the path of integrity.

It is okay to feel lost from time to time. Anything new requires feeling the way rather than following an established path. Carried within are all the required resources for self-realisation. The most valuable resource is creativity. The inner world magnetically attracts all that is required to evolve to the next level.

The most important relationship is always with oneself, constantly present from the time of conception and incessantly aware of the Soul's desires. Balance is the key that unlocks the door to amicable cohabitation, with all the various personalities cohabitating internally. Acknowledging and embracing the special gifts within is what makes individuals divinely unique, leaving no room for comparisons.

Tapping into the wealth of resources residing at the core brings with it a realisation of the abundant source of life. There is an innate drive to constantly improve, utilising unlimited potential. Roadblocks along the way are evolutionary opportunities to divert and possibly find an even better route.

Once committed to the Spiritual journey, all needs are honoured, according to what has been 'put out there', as and when required. Every journey has a pot of gold at the end of the rainbow when fulfilling the heart's desires. Every body already possesses a very precious elixir called 'joy'. There is no need to keep searching for happiness. It happens when making things happen.

True worth comes from all the good that is done in the world!

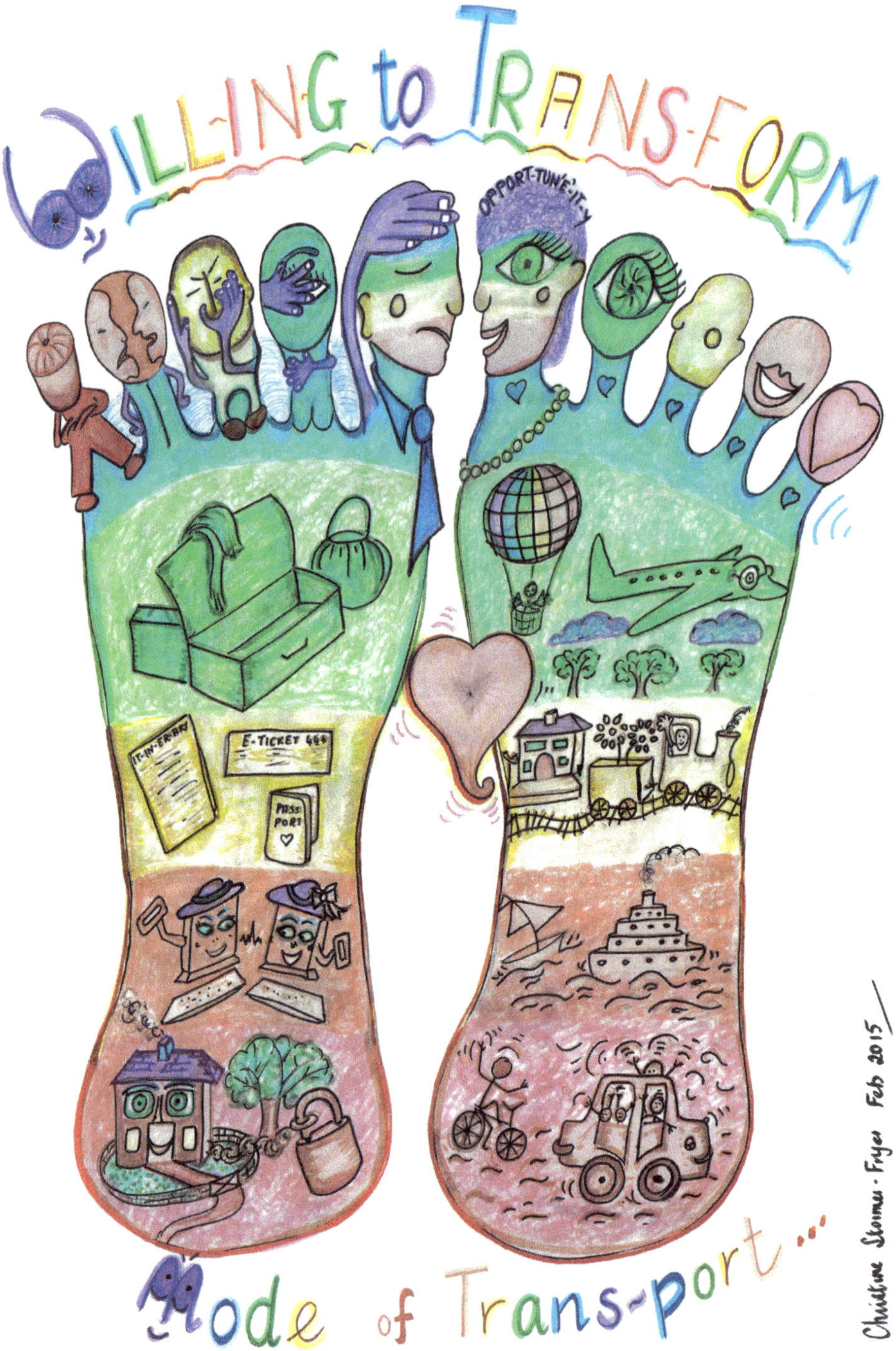
WILL-ING to TRANS-FORM
OPPORT-TUN'E-IT-Y
IT-IN-ER-ARY
E-TICKET
PASS PORT
Mode of Trans-port...
Christine Stormer-Fryer Feb 2015

WILLING TO TRANSFORM

Within every body is sacred geometric coding, instrumental in providing the courage to travel within, and along, the road of self-discovery. Although much personal pain, frustration, resentment, distress and so on are encountered, it is the only way to gain greater 'under-standing'. The subsequent healing and freedom make the journey more than worthwhile. Travelling may not always be comfortable, yet it is the discomfort that accelerates transformation. Taking mental flight to rise above mundane ways of thinking, fools the brain into conceiving ideas way beyond its wildest dreams.

As earthbound beings, there has always been a fascination in winged creatures, leading to the invention of hot air balloons, aeroplanes and a myriad of flying machines, offering the gift of being airborne. Flying high and looking back is to see life on Earth from a completely different perspective. Airlines do the body a huge favour, restricting the amount of baggage taken on board, and drastically reducing all the hefty 'e-motions' 'crammed into a suitcases' and lugged needlessly around.

With a whole universe of its own, the heart uses loving energies to embrace anything strange or foreign. With such a bountiful amount of heart energy, the mind can take flight and go anywhere its Soul desires.

The journey of 'nu-trients', 'new trends', always follows a 'train' of thought involving the whole body, even when 'going off the tracks'. But first, 'a ticket to ride' is required. 'Grilled' by the teeth when first embarking on a trip, a 'passport' is needed to 'cross borders' into foreign lands before being checked by 'customs'. Once permitted to pass onto the next adventure, based on personal identification, access is gained to other realms of possibility. A life rich in opportunities, good or bad, relieves the monotony of a dull routine.

Every body is 'in the same boat'. All human vehicles riding the 'waves of the storm' and sailing from the unfamiliar to the familiar parts of the self. The ideal opportunity to recognise, acknowledge and honour differences mirrored by strangers, yet also appreciating the similarities to stay grounded. Exploring the 'four corners of the world', immersed in mystery and unfamiliar energy, the simplest of joys can be the most profound.

Waving 'bye-bye' to anything wasting time and energy in the body is a massive relief and clears the way for a whole new chapter in life. For any transition to take place, a part needs to die for another part to come alive. It helps to feel secure within when this happens. Leaving the home under 'lock and key' provides 'peace of mind', although 'peace within' is far more dependable.

Transient times involve movement. The messengers that relay this shift are 'confusion' and 'disorientation'. There is always a transition 'bridging the gap' between the time a decision is made and the time it actually happens.

Spiritual flight is inevitable when freed from the constraints of linear time. The wider the wings spread, the higher and deeper the meaning of life and the inspiration to transcend the 'norm'. Every event, and all experiences, individually and collectively attract opportunities to raise consciousness and promote Spiritual awareness.

Wherever travels may lead, paradise is always there!

208 - CHRISTINE LYNNE STORMER-FRYER

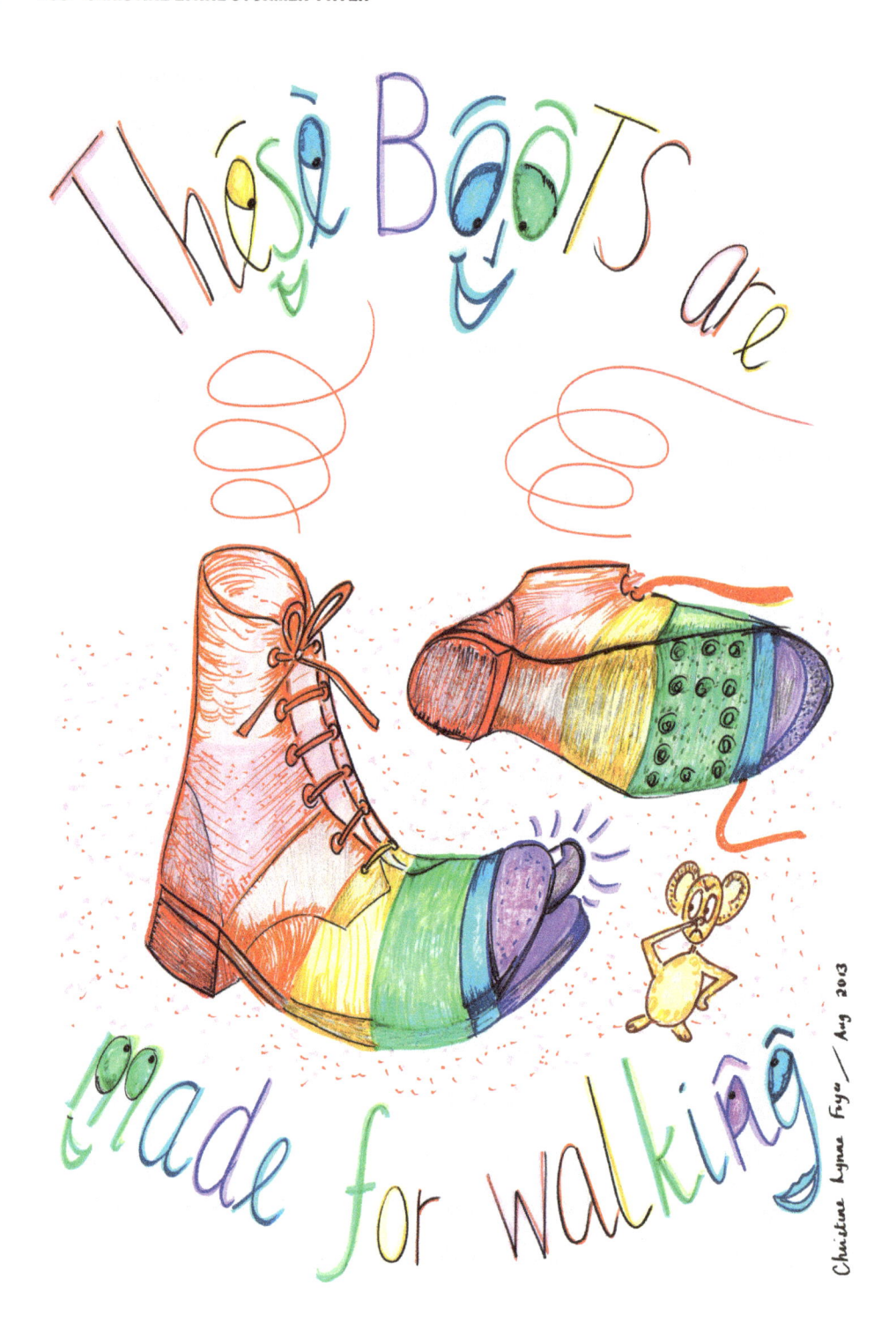

These Boots are made for walking

Christine Lynne Frye — Aug 2013

BOOTS MADE FOR WALKING

Whether 'tough as old boots' or 'shaking in the boots', 'pulling oneself up by the bootstraps' and getting on with life without relying on others is so much better. 'Giving the boot' to old energies and 'kicking off the boots' from time to time to relax and put the feet up is a great way to 'boot up' and recharge the batteries.

'To boot', 'betting the boots' when discouraged and terrified, with the 'heart in the boots' or being a 'bootlicker' and sucking up to others to get ahead, is not an option. Nor is being 'too big for one's boots'. 'Hanging up the old boots' and retiring is an ideal opportunity to put the most into what is left of life, until 'dying with the boots on'.

Full of symbolism, footwear changes the demeanour. From the time when only the rich could adorn their feet, footgear represents anything from authority and power to vanity and arrogance, to servitude and poverty. Removing footgear when entering a home or a place of worship is a sign of respect and humility.

Gender differences in shoes only happened in the eighteenth century when high heels became popular among rich men as a means of raising them above the filth of the streets and the poor. Women started wearing them as a sign of rebellion in an attempt to gain some equality with men, with shoes representing the vagina and the foot the penis. In China, the tighter the bondage and subservience of women, the more the vagina shrank to fit into exceptionally demeaning circumstances. To even the score, penises started shrivelling almost into oblivion.

Although menswear is traditionally more supportive, practical, and sensible, a tremendous amount of male potential is concealed from having to conform and 'fit in'. Meanwhile, ladieswear undergoes endless fashion crazes in a desperate attempt to 'find the feet' and choose what suits them best. Children prefer to go barefoot, uninhibited and unrestricted when exploring the wonders of life.

Old, worn-out shoes are like old friends. Invariably the most comfortable and often the most difficult to throw out. Symbolic of hard graft challenges and struggles, it is often a matter of 'the devil you know is better than the devil you don't'. Spelt backwards, 'devil' becomes 'lived'. Inappropriate or impractical shoes highlight feeling like a misfit and the difficulty of having to conform to rigid social boundaries.

Ultimately, footwear is not the cause of foot disorders. It does, however, effectively accentuate tense and painful aspects in moving 'a-head' in life that require attention. 'Worn-out' soles speak for themselves and are more likely 'to fall apart' when the Soul can take no more.

The numerous benefits of walking are frequently taken for granted. It is the ideal way of existing in the moment. The simplicity and ease of it creates time and space. A mindfulness of innermost feelings. An awareness of the wonders within while appreciating the beauty of the surrounding environment. Walking softly on this Earth and listening to her heartbeat puts everything into perspective.

Those who walk in and out of life leave footprints in the heart!

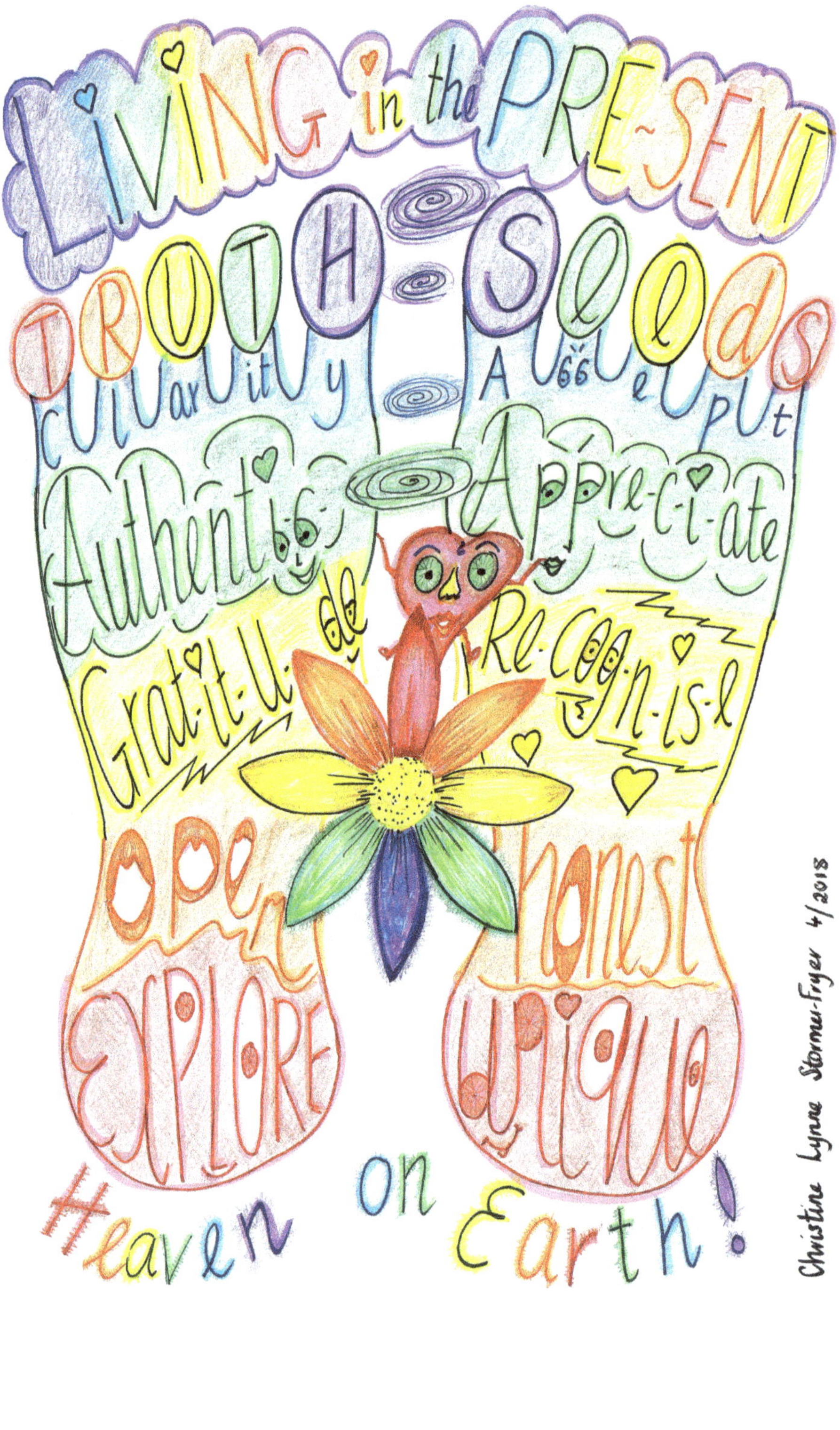
LIVING in the PRE-SENT
TRUTH SEEDS
Authentic
Appre-ci-ate
Grat-it-ude
Re-cog-n-is-e
open
honest
EXPLORE
Heaven on Earth!
Christine Lynne Stormer-Fryer 4/2018

LIVING IN THE PRESENT

There is a reason for remembering certain events. Residing memories have a profound impact on decision-making, subsequent choices, and eventual experiences. Whether hurtful or helpful, either way, enduring lessons shape life. As such, the present is a good time as any to embrace, thank, and release perceived mistakes, past regrets, and previous problems.

Thoughts leave a legacy that lives forever. Every thought ever thought is still here. As consciousness raises ultra-violet levels of enlightenment from the Divine source, accessed through the hole in the ozone layer, thoughts evolve, to the benefit of all humanity. The force of thought is a means to personal power, with adjustments possible at any given moment to improve circumstances.

Along with thought comes truth and trust, two extremely valuable assets and precious possessions to be cherished always, with no rehearsal required for either. Both are completely honest reflections of the Spirit opening a magnificent doorway to a fathomless understanding of the source of life. Faith is the key to walk through it and enjoy all the treasures within.

Magnificent co-creations with the Universe, thoughts are the seeds of the mind. Cultivated well, the body flourishes. In such a chaotic and noisy world, locating and cultivating the seed of peace to become a reliable source of serenity provides an inner calm, and the 'clarity' to 'accept' Universal gifts and physically manifest them. 'As above so below'.

With each heartbeat and every breath comes a choice of how to direct Spiritual energy. A time to resolve conflicts between the mind and the heart, putting aside hurtful 'e-motions' and replacing them with the power of acceptance. A time to embrace reality and the uncertainty of the future. A time for pure love, 'authenticity' and 'appreciation'.

Being fully present in daily activities is to appreciate personal talents and opportunities. With undivided attention and absolute integrity focused on the 'task at hand', each moment becomes a truly powerful experience. 'Recognising' the feeling of being completely alive and showing 'gratitude' for being so invigorated is to witness reality opening up before the very eyes.

All life experiences are greatly influenced by relationships, with the 'pre-sent' being a time to grow out of painful associations and augment beneficial ones. Being fully present is to give and receive vibrancy in equal measures. Being 'open' and 'honest' is a way of honouring the gift of companionship.

Once past perceptions are seen through a 'different set of lenses', endless opportunities to heal and get better at being oneself present themselves. Every moment becomes yet another chance to re-evaluate choices and decisions.

Each present moment is completely new and a time to explore. Nothing like this has ever happened before, nor will it ever happen again. It is a time to fully embrace destiny and experience being completely alive, knowing that 'heaven does exist on Earth'.

Being present is to experience a life that cannot be fully lived through memory or fantasy!

ABOUT THE AUTHOR

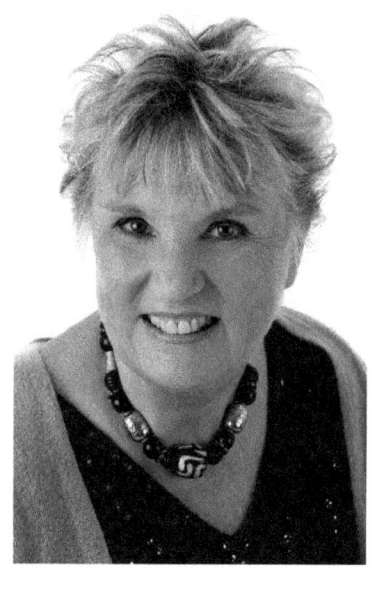

Affectionately known as the 'Universal Foot Lady', Christine Lynne Stormer-Fryer is renowned globally for her innovative and pioneering Spirit. Having a more wholistic and visionary approach to healing and health makes sure that natural remedies keep pace with the phenomenal strides in human evolution. Worldwide media coverage on television and radio, as well as frequent articles in newspapers and magazines, has enabled Christine to share the vital link between orthodox and natural healing.

Considered a renowned authority on natural healing and health, Christine constantly receives invitations to be a guest or keynote speaker at International Congresses and Conferences, as well as give seminars, workshops and presentations throughout the world, which she has been doing since 1992. In 2000, and again in 2009, Christine had hoped to 'put her feet up' to write more books, but the requests for her to continue presenting this phenomenal Universal wisdom grew so much that her presentations are now more popular than ever. It took the 'lockdown'' to allow this to finally happen! With the ever-increasing demand for new books, more courses and videos, Christine feels honoured to share the wealth of universal knowledge entrusted to her, realising how much it adds meaning to life.

Now married to her wonderful husband, John Fryer, Christine's two brilliant sons, Andrew and David, have long since left home to pursue successful careers in London, United Kingdom. Becoming a grandmother to William Stormer at the age of 69 is such a Divine Gift.

Christine feels that her Soul journey is only just beginning, despite having already encouraged thousands of individuals worldwide to 'stand on their own two feet'.

To get in touch with Chris, please email her at inspired@worldonline.co.za, or visit her online at www.alwaysb.com

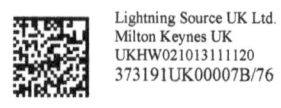

Lightning Source UK Ltd.
Milton Keynes UK
UKHW021013111120
373191UK00007B/76